AF598105

Merkel Cell Carcinoma

Murad Alam • Jeremy S. Bordeaux
Siegrid S. Yu
Editors

Merkel Cell Carcinoma

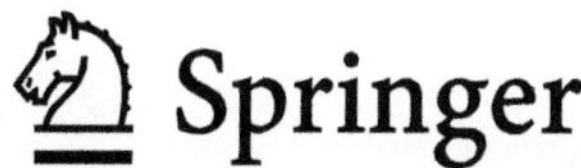

Editors
Murad Alam, MD
Department of Dermatology
Northwestern University
Chicago, IL, USA

Siegrid S. Yu, MD
Department of Dermatology
University of California, San Francisco
San Francisco, CA, USA

Jeremy S. Bordeaux, MD, MPH
Department of Dermatology
University Hospitals Case Medical Center
Case Western Reserve University
Cleveland, OH, USA

ISBN 978-1-4614-6607-9 ISBN 978-1-4614-6608-6 (eBook)
DOI 10.1007/978-1-4614-6608-6
Springer New York Heidelberg Dordrecht London

Library of Congress Control Number: 2013935215

Printed on acid-free paper

Springer is part of Springer Science+Business Media (www.springer.com)

To my husband, Ron, who continues to provide enduring companionship, encouragement, and support during our life's journey together.

Siegrid S. Yu

I dedicate this book to my loving wife, Jen, and my kind, caring, curious sons, Tyler and Nathan. Thank you for providing meaning in life.

Jeremy S. Bordeaux

To Noor and Ali, my only niece and nephew, respectively, and to MP and BT, who were patient.

Murad Alam

Preface

Poorly understood with regard to etiology, risk factors, and treatment, Merkel cell carcinoma is growing in incidence. Compared to other nonmelanoma skin cancers, Merkel cell is aggressive and frequently deadly. Yet the dissemination of information about this tumor remains inadequate even among specialists.

The purpose of this volume is to provide an accessible introduction to the clinical management of Merkel cell carcinoma for the interested specialist in dermatology, oncology, surgical oncology, plastic surgery, and allied disciplines. Practical elements of presentation and epidemiology are described, and the need for multimodal treatment is highlighted. Chapters on particular therapeutic approaches are written by experts in the relevant specialties. Treatment algorithms and case studies are provided to coalesce the large quantity of detailed information into a manageable, usable form. Finally, chapters on basic science and future research directions are included since ongoing investigations are crucial to battling this tumor.

Much remains to be done to better manage Merkel cell carcinoma. Here, we provide a starting point that cumulates the knowledge that we have, suggests guidance for treatment, and offers hope for the future.

Chicago, IL, USA — Murad Alam
Cleveland, OH, USA — Jeremy S. Bordeaux
San Francisco, CA, USA — Siegrid S. Yu

Acknowledgements

We are particularly thankful that Springer initially recognized the need for a book on this important topic, a life-threatening disease seen increasingly often. We are very grateful to Rebekah Amos, our editor at Springer, who allowed us to proceed with this book, and who provided constant support and reassurance to move it to completion. Michael D. Sova, our Developmental Editor, was similarly exceedingly helpful in making sure that the many chapters came together and the production met Springer's high standards.

Contents

Part IV Expert Opinions and Future Directions

Contributors

Olga Afanasiev, BA Department of Pathology and Dermatology, University of Washington School of Medicine, Seattle, WA, USA

Iris Ahronowitz, MD Department of Dermatology, University of California, San Francisco, San Francisco, CA, USA

Murad Alam, MD Department of Dermatology, Northwestern University, Chicago, IL, USA

Jeremy S. Bordeaux, MD, MPH Department of Dermatology, University Hospitals Case Medical Center, Case Western Reserve University, Cleveland, OH, USA

Jerry D. Brewer, MD Department of Dermatology, Mayo Clinic, Rochester, MN, USA

Sandra Y. Han, MD Department of Dermatology, University of California, San Francisco, San Francisco, CA, USA

Chase M. Heaton, MD Department of Dermatology, University of California, San Francisco, San Francisco, CA, USA

Sherrif F. Ibrahim, MD, PhD Department of Dermatology, University of Rochester Medical Center, Rochester, NY, USA

Julian Kim, MD, MS Department of Surgery, University Hospitals Case Medical Center, Cleveland, OH, USA

Nancy Kim, MD Department of Dermatology, UCSF Dermatologic Surgery & Laser Center, San Francisco, CA, USA

Timothy M. Kuzel, MD Division of Hematology/Oncology, Department of Medicine, Feinberg School of Medicine of Northwestern University, Chicago, IL, USA

Garrett C. Lowe, MD Department of Dermatology, Mayo Clinic, Rochester, MN, USA

Stephen Michael Maricich, MD, PhD Department of Pediatrics, Division of Neurology, University of Pittsburgh School of Medicine, Children's Hospital of Pittsburgh of UPMC, Pittsburgh, PA, USA

Timothy H. McCalmont, MD Department of Pathology and Dermatology, University of California, San Francisco, San Francisco, CA, USA

Paul Nghiem, MD, PhD Department of Dermatology Medicine, University of Washington School of Medicine & Fred Hutchinson Cancer Research Center, Seattle, WA, USA

Jeffrey North, MD Department of Dermatology, University of Missouri, Columbus, MO, USA

Stephen M. Ostrowski, MD, PhD Department of Dermatology, University Hospitals Case Medical Center, Cleveland, OH, USA

Rupali Roy, MD Division of Hematology/Oncology, Department of Internal Medicine, University of Michigan Hospital, Ann Arbor, MI, USA

Adam R. Schmitt, BA Case Western Reserve University School of Medicine, Cleveland, OH, USA

William R. Silveira, MD, PhD Department of Radiation Oncology, University of California, San Francisco, San Francisco, CA, USA

Seaver Soon, MD Division of Dermatology & Dermatologic Surgery, Scripps Clinic, La Jolla, CA, USA

Natalie Vandeven, BS Department of Medicine, University of Washington, Seattle, WA, USA

Steven J. Wang, MD Department of Otolaryngology-Head and Neck Surgery, University of California, San Francisco, San Francisco, CA, USA

Melanie Warycha, MD Mount Kisco Medical Group, Department of Dermatology, Mount Kisco, NY, USA

Douglas Winstanley, DO Division of Dermatology & Dermatologic Surgery, Scripps Clinic, La Jolla, CA, USA

Sue S. Yom, MD, PhD Department of Radiation Oncology, University of California, San Francisco, San Francisco, CA, USA

Siegrid S. Yu, MD Department of Clinical Dermatology, UCSF Dermatologic Surgery & Laser Center, San Francisco, CA, USA

Part I

Basic Science and Epidemiology

Basic Science of the Merkel Cell

1

Stephen M. Ostrowski
and Stephen Michael Maricich

Merkel Cell Structure

Ultrastructure

Merkel cells are a distinct epidermal cell type found at the dermal/epidermal junction just below the basal layer of the epidermis. They are roughly the same size as keratinocytes, with oval or round cell somata ~10 μm in diameter and large, lobulated nuclei (Fig. 1.1a) [1–4]. Merkel cell cytoplasm is relatively clear and contains intermediate filaments that are thinner, less dense, and ultrastructurally distinct from those of other skin cells. These filaments are most abundant near desmosomal contacts that link Merkel cells with adjacent keratinocytes (Fig. 1.1b, c) [5]. Each Merkel cell extends many fine, spine-like microvilli that contact nearby keratinocytes and may allow increased sensitivity for detecting mechanical stimuli (Fig. 1.1d, e) [6]. Typical cytokeratins (CK) found in immature (CK5, CK14) and mature (CK1, CK10) epidermal cells are absent from Merkel cells. Instead, CK8, 18, 19, and 20 constitute the building blocks of Merkel cell intermediate filaments [7, 8], and three of these cytokeratins (CK8, 18, and 20) are highly specific for Merkel cells in humans and other mammals (Fig. 1.1e) [9].

A defining feature of Merkel cells across species is the presence of electron dense granules unlike any others seen in the epidermis. These structures, 80–120 nm in size, are concentrated at the basal surface opposite to Merkel cell-associated nerve termini (see below) (Fig. 1.1a). Merkel cell granules likely derive from the Golgi apparatus classical secretory pathway and are similar in size and appearance to those found in neurosecretory and neuroepithelial cell types present in other tissues [10]. The physical location and appearance of these granules suggest that they may function as key mediators of Merkel cell–nerve interactions.

Organization and Anatomic Distribution

Using basic histochemical staining methods, Merkel and others identified expanded nerve endings associated with the majority of Merkel cells (Fig. 1.2a) [11–13]. These Merkel cell–neurite complexes are present in almost all vertebrates including mammals, birds, reptiles, amphibians, and some classes of fish [11, 14, 15]. Merkel cells are innervated by neurites derived from large, heavily myelinated Aβ

S.M. Ostrowski
Department of Dermatology, University Hospitals Case Medical Center, 11100 Euclid Avenue, 44106, Cleveland, OH, USA
e-mail: stephen.ostrowski@uhhospitals.org

S.M. Maricich (✉)
Department of Pediatrics, Division of Neurology, University of Pittsburgh School of Medicine, Children's Hospital of Pittsburgh of UPMC, Rangos Research Building Room 8129, One Children's Hospital Drive, Pittsburgh, 15224, PA, USA
e-mail: stephen.maricich@chp.edu

M. Alam et al. (eds.), *Merkel Cell Carcinoma*, DOI 10.1007/978-1-4614-6608-6_1,

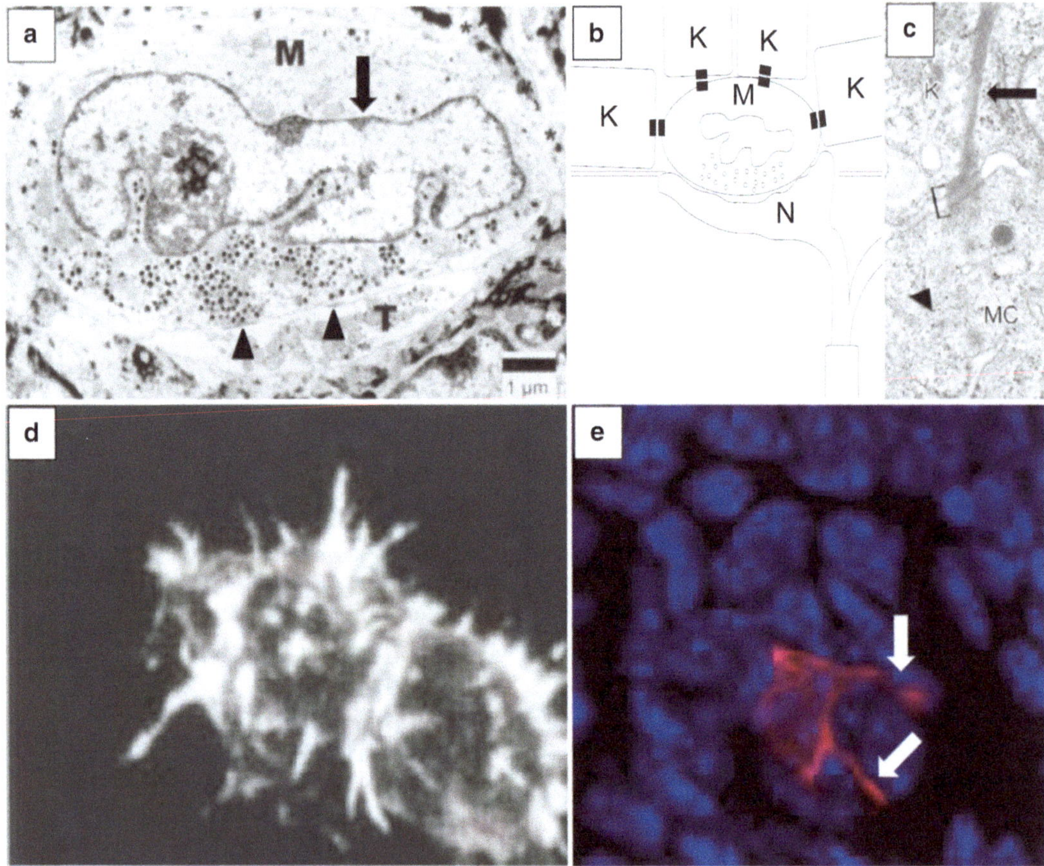

Fig. 1.1 Merkel cell structure. (**a**) Electron microscopic image of a Merkel cell (M). Note the lobulated nucleus (*arrow*) and numerous electron dense granules (*arrowheads*) positioned across from an adjacent nerve terminal (T). (**b**) Diagram showing relationship of a Merkel cell (M) to surrounding keratinocytes (K) and sensory nerve (N). Desmosomes (*dark rectangles*) attach adjacent cells. (**c**) Electron micrograph of a desmosome (*bracket*) and intermediate filaments in a keratinocyte (*arrow*) and Merkel cell (*arrowhead*). (**d**) 3D confocal microscopic reconstruction of a Merkel cell stained with an antibody against villin, demonstrating numerous spike-like villi projecting from the cell surface. (**e**) Merkel cell in the mouse footpad stained with an antibody against cytokeratin 8. Villous projections (*arrows*) intercalate with surrounding keratinocytes (**a**: Reprinted from Halata Z, Grim M, Bauman KI. Friedrich Sigmund Merkel and his "Merkel cell", morphology, development, and physiology: review and new results. The anatomical record. 2003;271, 225–239. With permission from John Wiley & Sons.). (**c**: Reprinted from Rickelt S, Moll I, Franke WW. Intercellular adhering junctions with an asymmetric molecular composition: desmosomes connecting Merkel cells and keratinocytes. Cell and tissue research 2011;346, 65–77. With permission from Springer Science + Business Media.). (**d**: Reprinted from Toyoshima K, Seta Y, Takeda S, Harada H. Identification of Merkel Cells by an Antibody to Villin. Journal of Histochemistry & Cytochemistry 1998;46, 1329–1334. With permission from Sage Publications)

sensory nerves whose cell bodies are located in dorsal root ganglia next to the spinal cord. The terminal branches of these neurites, which are unmyelinated, form a flattened nerve plate that closely apposes the basal surface of the Merkel cell [16] (Fig. 1.1a, b). In certain areas the nerve plasma membrane thickens and runs parallel to that of the Merkel cell. These points of contact possess many of the morphological characteristics of chemical synapses found in the central and peripheral nervous systems [17], suggesting a potential mechanism by which Merkel cells communicate with the neurons that contact them.

The best characterized Merkel cell–neurite complexes are found in epidermal structures of the hairy skin first described by Pinkus as

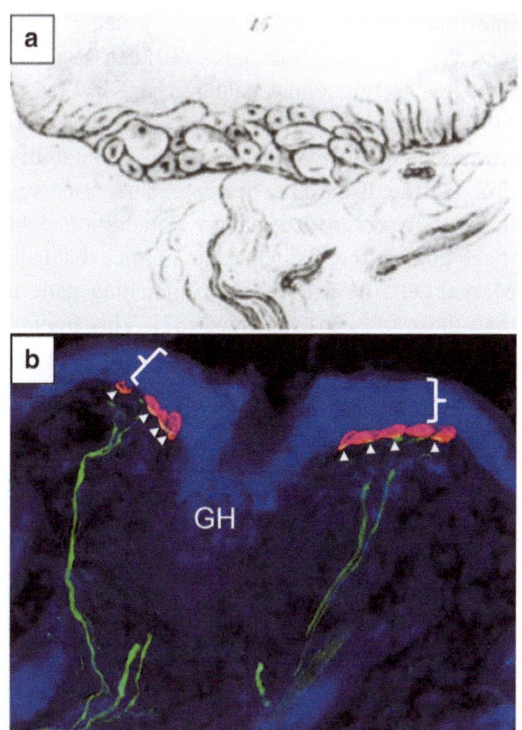

Fig. 1.2 Organization of Merkel cells in the touch dome. (**a**) One of Merkel's original touch dome illustrations. (**b**) Mouse touch dome viewed under fluorescence. Merkel cells, immunostained with anti-CK8 (*red*), are innervated by branching sensory nerves immunostained with NF200 (*green*); nerve terminals are shown by *arrowheads*. Brackets mark thickened touch dome epidermis. A single guard hair follicle (GH) sits in the middle of the touch dome. Cell nuclei are stained with TOTO-3 (*blue*) (**a**: Reprinted from Halata Z, Grim M, Bauman KI. Friedrich Sigmund Merkel and his "Merkel cell", morphology, development, and physiology: review and new results. The anatomical record. 2003;271, 225–239. With permission from John Wiley & Sons, Inc.)

"Haarschibe" and subsequently termed "touch domes" [16, 18]. Each of these dome-shaped elevations of the epidermis measures 100–400 μm in diameter and is typically composed of more than 50 Merkel cells, the nerve that innervates them, a keratinocyte layer 1–2 cell layers thicker than the surrounding epidermis, and a single guard hair (tylotrich) follicle (Fig. 1.2b). Human touch domes are somewhat rarer and more irregular in shape than those found in other mammals and are most highly concentrated on the neck, abdomen, and arms [1, 19].

Large numbers of Merkel cells are also found in glabrous (hairless) skin of the plantar and palmar surfaces, being most highly concentrated at the fingertips [2, 8]. In these regions, Merkel cell–neurite complexes occupy the base of epidermal (rete) ridges near the penetration of sweat gland ducts [20]. Merkel cells are highly concentrated in mammalian sensory vibrissal (whisker) hairs, where several hundred are found in each follicle [20], as well as in human terminal and vellus hair follicles [21, 22]. Merkel cells in these structures are identical in ultrastructure to those found in touch domes [23]. Merkel cells are also found in the oral mucosa, esophagus, and anus, singly or in groups of two to three sporadically located throughout interfollicular areas of hairy skin and rarely in the dermis [20, 24–26]. These Merkel cells are not associated with nerve endings, and their function is unknown.

Merkel Cell Function

The Sense of Touch

Merkel himself first proposed that Merkel cells must be involved in cutaneous mechanosensation based on their intimate association with cutaneous nerves. The accuracy of this claim has been debated for over 130 years, with various lines of evidence either supporting or refuting his hypothesis.

Several types of electrophysiological responses are elicited from cutaneous nerves following mechanical deformation of the skin surface. The slowly adapting type I (SAI) response was among the first to be associated with a defined anatomical structure. Nerve fibers that exhibit SAI responses have small receptive fields that center around small, distinct areas of the skin originally termed "touch spots" [27]. Intricate electrophysiological studies demonstrated that these "touch spots" were in fact touch domes [16]. Subsequent psychophysical experiments conducted on humans and other primates correlated SAI responses to the detection of curvature, shape, size, texture, and two-point discrimination, implicating Merkel cell–neurite complexes in these processes [28–31]. However, the question remained as to whether the SAI nerve fibers that innervate touch domes were sufficient to detect these stimuli or whether Merkel cells were required for mechanotransduction (transformation of mechanical to electrical stimuli).

Recently, this question was definitively addressed in genetically engineered mice. The gene encoding the transcription factor *Atoh1*, which is required for specification of Merkel cells, was conditionally (specifically) deleted from the skin of transgenic mice [32]. Touch dome ultrastructure and innervation were preserved in these animals, allowing the opportunity to test peripheral nerve responses to mechanical stimulation in the absence of Merkel cells. These mice completely lacked SAI responses to light touch stimuli, demonstrating that Merkel cells are necessary for the generation of these signals. These data also demonstrate that Merkel cells are not required for general development or maintenance of touch dome innervation and structure but instead play a direct role in mechanotransduction.

Despite this advance, it is still unclear how Merkel cells detect and transduce mechanical stimuli. It seems most likely that Merkel cells respond to and convert primary mechanical stimuli into chemical signals that initiate electrical impulses in associated nerve endings. In support of this view, Merkel cells express a number of presynaptic molecules such as piccolo, Rab3C, synapsins, synaptotagmins, and the vesicular glutamate transporter VGLUT2 [33], suggesting that they signal innervating neurites via classical synaptic transmission. Alternatively, Merkel cells may act as physical amplifiers allowing mechanical cues to more efficiently stimulate nerve terminals and activate mechanosensitive channels on neuronal membranes [34]. An ongoing area of research is to identify the mechanosensitive channels directly involved in these processes [35].

Merkel cells may also serve neuromodulatory and/or developmental functions. Merkel cell granules contain a wide variety of neuroactive peptides including bombesin, calcitonin gene-related peptide (CGRP), met-enkephalin, serotonin, somatostatin, substance P, and vasoactive intestinal peptide (VIP) [36–42]. Release of at least one of these molecules (VIP) can be regulated by acetylcholine, calcium, and histamine [43]. This suggests that Merkel cell-derived neuropeptides could modulate neuronal excitability of SAI afferents or other nearby cutaneous nerves in a locally controlled manner. In addition, SAI touch dome afferents in the skin of mice that lack Merkel cells have a different branching pattern than those of wild-type mice [32]. This finding implies that Merkel cells may be instructive for axon branching and terminal refinement, although the identity of putative Merkel cell-derived cues is currently unknown.

Neuroendocrine Function

Several lines of circumstantial evidence point to a potential neuroendocrine function of Merkel cells. First, they express neuropeptides (above) and other general markers of neuroendocrine cells such as cholecystokinin, chromogranin A, neuron-specific enolase, protein gene product 9.5 (PGP9.5), and synaptophysin [33, 41, 44–46]. Second, granules similar in ultrastructure to Merkel cell granules are found in cells with defined neuroendocrine functions such as intestinal secretory cells and pulmonary neuroepithelial cells [47]. Interestingly, intestinal secretory cells also require *Atoh1* for development, suggesting developmental homology with Merkel cells [48]. Third, some Merkel cells in the skin and other areas are not associated with nerves, suggesting that they are not involved in mechanosensation but instead serve other functions.

Despite these findings, the mechanisms by which Merkel cell-derived signals might influence skin homeostasis are unclear. What is known is that neuropeptides expressed by Merkel cells have well-characterized functions in the skin [49, 50]. For example, CGRP modulates Langerhans cell function [51], increases keratinocyte proliferation [52], and stimulates T-cell migration [53], while substance P stimulates keratinocyte and T-cell proliferation [54, 55]. Altered sensory innervation and increased neuropeptide expression are found in psoriasis and other skin diseases

[56, 57], and CGRP and substance P play key roles in maintenance of skin disease in a mouse model of psoriasiform dermatitis [58]. Thus, it is possible that neuropeptides produced by Merkel cells take part in skin homeostasis and disease.

Merkel Cell Origins

During embryogenesis, CK18- and CK20-positive cells can be identified in human skin as early as 8–12 weeks gestation, and cells with the characteristic ultrastructure of Merkel cells can be seen as early as 13 weeks gestation [59, 60]. By 18–24 weeks, Merkel cells reach particularly high concentrations of up to 1,700 cells/mm [2] in the glandular ridges of palmar skin, then show dramatic decreases in number over subsequent weeks [8]. This observation suggests that Merkel cell production is dynamically regulated during development. Most of these studies were carried out in human plantar skin where Merkel cells are at the highest density; the embryology of Merkel cells in human hairy skin has not been well characterized.

Adult Merkel cells are post-mitotic but are replaced after injury and during hair cycle progression [61–66]. From what tissue lineage do these Merkel cells arise? This question has been hotly debated and has obvious relevance for understanding the pathogenesis of Merkel cell carcinoma (MCC). Expression of neuropeptides, presynaptic machinery components, and transcription factors implicated in neuronal cell fate determination supported the hypothesis that Merkel cells descended from the neural crest, a migratory precursor cell population derived from the neural tube that gives rise to multiple cell types including skin melanocytes [67]. On the other hand, expression of epidermal-type cytokeratins, formation of desmosomal structures, and early appearance of Merkel cells in embryonic skin argued that Merkel cells had an epidermal origin [59, 68]. Experimental evidence from animal models supported both assertions to varying degrees [69, 70]. However, recent genetic studies have finally resolved this controversy. Fate-mapping studies in transgenic mice explicitly demonstrated that Merkel cells are derived from the skin, specifically from the epidermal lineage [71, 72]. However, whether adult Merkel cell precursors are multipotent or committed to the Merkel cell lineage is not clear, and the factors that directly control Merkel cell specification and differentiation are unknown. Answers to these questions are important as it is tempting to speculate that these precursor cells are directly involved in the pathogenesis of MCC.

The Biology of Merkel Cell Carcinoma

MCC is a rare and aggressive skin cancer that was initially described as "trabecular carcinoma" by Toker in 1972 [73]. The incidence of MCC has increased steadily over the years and is currently >1,500 cases/year in the United States. Treatment for localized disease involves liberal surgical resection with or without adjuvant radiotherapy; unfortunately, a high rate of local recurrence is the rule [74–76]. Tumors grow rapidly and are highly aggressive with ~1/3 of patients presenting with metastatic disease, a particularly dire diagnosis with a median survival of less than 7 months [77, 78]. As in other cancers, immune surveillance plays a role in MCC prevention, and immunosuppression markedly increases MCC risk and typically heralds a more aggressive clinical course [79–81]. Insights into the basic biology of MCC might provide clues to the origins of this cancer as well as possible therapeutic targets for anticancer agents.

Ultrastructural and Cell Biological Features of MCC

Based on cell size, MCC can be classified into three histological subtypes (trabecular, intermediate, and small cell), with admixture of the three being common [82]. Microscopically, MCC appears as sheets of poorly differentiated small basophilic cells with vesicular nuclei that fill the dermis, sometimes forming poorly defined clusters and cords of cells (Fig. 1.3a) [73, 83]. There are no specific histological features that distinguish MCC from other tumors composed of

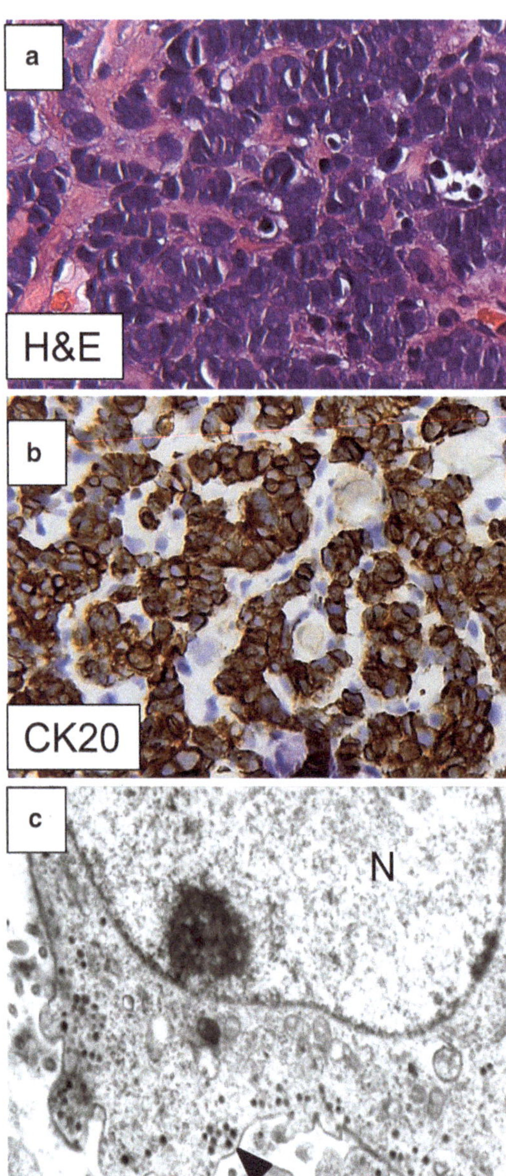

Fig. 1.3 Merkel cell carcinoma cells share key immunohistochemical and structural features of Merkel cells. (**a**, **b**) MCC cells exist as sheets of small round blue cells that stain specifically with an antibody directed against cytokeratin 20. (**c**) Electron micrograph of MCC small cell variant reveals numerous peripherally located dense-core granules (*arrowhead*) identical to those found in Merkel cells (**a**, **b**: Courtesy of Dr. Kord Honda, Case Western). (**c**: Reprinted from Llombart B, et al. Clinicopathological and immunohistochemical analysis of 20 cases of Merkel cell carcinoma in search of prognostic markers. Histopathology 2005; 46: 622–34. With permission from John Wiley and Sons, Inc.)

small, round blue cells such as Ewing's sarcoma, lymphoma, neuroblastoma, and small cell carcinoma of the lung.

The hypothesis that Merkel cells or their precursors gives rise to MCC stems from several observations. First, ultrastructural studies revealed that MCC tumor cells share many morphological similarities with Merkel cells, including dense-core granules and desmosome-type intercellular junctions (Fig. 1.3c) [84, 85]. Trabecular variants appear to be the most differentiated and always have well-formed desmosomes and many granules, while intermediate and small cell types have more primitive junctions and fewer granules. MCC cells also contain intermediate filament proteins composed of simple cytokeratins, although these are typically arranged in whorled or ball-like configurations rather than the loose homogenous arrangement found in normal Merkel cells [86, 87]. Second, MCC cells and Merkel cells express many of the same markers including bombesin, chromogranin, met-enkephalin, neuron-specific enolase, substance P, synaptophysin, VIP, and, occasionally, neurofilament protein [9, 88–93]. The mature Merkel cell marker CK20 is also expressed by most MCC tumors, allowing them to be distinguished from other tumors such as small cell carcinoma and lymphoma (Fig. 1.3b) [94]. Further evidence for a common link between Merkel cells and MCC is derived from gene expression analyses of Merkel cells and MCC cells which show that certain mRNA transcripts are enriched in both cell types [33, 95]. For example, *Atoh1*, which is required for normal Merkel cell development, is also expressed by many MCC cells, although there is conflicting evidence regarding whether it promotes or suppresses tumor formation [96–98].

DNA Damage and Chromosomal Abnormalities

Ultraviolet (UV) light exposure is thought to be a key MCC risk factor because tumors show a predilection for sun-exposed sites and a slightly increased incidence on the left side of the body, implicating driver-side automobile sun exposure as a likely contributing factor [99, 100]. Furthermore, increased incidence of MCC has been reported in patients who received the photosensitizer psoralen plus ultraviolet A (PUVA) therapy to treat skin diseases such as psoriasis [101], an association previously demonstrated with other cutaneous malignancies such as squamous cell carcinoma and melanoma [102, 103]. While this epidemiological data links MCC to UV exposure, direct evidence for UV-induced pathogenesis is limited. Some MCC tumor cell lines possess characteristic UV light-induced mutations (CC to TT) in the tumor suppressor gene *p53* and oncogene *h-Ras*, but the extent and functional significance of these mutations is uncertain [104]. This is in stark contrast to melanoma tumor cells, where genomic sequencing has revealed extensive UV-type mutations [105]. UV light could also contribute to MCC pathogenesis by suppressing immune surveillance [106].

Cancer cell karyotypes are often abnormal in chromosome structure and number, and analysis of these changes has been used to identify genes involved in tumorigenesis. Human MCC cells can have extrachromosomal copies of chromosome 1, 3p, and 5p regions and/or loss of 3p, 5q, 10, and 13 regions [107, 108]. Of particular note is deletion of 13q14–21, which occurs in 26 % of MCC tumors and contains the locus for the well-characterized *Retinoblastoma* (*Rb*) tumor suppressor gene [107, 108], and focal amplification at 1p34, which is found in 39 % of tumors and contains the *L-Myc* locus [107]. The proteins encoded by these genes play important roles in cell cycle regulation and are mutated in many human cancers.

Cell Cycle Pathways

In normal cells, the transition from quiescence to cell cycle entry is tightly regulated. The Rb protein plays an important role in this process (Fig. 1.4A). In non-cycling cells, Rb and the Rb-related proteins p107 and p130 are hypophosphorylated and thus are capable of binding and repressing members of the pro-growth E2F transcription factor family [109–111]. Cell cycle entry occurs only when growth signals activate cyclin-dependent kinases (CDKs), resulting in Rb phosphorylation and E2F release [109, 112, 113]. In many human cancers, this gatekeeper function is eliminated by mutations or deletions of the *Rb* gene, leading to the unchecked cell proliferation that is a key feature of cancer cells [114] (Fig. 1.4A). Oncogenic viruses such as adenovirus, human papillomavirus (HPV), and SV40 act similarly by targeting and inhibiting Rb [115]. There is conflicting evidence for Rb mutation or deletion in MCC [104, 116]. However, as detailed below, the Merkel cell polyomavirus (MCPyV) may contribute to MCC pathogenesis through perturbation of the Rb pathway.

Growth Factor Pathways

Extracellular growth factors stimulate cell division that is required for normal development and maintenance of tissues. Overexpression of these factors or constitutively active mutations in their receptors and/or downstream signaling components occurs in many human cancers (Fig. 1.4B). There is evidence that at least one of these pathways may be involved in MCC. Platelet-derived growth factors (PDGFs) are soluble peptides that signal cell surface receptors (PDGFRs) to modulate cell proliferation and differentiation. PDGF is a key player in many cancers, acting both as an autocrine growth factor and as a signal to the stroma and vasculature to stimulate angiogenesis [117]. One study found increased PDGF and PDGFR expression in over 80 % of MCC cells [118], while another identified a single novel base pair substitution in the *PDGFR* gene in three of ten MCCs examined [119]. These findings suggest that PDGF signaling may play a role in MCC.

Mitogen-activated protein kinases (MAPKs) such as Erk, Raf, and Ras constitute a common intracellular signaling pathway that is the effector arm of PDGF and other growth factor receptor signaling pathways. Mutations and/or upregulation of MAPK signaling occur in a high

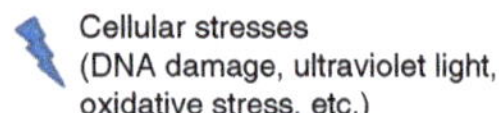

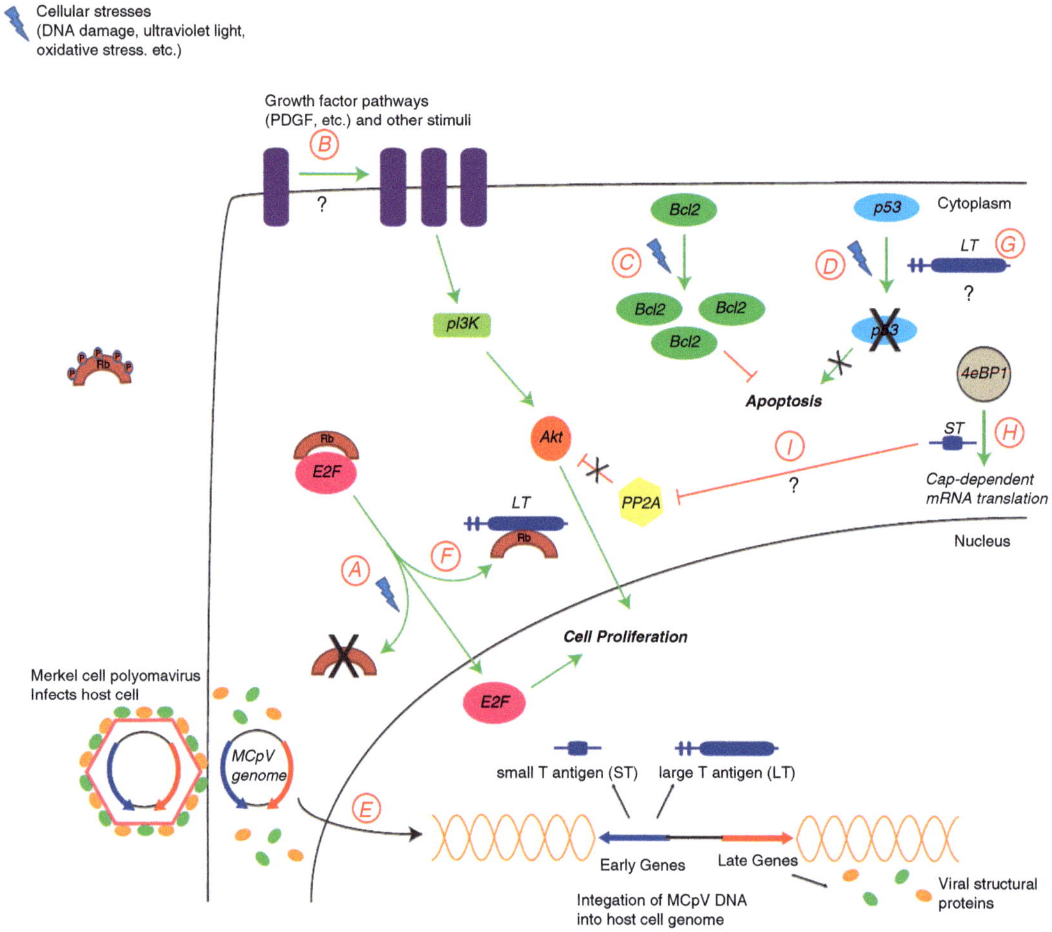

Fig. 1.4 Potential mechanisms of MCC pathogenesis—(A, F) Inactivation of Rb leads to E2F release and gene expression that promotes cell proliferation. (B) Growth factor signaling and other stimuli promote tumor cell survival and proliferation through multiple mechanisms, including the PI3K/Akt pathway. (C, D, G) Apoptosis is inhibited by Bcl-2 or interference with p53 function. (E) Entry of MCPyV and DNA integration into the host genome leads to production of LT, ST, and viral structural proteins. (H) Cap-dependent translation is regulated by 4eBP1 and contributes to tumorigenesis. (I) SV40 (and possibly MCPyV) ST can bind and inhibit PP2A, leading to release of Akt inhibition and increased cell proliferation. *Green arrows*—activation, *red arrows*—repression, ?—possible interaction

percentage of melanomas [120] but not in MCCs [121]. Instead, MAPK pathway activation in MCC cells induces apoptosis [122], suggesting that PDGF signaling might impact pathogenesis by acting through other cellular pathways. Interestingly, PDGF can stimulate the PI3K pathway, resulting in activation of downstream effectors such as Akt kinase [123, 124] (Fig. 1.4B). This pathway is targeted in a number of human cancers but has not been explored in detail in MCC [125].

Apoptotic Pathways

Apoptosis, or programmed cell death, is a critical defense mechanism that destroys aging and damaged cells. Predictably, evasion of apoptotic pathways is a hallmark of many cancers. Two antiapoptotic factors have been implicated in MCC. The first, Bcl-2, was identified at the site of a chromosomal translocation associated with human follicular B-cell lymphoma [126]. This translocation causes Bcl-2 overexpression;

overexpression of Bcl-2 occurs in many tumor cell types including MCC [127, 130]. Bcl-2 overexpression is thought to act as a key step in tumorigenesis by blocking tumor cell death [131, 132] (Fig. 1.4C). Conversely, disruption of Bcl-2 leads to cell death [133], an observation whose clinical significance to MCC is suggested by an in vivo mouse xenograft model where knockdown of *Bcl-2* expression by antisense oligonucleotides resulted in MCC tumor shrinkage [134]. Unfortunately, this same strategy showed no benefit in nine human patients with advanced MCC [135]. A second antiapoptotic factor, survivin, is also upregulated in many cancers [136] including MCC, and its expression is associated with poor clinical prognosis [137, 138]. The specific mechanism by which survivin acts in MCC is unknown.

The well-characterized transcription factor p53 plays several roles in carcinogenesis (Fig. 1.4D). In response to cellular stressors including DNA damage, hypoxia, and oxidative stress, the p53 protein is stabilized and p53-dependent gene expression increases. Low levels of stress cause p53 to halt the cell cycle and promote repair of DNA damage, while severe stress causes increased expression of proapoptotic genes that initiate cell death [139]. This latter mechanism presumably eliminates cells that might otherwise progress to cancer. Mutation of p53 occurs in up to 50 % of human cancers [140], and mice deficient in p53 develop multiple types of spontaneous tumors [141]. Other alterations in p53 activity, including epigenetic silencing of the *p53* gene, posttranslational modification of p53 protein, and increased expression of the p53 inhibitor Mdm2, can also cause disease [142–144] [145]. However, p53 mutation occurs rarely in MCC [146–148], and the contribution of alternative mechanisms to MCC genesis has not been studied.

Merkel Cell Polyomavirus and MCC

In 2008 it was reported that a novel virus termed Merkel cell polyomavirus (MCPyV) was clonally integrated into the genome of MCC cells [149]. Several lines of evidence suggest that MCPyV is involved in MCC pathogenesis, and further understanding of the pathogenic mechanisms by which the virus operates holds the hope of producing novel MCC therapies.

Basic Biology of Polyomaviruses and MCPyV

Polyomaviruses are double-stranded DNA viruses with an icosahedral capsid [150]. Their genomes can be divided into early-expressed genes that encode T-antigens and late-expressed genes that encode viral coat proteins and proteins that cause host cell lysis [151] (Fig. 1.4E). T-antigens (so named because host T-cell responses are primarily directed at these proteins) bind to multiple cellular proteins, hijacking the host replication machinery to force S-phase cells to allow viral replication (detailed below).

Advances in high throughput DNA sequencing have facilitated the discovery of viruses integrated into the human genome, resulting in an explosion of human polyomaviruses identified since 2006. There are now nine known human polyomaviruses (MCPyV, BKV, JCV, KIV, WUV, TSPyV, HPyV6, HPyV7, and HPyV9) [152]. The monkey LPV and SV40 polyomaviruses are also thought to infect human populations [152]. BKV, JCV, and SV40 induce tumors in animal models, but their carcinogenic potential in humans is controversial [153–155].

The MCPyV genome is ~5,400 base pairs in size and encodes sequences similar to other polyomaviruses including T-antigens, viral protein (VP)1, VP2/3, and replication origin sequences [149]. Similar to other polyomaviruses, the MCPyV T-antigen sequence undergoes alternative splicing to produce three transcripts: large T-antigen (LT), small T-antigen (ST), and 57kd T-antigen (57kT). The MCPyV T-antigens share only ~30 % amino acid homology to those produced by other polyomaviruses, but there is marked conservation of key structural domains [156].

Evidence for a Role of MCPyV in MCC Pathogenesis

Current evidence suggests that MCPyV infection is highly specific to MCC and that it plays a role in tumorigenesis. MCPyV sequences are found in ~80 % of MCC tumors but are present at much lower percentages (<15 %) in other tumors and normal tissue [149, 157–159]. In most cases, MCPyV DNA is integrated into the MCC tumor genome in a clonal pattern, suggesting that MCPyV infection and integration precede clonal expansion and metastasis of tumor cells [149]. MCPyV LT protein is detectable only in MCC cells and not in other skin cancers such as basal or squamous cell carcinomas, even in patients with both types of tumors [160, 161]. Serum levels of MCC patient antibodies directed against the common T-antigen sequence appear to correlate with MCC tumor load and increase with cancer recurrence [156, 162].

Importantly, MCC-derived MCPyV contains mutations that result in truncation of the LT-antigen protein; in contrast, MCPyV from non-tumor sources lacks these mutations [156, 163]. These truncating mutations cause loss of the LT helicase and origin binding domains, leading to loss of viral replication capacity. It has been suggested that LT that retains these domains after viral DNA integration mediates unchecked DNA synthesis at the integrated DNA site, causing replication fork collisions and ultimately host cell death [164, 165]. Thus, loss of viral replication capacity appears to be a key step in viable host integration and, ultimately, carcinogenesis caused by tumor viruses. As independent viral integration and mutation are individually rare events, it could explain why MCC is uncommon even though MCPyV infection (as assayed by VP1 and VP2 seropositivity) appears to occur in 25–80 % of the population [166, 167]. It has also been speculated that truncated LT may have decreased antigenicity and thus help promote immune evasion of infected cells.

While some studies have shown that MCPyV-positive tumors are clinically more aggressive than MCPyV-negative tumors, others have demonstrated that MCC tumors display similar clinical behavior and prognosis regardless of MCPyV status [168, 169]. Likewise, in vitro evidence is mixed regarding whether MCC cell morphology or growth characteristics can predict MCPyV status [170]. Some common pathways are likely to be involved in MCPyV-positive and negative MCC, but how these pathways are activated likely differs. For example, MCPyV-positive tumors may result from MCPyV activation of cellular growth pathways, while MCPyV-negative tumors may require increased UV-induced mutations or other genetic initiating factors. MCPyV-negative tumor cells typically contain more chromosomal aberrations than MCPyV-positive cells [107], and MCPyV-negative tumor cells can contain p53 mutations, whereas MCPyV-positive tumor cells do not [163]. The association of alterations in Rb expression and phosphorylation status with MCPyV infection is less clear [162, 171, 172]. Further studies are needed to clarify the carcinogenic pathways in MCPyV-positive and MCPyV-negative tumors.

Potential Mechanisms of MCPyV Tumorigenesis

The simian virus 40 (SV40) polyomavirus causes tumor formation in many animal and cellular models [153, 173]. Study of this and other polyomaviruses has provided great insight into polyomavirus biology and general mechanisms involved in human carcinogenesis, including the discovery of the p53 protein and information relating to the function of the Rb and phosphatidylinositol 3-kinase (PI3K) signaling pathways [115, 174, 175]. SV40 T-antigens modulate these and other pathways to facilitate viral integration and/or proliferation with the unintended side effect of carcinogenesis. Current evidence suggests that MCPyV may contribute to MCC carcinogenesis through both similar and novel mechanisms.

Large T-Cell Antigen

The MCPyV large T (LT) antigen shares several domains (DnaJ, Rb-binding, p53-binding, origin binding, and helicase) that are highly homologous to those of SV40 LT [176]. These domains are well-characterized with respect to their role in SV40-mediated tumorigenesis; therefore, it is possible that MCPyV and SV40 LT function similarly to promote carcinogenesis.

The Rb protein is a key cell cycle regulator (see above). The SV40 LT Rb-binding domain binds and inactivates Rb, causing unchecked cell proliferation and cellular transformation [115, 177]. Similar mechanisms appear to be involved in MCPyV-mediated pathogenesis. MCPyV LT binds Rb in vitro [156], and knockdown of MCPyV LT antigen by short-hairpin RNA (shRNA) impairs growth of MCPyV-positive but not MCPyV-negative MCC tumor cells [178], an effect that requires an intact Rb-binding domain [179]. Furthermore, truncating mutations found in MCC-derived MCPyV retain an intact Rb-binding domain [156]. These data suggest that MCPyV LT binding to Rb is required for the transforming properties of the virus (Fig. 1.4F). The Rb-binding and DnaJ domains of SV40 cooperate with heat shock protein 70 (Hsp70) to trigger phosphorylation and dissociation of Rb-related proteins p107 and p130 from the E2F4 transcription factor [180, 181]; it is unclear if MCPyV acts by similar mechanisms.

As detailed above, p53, a critical regulator of cell proliferation and apoptosis, is mutated in many human cancers. SV40 LT binds directly to p53, abrogating its ability to bind DNA and enhancing cancerous transformation [182]. SV40 LT also blocks p53 association with cofactors p300 and CBP [183], promoting p53 phosphorylation and subsequent inactivation [184] (Fig. 1.4G). However, it is unclear whether MCPyV-dependent inactivation of p53 is a mechanism in MCC genesis because MCPyV integrated into MCC cells contains nonsense mutations that truncate the LT antigen, often (~50 %) resulting in loss of the predicted p53-binding domain [156, 176]. One intriguing new observation is that p53 is mutated in MCPyV-negative but not MCPyV-positive tumors [185]. If p53 inactivation were required for MCC pathogenesis, this would suggest that MCPyV may inhibit p53, perhaps through a novel mechanism.

Small T-Cell Antigen

SV40 small T-cell (ST) antigen alone is insufficient to cause transformation, but it facilitates transformation by LT [186, 187]. In contrast, MCPyV ST alone is sufficient to transform rodent cells, and knockdown of ST protein levels in MCC tumor cells slows their growth [188]. MCPyV ST also causes hyperphosphorylation of eIF4E-binding protein (4E-BP1), a key regulator of protein translation. 4E-BP1 phosphorylation releases it from the mRNA cap, allowing cap-dependent translation (protein synthesis) to proceed [189] (Fig. 1.4H). Hyperphosphorylation of 4E-BP1 is thought to be important in the pathogenesis of a number of different cancers [190].

The major target of SV40 ST is the multifunctional serine–threonine protein phosphatase A (PP2A), which it binds and functionally inhibits [191]. SV40 ST-mediated inhibition of PP2A allows Akt kinase to be maintained in a phosphorylated and activated state, leading to stabilization of Myc and, ultimately, cell cycle entry [192] (Fig. 1.4I). Interestingly, MCPyV ST-induced transformation and 4E-BP1 phosphorylation does not appear to depend on PP2A interaction as it also occurs with mutant MCPyV ST proteins that have lost the ability to bind PP2A [188]. Whether other MCPyV ST-PP2A interactions contribute to MCC pathogenesis remains an open question.

Other Potential Mechanisms of Carcinogenesis

As noted above, the T-antigen domains of MCPyV are partially conserved among polyomaviruses. However, MCPyV T-antigen also contains a novel 200 amino acid N-terminal domain termed the MCPyV T-antigen unique region (MUR). MUR is conserved among all tumor-derived MCPyV strains [193]. A recent study identified hVamp6, a protein that causes lysosomal clustering, as a MUR-binding partner [193]. Wild-type, but not truncated, MCC-derived MCPyV LT causes nuclear localization of hVAM6P suggesting that if this interaction is physiologically relevant, it is unlikely to play a role in tumorigenesis. However, MUR may induce tumorigenesis through other mechanisms.

Analysis of the MCPyV genome reveals a predicted novel microRNA species (MCV-miR-M1-5p) [194], and this microRNA has since been detected in 50 % of MCC cell lines but not in control tissues [195]. Similar to microRNAs produced by other polyomaviruses, MCV-miR-M1-5p downregulates T-antigen expression in cultured cells [194] and may thus contribute to MCC pathogenesis through promotion of immune evasion [196].

References

1. Smith KR. The ultrastructure of the human Haarscheibe and Merkel cell. J Invest Dermatol. 1970;54:150–9.
2. Hashimoto K. The ultrastructure of the skin of human embryos. X. Merkel tactile cells in the finger and nail. J Anat. 1972;111:99–120.
3. Kurosumi K, Kurosumi U, Suzuki H. Fine structures of Merkel cells and associated nerve fibers in the epidermis of certain mammalian species. Arch Histol Jpn. 1969;30:295–313.
4. Halata Z, Grim M, Bauman KI. Friedrich Sigmund Merkel and his "Merkel cell", morphology, development, and physiology: review and new results. Anat Rec. 2003;271:225–39.
5. Rickelt S, Moll I, Franke WW. Intercellular adhering junctions with an asymmetric molecular composition: desmosomes connecting Merkel cells and keratinocytes. Cell Tissue Res. 2011;346:65–77.
6. Toyoshima K, Seta Y, Takeda S, Harada H. Identification of Merkel cells by an antibody to villin. J Histochem Cytochem. 1998;46:1329–34.
7. Saurat JH, Didierjean L, Skalli O, Siegenthaler G, Gabbiani G. The intermediate filament proteins of rabbit normal epidermal Merkel cells are cytokeratins. J Invest Dermatol. 1984;83:431–5.
8. Moll R, Moll I, Franke WW. Identification of Merkel cells in human skin by specific cytokeratin antibodies: changes of cell density and distribution in fetal and adult plantar epidermis. Differentiation. 1984;28:136–54.
9. Moll I, Kuhn C, Moll R. Cytokeratin 20 is a general marker of cutaneous Merkel cells while certain neuronal proteins are absent. J Invest Dermatol. 1995;104:910–5.
10. Salomon D, Carraux P, Mérot Y, Saurat JH. Pathway of granule formation in Merkel cells: an ultrastructural study. J Invest Dermatol. 1987;89:362–5.
11. Merkel F. Tastzellen und Tastkorperchen bei den Hausthieren und beim Menschen. Archiv für mikroskopische Anatomie. 1875;11:636–52.
12. Ranvier L. De la terminaison des nerfs dans le corpuscles du tact. Comptes Rendus de l'Académie des Sciences. 1877;85:1020–30.
13. Botezat E. Die Nerven der Epidermis. Anat Anz. 1908;33:45.
14. Whitear M. Merkel cells in lower vertebrates. Arch Histol Cytol. 1989;52(Suppl):415–22.
15. Lane EB, Whitear M. On the occurrence of Merkel cells in the epidermis of teleost fishes. Cell Tissue Res. 1977;182:235–46.
16. Iggo A, Muir AR. The structure and function of a slowly adapting touch corpuscle in hairy skin. J Physiol. 1969;200:763–96.
17. Hartschuh W, Weihe E. Fine structural analysis of the synaptic junction of Merkel cell-axon-complexes. J Invest Dermatol. 1980;75:159–65.
18. Pinkus F. Uber einen bisher unbekannten Nebenapparat am Haarsystem des Menschen: Haarscheiben. Dermatol Zeitschr. 1902;9:465–9.
19. Kawamura T, Nishiyama S, Ikeda S, Tajima K. The human haarscheibe, its structure and function. J Invest Dermatol. 1964;42:87–90.
20. Halata Z. The mechanoreceptors of the mammalian skin ultrastructure and morphological classification. Adv Anat Embryol Cell Biol. 1975;50:3–77.
21. Narisawa Y, Hashimoto K, Kohda H. Merkel cells of the terminal hair follicle of the adult human scalp. J Invest Dermatol. 1994;102:506–10.
22. Santa Cruz DJ, Bauer EA. Merkel cells in the outer follicular sheath. Ultrastruct Pathol. 1982;3:59–63.
23. Munger BL, Pubols LM, Pubols BH. The Merkel rete papilla—a slowly adapting sensory receptor in mammalian glabrous skin. Brain Res. 1971;29:47–61.
24. Mahrle G, Orfanos CE. Merkel cells as human cutaneous neuroreceptor cells. Their presence in dermal neural corpuscles and in the external hair root sheath of human adult skin. Arch Dermatol Forsch. 1974;251:19–26.
25. Moll I, Bladt U, Jung EG. Presence of Merkel cells in sun-exposed and not sun-exposed skin: a quantitative study. Arch Dermatol Res. 1990;282:213–6.
26. Hashimoto K. Fine structure of Merkel cell in human oral mucosa. J Invest Dermatol. 1972;58:381–7.
27. Frankenhauser B. Impulses from a cutaneous receptor with slow adaptation and low mechanical threshold. Acta Physiol Scand. 1949;18:68–74.
28. Goodwin AW, Macefield VG, Bisley JW. Encoding of object curvature by tactile afferents from human fingers. J Neurophysiol. 1997;78:2881–8.
29. LaMotte RH, Srinivasan MA, Lu C, Klusch-Petersen A. Cutaneous neural codes for shape. Can J Physiol Pharmacol. 1994;72:498–505.
30. Yoshioka T, Gibb B, Dorsch AK, Hsiao SS, Johnson KO. Neural coding mechanisms underlying perceived roughness of finely textured surfaces. J Neurosci. 2001;21:6905–16.

31. Johnson KO, Lamb GD. Neural mechanisms of spatial tactile discrimination: neural patterns evoked by braille-like dot patterns in the monkey. J Physiol. 1981;310:117–44.
32. Maricich SM et al. Merkel cells are essential for light-touch responses. Science. 2009;324:1580–2.
33. Haeberle H et al. Molecular profiling reveals synaptic release machinery in Merkel cells. Proc Natl Acad Sci U S A. 2004;101:14503–8.
34. Gottschaldt KM, Vahle-Hinz C. Merkel cell receptors: structure and transducer function. Science. 1981;214:183–6.
35. Delmas P, Hao J, Rodat-Despoix L. Molecular mechanisms of mechanotransduction in mammalian sensory neurons. Nat Rev Neurosci. 2011;12:139–53.
36. Hartschuh W, Weihe E, Yanaihara N, Reinecke M. Immunohistochemical localization of vasoactive intestinal polypeptide (VIP) in Merkel cells of various mammals: evidence for a neuromodulator function of the Merkel cell. J Invest Dermatol. 1983;81:361–4.
37. Chew SB, Leung PY. Immunocytochemical evidence of a met-enkephalin-like substance in the dense-core granules of mouse Merkel cells. Cell Tissue Res. 1991;265:611–4.
38. Fantini F, Johansson O. Neurochemical markers in human cutaneous Merkel cells. An immunohistochemical investigation. Exp Dermatol. 1995;4:365–71.
39. English KB et al. Serotonin-like immunoreactivity in Merkel cells and their afferent neurons in touch domes from the hairy skin of rats. Anat Rec. 1992;232:112–20.
40. García-Caballero T, Gallego R, Rosón E, Fraga M, Beiras A. Calcitonin gene-related peptide (CGRP) immunoreactivity in the neuroendocrine Merkel cells and nerve fibres of pig and human skin. Histochemistry. 1989;92:127–32.
41. Hartschuh W, Weihe E, Yanaihara N. Immunohistochemical analysis of chromogranin A and multiple peptides in the mammalian Merkel cell: further evidence for its paraneuronal function? Arch Histol Cytol. 1989;52(Suppl):423–31.
42. Alvarez FJ et al. Immunocytochemical analysis of calcitonin gene-related peptide and vasoactive intestinal polypeptide in Merkel cells and cutaneous free nerve endings of cats. Cell Tissue Res. 1988;254:429–37.
43. Boulais N et al. Merkel cells as putative regulatory cells in skin disorders: an in vitro study. PLoS One. 2009;4:9.
44. Casasco A et al. Immunocytochemical labelling of Merkel cells of human oral mucosa by means of antibodies to protein gene product 9.5. Bull Group Int Rech Sci Stomatol Odontol. 1990;33:61–4.
45. Gu J, Polak JM, Tapia FJ, Marangos PJ, Pearse AG. Neuron-specific enolase in the Merkel cells of mammalian skin. The use of specific antibody as a simple and reliable histologic marker. Am J Pathol. 1981;104:63–8.
46. Ortonne JP et al. Normal Merkel cells express a synaptophysin-like immunoreactivity. Dermatologica. 1988;177:1–10.
47. Winkelmann RK. The Merkel cell system and a comparison between it and the neurosecretory or APUD cell system. J Invest Dermatol. 1977;69:41–6.
48. Yang Q, Bermingham NA, Finegold MJ, Zoghbi HY. Requirement of Math1 for secretory cell lineage commitment in the mouse intestine. Science. 2001;294:2155–8.
49. Seiffert K, Granstein RD. Neuroendocrine regulation of skin dendritic cells. Ann N Y Acad Sci. 2006;1088:195–206.
50. Scholzen T et al. Neuropeptides in the skin: interactions between the neuroendocrine and the skin immune systems. Exp Dermatol. 1998;7:81–96.
51. Hosoi J et al. Regulation of Langerhans cell function by nerves containing calcitonin gene-related peptide. Nature. 1993;363:159–63.
52. Yu X-J, Li C-Y, Xu Y-H, Chen L-M, Zhou C-L. Calcitonin gene-related peptide increases proliferation of human HaCaT keratinocytes by activation of MAP kinases. Cell Biol Int. 2009;33:1144–8.
53. Talme T, Liu Z, Sundqvist K-G. The neuropeptide calcitonin gene-related peptide (CGRP) stimulates T cell migration into collagen matrices. J Neuroimmunol. 2008;196:60–6.
54. Tanaka T, Danno K, Ikai K, Imamura S. Effects of substance P and substance K on the growth of cultured keratinocytes. J Invest Dermatol. 1988;90:399–401.
55. Payan DG, Brewster DR, Goetzl EJ. Specific stimulation of human T lymphocytes by substance P. J Immunol. 1983;131:1613–5.
56. Farber EM, Nickoloff BJ, Recht B, Fraki JE. Stress, symmetry, and psoriasis: possible role of neuropeptides. J Am Acad Dermatol. 1986;14:305–11.
57. Saraceno R, Kleyn CE, Terenghi G, Griffiths CEM. The role of neuropeptides in psoriasis. Br J Dermatol. 2006;155:876–82.
58. Ostrowski SM, Belkadi A, Loyd CM, Diaconu D, Ward NL. Cutaneous denervation of psoriasiform mouse skin improves acanthosis and inflammation in a sensory neuropeptide-dependent manner. J Invest Dermatol. 2011;131:1530–8.
59. Moll I, Moll R, Franke WW. Formation of epidermal and dermal Merkel cells during human fetal skin development. J Invest Dermatol. 1986;87:779–87.
60. Kim D-K, Holbrook KA. The appearance, density, and distribution of Merkel cells in human embryonic and fetal skin: their relation to sweat gland and hair follicle development. J Invest Dermatol. 1995;104:411–6.
61. Vaigot P, Pisani A, Darmon YM, Ortonne JP. The majority of epidermal Merkel cells are non-proliferative: a quantitative immunofluorescence analysis. Acta Derm Venereol. 1987;67(6):517–20.

62. Moll I, Zieger W, Schmelz M. Proliferative Merkel cells were not detected in human skin. Arch Dermatol Res. 1996;288:184–7.
63. Tachibana T, Fujiwara N, Nawa T. Postnatal differentiation of Merkel cells in the rat palatine mucosa, with special reference to the timing of peripheral nerve development and the potency of cell mitosis. Anat Embryol. 2000;202:359–67.
64. Fradette J et al. Normal human Merkel cells are present in epidermal cell populations isolated and cultured from glabrous and hairy skin sites. J Invest Dermatol. 2003;120:313–7.
65. Nakafusa J et al. Changes in the number of Merkel cells with the hair cycle in hair discs on rat back skin. Br J Dermatol. 2006;155:883–9.
66. Nurse CA, Macintyre L, Diamond J. Reinnervation of the rat touch dome restores the Merkel cell population reduced after denervation. Neuroscience. 1984;13:563–71.
67. Grim M, Halata Z. Developmental origin of avian Merkel cells. Anat Embryol. 2000;202:401–10.
68. Ochiai T, Suzuki H. Fine structural and morphometric studies of the Merkel cell during fetal and postnatal development. J Invest Dermatol. 1981;77: 437–43.
69. Moll I, Lane AT, Franke WW, Moll R. Intraepidermal formation of Merkel cells in xenografts of human fetal skin. J Invest Dermatol. 1990;94:359–64.
70. Szeder V, Grim M, Halata Z, Sieber-Blum M. Neural crest origin of mammalian Merkel cells. Dev Biol. 2003;253:258–63.
71. Morrison KM, Miesegaes GR, Lumpkin EA, Maricich SM. Mammalian Merkel cells are descended from the epidermal lineage. Dev Biol. 2009;336:76–83.
72. Van Keymeulen A et al. Epidermal progenitors give rise to Merkel cells during embryonic development and adult homeostasis. J Cell Biol. 2009;187: 91–100.
73. Toker C. Trabecular carcinoma of the skin. Arch Dermatol. 1972;105:107–10.
74. Lewis KG, Weinstock MA, Weaver AL, Otley CC. Adjuvant local irradiation for Merkel cell carcinoma. Arch Dermatol. 2006;142:693–700.
75. O'Connor WJ, Roenigk RK, Brodland DG. Merkel cell carcinoma. Comparison of Mohs micrographic surgery and wide excision in eighty-six patients. Dermatol Surg. 1997;23:929–33.
76. Yiengpruksawan A, Coit DG, Thaler HT, Urmacher C, Knapper WK. Merkel cell carcinoma: prognosis and management. Arch Surg. 1991;126:1514–9.
77. Akhtar S, Oza KK, Wright J. Merkel cell carcinoma: report of 10 cases and review of the literature. J Am Acad Dermatol. 2000;43:755–67.
78. Allen PJ et al. Merkel cell carcinoma: prognosis and treatment of patients from a single institution. J Clin Oncol. 2005;23:2300–9.
79. Ziprin P, Smith S, Salerno G, Rosin RD. Two cases of Merkel cell tumour arising in patients with chronic lymphocytic leukaemia. Br J Dermatol. 2000;142: 525–8.
80. Engels EA, Frisch M, Goedert JJ, Biggar RJ, Miller RW. Merkel cell carcinoma and HIV infection. Lancet. 2002;359:497–8.
81. Penn I, First MR. Merkel's cell carcinoma in organ recipients: report of 41 cases. Transplantation. 1999; 68:1717–21.
82. Gould VE, Moll R, Moll I, Lee I, Franke WW. Neuroendocrine (Merkel) cells of the skin: hyperplasias, dysplasias, and neoplasms. Lab Invest. 1985;52: 334–53.
83. Sidhu GS et al. Merkel cell neoplasms. Histology, electron microscopy, biology, and histogenesis. Am J Dermatopathol. 1980;2:101–19.
84. Tang CK, Toker C. Trabecular carcinoma of the skin: an ultrastructural study. Cancer. 1978;42: 2311–21.
85. Llombart B et al. Clinicopathological and immunohistochemical analysis of 20 cases of Merkel cell carcinoma in search of prognostic markers. Histopathology. 2005;46:622–34.
86. Moll I et al. Establishment and characterization of two Merkel cell tumor cultures. J Invest Dermatol. 1994;102:346–53.
87. Wick MR et al. Primary neuroendocrine carcinomas of the skin (Merkel cell tumors). a clinical, histologic, and ultrastructural study of thirteen cases. Am J Clin Pathol. 1983;79:6–13.
88. Furuno K, Wakakura M, Shimizu K, Iwabuchi K, Kameya T. Immunohistochemical studies of Merkel cell carcinoma of the eyelid. Jpn J Ophthalmol. 1992;36:348–55.
89. Visscher D, Cooper PH, Zarbo RJ, Crissman JD. Cutaneous neuroendocrine (Merkel cell) carcinoma: an immunophenotypic, clinicopathologic, and flow cytometric study. Mod Pathol. 1989;2:331–8.
90. Gu J et al. Immunostaining of neuron-specific enolase as a diagnostic tool for Merkel cell tumors. Cancer. 1983;52:1039–43.
91. Green WR, Linnoila RI, Triche TJ. Neuroendocrine carcinoma of skin with simultaneous cytokeratin expression. Ultrastruct Pathol. 1984;6:141–52.
92. Leong AS, Phillips GE, Pieterse AS, Milios J. Criteria for the diagnosis of primary endocrine carcinoma of the skin (Merkel cell carcinoma). A histological, immunohistochemical and ultrastructural study of 13 cases. Pathology. 1986;18:393–9.
93. Narisawa Y, Hashimoto K, Kohda H. Immunohistochemical demonstration of the expression of neurofilament proteins in Merkel cells. Acta Derm Venereol. 1994;74:441–3.
94. Moll R, Löwe A, Laufer J, Franke WW. Cytokeratin 20 in human carcinomas. A new histodiagnostic marker detected by monoclonal antibodies. Am J Pathol. 1992;140:427–47.
95. Van Gele M et al. Gene-expression profiling reveals distinct expression patterns for classic versus variant Merkel cell phenotypes and new classifier genes to

distinguish Merkel cell from small-cell lung carcinoma. Oncogene. 2004;23:2732–42.
96. Heiskala K, Arola J, Heiskala M, Andersson LC. Expression of Reg IV and Hath1 in neuroendocrine neoplasms. Histol Histopathol. 2010;25:63–72.
97. Flora A, Klisch TJ, Schuster G, Zoghbi HY. Deletion of Atoh1 disrupts Sonic Hedgehog signaling in the developing cerebellum and prevents medulloblastoma. Science. 2009;326:1424–7.
98. Bossuyt W et al. Atonal homolog 1 is a tumor suppressor gene. PLoS Biol. 2009;7:e39.
99. Agelli M, Clegg LX. Epidemiology of primary Merkel cell carcinoma in the United States. J Am Acad Dermatol. 2003;49:832–41.
100. Paulson KG, Iyer JG, Nghiem P. Asymmetric lateral distribution of melanoma and Merkel cell carcinoma in the United States. J Am Acad Dermatol. 2011;65: 35–9.
101. Lunder EJ, Stern RS. Merkel-cell carcinomas in patients treated with methoxsalen and ultraviolet A radiation. N Engl J Med. 1998;339:1247–8.
102. Stern RS, Lunder EJ. Risk of squamous cell carcinoma and methoxsalen (psoralen) and UV-A radiation (PUVA). A meta-analysis. Arch Dermatol. 1998;134:1582–5.
103. Stern RS. The risk of melanoma in association with long-term exposure to PUVA. J Am Acad Dermatol. 2001;44:755–61.
104. Popp S, Waltering S, Herbst C, Moll I, Boukamp P. UV-B-type mutations and chromosomal imbalances indicate common pathways for the development of Merkel and skin squamous cell carcinomas. Int J Cancer. 2002;99:352–60.
105. Pleasance ED et al. A comprehensive catalogue of somatic mutations from a human cancer genome. Nature. 2010;463:191–6.
106. Schwarz T, Schwarz A. Molecular mechanisms of ultraviolet radiation-induced immunosuppression. Eur J Cell Biol. 2011;90:560–4.
107. Paulson KG et al. Array-CGH reveals recurrent genomic changes in Merkel cell carcinoma including amplification of L-Myc. J Invest Dermatol. 2009;129:1547–55.
108. Van Gele M, Speleman F, Vandesompele J, Van Roy N, Leonard JH. Characteristic pattern of chromosomal gains and losses in Merkel cell carcinoma detected by comparative genomic hybridization. Cancer Res. 1998;58:1503–8.
109. Chellappan SP, Hiebert S, Mudryj M, Horowitz JM, Nevins JR. The E2F transcription factor is a cellular target for the RB protein. Cell. 1991;65:1053–61.
110. Cao L et al. Independent binding of the retinoblastoma protein and p107 to the transcription factor E2F. Nature. 1992;355:176–9.
111. Cobrinik D, Whyte P, Peeper DS, Jacks T, Weinberg RA. Cell cycle-specific association of E2F with the p130 E1A-binding protein. Genes Dev. 1993;7:2392–404.
112. Hiebert SW, Chellappan SP, Horowitz JM, Nevins JR. The interaction of RB with E2F coincides with an inhibition of the transcriptional activity of E2F. Genes Dev. 1992;6:177–85.
113. Bandara LR, Adamczewski JP, Hunt T, La Thangue NB. Cyclin A and the retinoblastoma gene product complex with a common transcription factor. Nature. 1991;352:249–51.
114. Harbour JW et al. Abnormalities in structure and expression of the human retinoblastoma gene in SCLC. Science. 1988;241:353–7.
115. DeCaprio JA et al. SV40 large tumor antigen forms a specific complex with the product of the retinoblastoma susceptibility gene. Cell. 1988;54:275–83.
116. Leonard JH, Hayard N. Loss of heterozygosity of chromosome 13 in Merkel cell carcinoma. Genes Chromosomes Cancer. 1997;20:93–7.
117. Yu J, Ustach C, Kim H-RC. Platelet-derived growth factor signaling and human cancer. J Biochem Mol Biol. 2003;36:49–59.
118. Kartha RV, Sundram UN. Silent mutations in KIT and PDGFRA and coexpression of receptors with SCF and PDGFA in Merkel cell carcinoma: implications for tyrosine kinase-based tumorigenesis. Mod Pathol. 2008;21:96–104.
119. Swick BL, Ravdel L, Fitzpatrick JE, Robinson WA. Platelet-derived growth factor receptor alpha mutational status and immunohistochemical expression in Merkel cell carcinoma: implications for treatment with imatinib mesylate. J Cutan Pathol. 2008;35:197–202.
120. Davies H et al. Mutations of the BRAF gene in human cancer. Nature. 2002;417:949–54.
121. Houben R et al. Absence of classical MAP kinase pathway signalling in Merkel cell carcinoma. J Invest Dermatol. 2006;126:1135–42.
122. Houben R et al. Activation of the MAP kinase pathway induces apoptosis in the Merkel cell carcinoma cell line UISO. J Invest Dermatol. 2007;127: 2116–22.
123. Franke TF et al. The protein kinase encoded by the Akt proto-oncogene is a target of the PDGF-activated phosphatidylinositol 3-kinase. Cell. 1995;81:727–36.
124. Kazlauskas A, Cooper JA. Phosphorylation of the PDGF receptor beta subunit creates a tight binding site for phosphatidylinositol 3 kinase. EMBO J. 1990;9:3279–86.
125. Cantley LC. The phosphoinositide 3-kinase pathway. Science. 2002;296:1655–7.
126. Tsujimoto Y et al. Clustering of breakpoints on chromosome 11 in human B-cell neoplasms with the t(11;14) chromosome translocation. Nature. 1985; 315:340–3.
127. McDonnell TJ et al. bcl-2-immunoglobulin transgenic mice demonstrate extended B cell survival and follicular lymphoproliferation. Cell. 1989;57: 79–88.
128. Tsujimoto Y, Cossman J, Jaffe E, Croce CM. Involvement of the bcl-2 gene in human follicular lymphoma. Science. 1985;228:1440–3.
129. Feinmesser M et al. Expression of the apoptosis-related oncogenes bcl-2, bax, and p53 in Merkel cell

carcinoma: can they predict treatment response and clinical outcome? Hum Pathol. 1999;30:1367–72.
130. Kennedy MM, Blessing K, King G, Kerr KM. Expression of bcl-2 and p53 in Merkel cell carcinoma. An immunohistochemical study. Am J Dermatopathol. 1996;18:273–7.
131. Hockenbery D, Nuñez G, Milliman C, Schreiber RD, Korsmeyer SJ. Bcl-2 is an inner mitochondrial membrane protein that blocks programmed cell death. Nature. 1990;348:334–6.
132. Martinou JC et al. Overexpression of BCL-2 in transgenic mice protects neurons from naturally occurring cell death and experimental ischemia. Neuron. 1994;13:1017–30.
133. Nicholson DW, Thornberry NA. Apoptosis. Life and death decisions. Science. 2003;299:214–5.
134. Schlagbauer-Wadl H et al. Bcl-2 antisense oligonucleotides (G3139) inhibit Merkel cell carcinoma growth in SCID mice. J Invest Dermatol. 2000;114: 725–30.
135. Shah MH et al. G3139 (Genasense) in patients with advanced Merkel cell carcinoma. Am J Clin Oncol. 2009;32:174–9.
136. Emens LA. Survivin' cancer. Cancer Biol Ther. 2004;3:180–3.
137. Kim J, McNiff JM. Nuclear expression of survivin portends a poor prognosis in Merkel cell carcinoma. Mod Pathol. 2008;21:764–9.
138. Tucci MG et al. Immunohistochemical study of apoptosis markers and involvement of chemokine CXCR4 in skin Merkel cell carcinoma. J Eur Acad Dermatol Venereol. 2006;20:1220–5.
139. Giono LE, Manfredi JJ. The p53 tumor suppressor participates in multiple cell cycle checkpoints. J Cell Physiol. 2006;209:13–20.
140. Vogelstein B, Lane D, Levine AJ. Surfing the p53 network. Nature. 2000;408:307–10.
141. Donehower LA et al. Mice deficient for p53 are developmentally normal but susceptible to spontaneous tumours. Nature. 1992;356:215–21.
142. Ito A et al. p300/CBP-mediated p53 acetylation is commonly induced by p53-activating agents and inhibited by MDM2. EMBO J. 2001;20:1331–40.
143. Onel K, Cordon-Cardo C. MDM2 and prognosis. Mol Cancer Res. 2004;2:1–8.
144. Hurt EM, Thomas SB, Peng B, Farrar WL. Reversal of p53 epigenetic silencing in multiple myeloma permits apoptosis by a p53 activator. Cancer Biol Ther. 2006;5:1154–60.
145. Bueso-Ramos CE et al. The human MDM-2 oncogene is overexpressed in leukemias. Blood. 1993;82: 2617–23.
146. Lassacher A, Heitzer E, Kerl H, Wolf P. p14ARF hypermethylation is common but INK4a-ARF locus or p53 mutations are rare in Merkel cell carcinoma. J Invest Dermatol. 2008;128:1788–96.
147. Lill C et al. P53 mutation is a rare event in Merkel cell carcinoma of the head and neck. Eur Arch Otorhinolaryngol. 2011;268:1639–46.
148. Van Gele M et al. Combined karyotyping. CGH and M-FISH analysis allows detailed characterization of unidentified chromosomal rearrangements in Merkel cell carcinoma. Int J Cancer. 2002;101:137–45.
149. Feng H, Shuda M, Chang Y, Moore PS. Clonal integration of a polyomavirus in human Merkel cell carcinoma. Science. 2008;319:1096–100.
150. Fauquet CM. Virus taxonomy: VIIIth report of the International Committee on Taxonomy of Viruses. Virus Res. 2005;83:221–2.
151. Stewart AR, Lednicky JA, Butel JS. Sequence analyses of human tumor-associated SV40 DNAs and SV40 viral isolates from monkeys and humans. J Neurovirol. 1998;4:182–93.
152. Moens U, Ludvigsen M, Van Ghelue M. Human polyomaviruses in skin diseases. Patholog Res Int. 2011;2011:123491.
153. Diamandopoulos GT. Leukemia, lymphoma, and osteosarcoma induced in the Syrian golden hamster by simian virus 40. Science. 1972;176:173–5.
154. Walker DL, Padgett BL, ZuRhein GM, Albert AE, Marsh RF. Human papovavirus (JC): induction of brain tumors in hamsters. Science. 1973;181:674–6.
155. Shah KV, Daniel RW, Strandberg JD. Sarcoma in a hamster inoculated with BK virus, a human papovavirus. J Natl Cancer Inst. 1975;54:945–50.
156. Shuda M et al. T antigen mutations are a human tumor-specific signature for Merkel cell polyomavirus. Proc Natl Acad Sci U S A. 2008;105: 16272–7.
157. Becker JC et al. MC polyomavirus is frequently present in Merkel cell carcinoma of European patients. J Invest Dermatol. 2009;129:248–50.
158. Kassem A et al. Frequent detection of Merkel cell polyomavirus in human Merkel cell carcinomas and identification of a unique deletion in the VP1 gene. Cancer Res. 2008;68:5009–13.
159. Garneski KM et al. Merkel cell polyomavirus is more frequently present in North American than Australian Merkel cell carcinoma tumors. J Invest Dermatol. 2009;129:246–8.
160. Shuda M et al. Human Merkel cell polyomavirus infection I. MCV T antigen expression in Merkel cell carcinoma, lymphoid tissues and lymphoid tumors. Int J Cancer. 2009;125:1243–9.
161. Reisinger DM, Shiffer JD, Cognetta AB, Chang Y, Moore PS. Lack of evidence for basal or squamous cell carcinoma infection with Merkel cell polyomavirus in immunocompetent patients with Merkel cell carcinoma. J Am Acad Dermatol. 2010;63:400–3.
162. Paulson KG et al. Antibodies to Merkel cell polyomavirus T antigen oncoproteins reflect tumor burden in Merkel cell carcinoma patients. Cancer Res. 2010;70:8388–97.
163. Laude HC et al. Distinct Merkel cell polyomavirus molecular features in tumour and Non tumour specimens from patients with Merkel cell carcinoma. PLoS Pathog. 2010;6:9.
164. Small MB, Gluzman Y, Ozer HL. Enhanced transformation of human fibroblasts by origin-defective simian virus 40. Nature. 1982;296:671–2.
165. Israel MA, Vanderryn DF, Meltzer ML, Martin MA. Characterization of polyoma viral DNA sequences

in polyoma-induced hamster tumor cell lines. J Biol Chem. 1980;255:3798–805.
166. Kean JM, Rao S, Wang M, Garcea RL. Seroepidemiology of human polyomaviruses. PLoS Pathog. 2009;5:e1000363.
167. Pastrana DV et al. Quantitation of human seroresponsiveness to Merkel cell polyomavirus. PLoS Pathog. 2009;5:e1000578.
168. Schrama D et al. Merkel cell polyomavirus status is not associated with clinical course of Merkel cell carcinoma. J Invest Dermatol. 2011;131:1631–8.
169. Asioli S et al. Expression of p63 is the sole independent marker of aggressiveness in localised (stage I-II) Merkel cell carcinomas. Mod Pathol. 2011;24:1451–61.
170. Fischer N, Brandner J, Fuchs F, Moll I, Grundhoff A. Detection of Merkel cell polyomavirus (MCPyV) in Merkel cell carcinoma cell lines: cell morphology and growth phenotype do not reflect presence of the virus. Int J Cancer. 2010;126:2133–42.
171. Sihto H et al. Merkel cell polyomavirus infection, large T antigen. Retinoblastoma protein and outcome in Merkel cell carcinoma. Clin Cancer Res. 2011;17:4806–13.
172. Houben R et al. Comparable expression and phosphorylation of the retinoblastoma protein in Merkel cell polyoma virus-positive and negative Merkel cell carcinoma. Int J Cancer. 2010;126:796–8.
173. Altstein AD, Vassiljeva NN, Sarycheva OF. Neoplastic transformation of rat embryo cells by simian papovavirus SV40. Nature. 1967;213:931–2.
174. Linzer DI, Levine AJ. Characterization of a 54 K dalton cellular SV40 tumor antigen present in SV40-transformed cells and uninfected embryonal carcinoma cells. Cell. 1979;17:43–52.
175. Kaplan DR et al. Common elements in growth factor stimulation and oncogenic transformation: 85 kd phosphoprotein and phosphatidylinositol kinase activity. Cell. 1987;50:1021–9.
176. Johnson EM. Structural evaluation of new human polyomaviruses provides clues to pathobiology. Trends Microbiol. 2010;18:215–23.
177. Chang LS, Pan S, Pater MM, Di Mayorca G. Differential requirement for SV40 early genes in immortalization and transformation of primary rat and human embryonic cells. Virology. 1985;146:246–61.
178. Houben R et al. Merkel cell polyomavirus-infected Merkel cell carcinoma cells require expression of viral T antigens. J Virol. 2010;84:7064–72.
179. Houben R et al. An intact retinoblastoma protein-binding site in Merkel cell polyomavirus large T antigen is required for promoting growth of Merkel cell carcinoma cells. Int J Cancer. 2011. doi:10.1002/ijc.26076.
180. Stubdal H, Zalvide J, DeCaprio JA. Simian virus 40 large T antigen alters the phosphorylation state of the RB-related proteins p130 and p107. J Virol. 1996;70:2781–8.
181. Stubdal H et al. Inactivation of pRB-related proteins p130 and p107 mediated by the J domain of simian virus 40 large T antigen. Mol Cell Biol. 1997;17:4979–90.
182. O'Reilly DR. p53 and transformation by SV40. Biol Cell. 1986;57:187–96.
183. Cho S, Tian Y, Benjamin TL. Binding of p300/CBP co-activators by polyoma large T antigen. J Biol Chem. 2001;276:33533–9.
184. Hein J et al. Simian virus 40 large T antigen disrupts genome integrity and activates a DNA damage response via Bub1 binding. J Virol. 2009;83:117–27.
185. Bhatia K, Goedert JJ, Modali R, Preiss L, Ayers LW. Merkel cell carcinoma subgroups by Merkel cell polyomavirus DNA relative abundance and oncogene expression. Int J Cancer. 2010;126:2240–6.
186. Sáenz-Robles MT, Sullivan CS, Pipas JM. Transforming functions of Simian Virus 40. Oncogene. 2001;20:7899–907.
187. Yu J, Boyapati A, Rundell K. Critical role for SV40 small-t antigen in human cell transformation. Virology. 2001;290:192–8.
188. Shuda M, Kwun HJ, Feng H, Chang Y, Moore PS. Human Merkel cell polyomavirus small T antigen is an oncoprotein targeting the 4E-BP1 translation regulator. J Clin Invest. 2011. doi:10.1172/JCI46323.
189. Beretta L, Gingras AC, Svitkin YV, Hall MN, Sonenberg N. Rapamycin blocks the phosphorylation of 4E-BP1 and inhibits cap-dependent initiation of translation. EMBO J. 1996;15:658–64.
190. She Q-B et al. 4E-BP1 is a key effector of the oncogenic activation of the AKT and ERK signaling pathways that integrates their function in tumors. Cancer Cell. 2010;18:39–51.
191. Pallas DC et al. Polyoma small and middle T antigens and SV40 small t antigen form stable complexes with protein phosphatase 2A. Cell. 1990;60:167–76.
192. Rodriguez-Viciana P, Collins C, Fried M. Polyoma and SV40 proteins differentially regulate PP2A to activate distinct cellular signaling pathways involved in growth control. Proc Natl Acad Sci U S A. 2006;103:19290–5.
193. Liu X et al. Merkel cell polyomavirus large T antigen disrupts lysosome clustering by translocating human VAM6P to the nucleus. J Biol Chem. 2011;286:17079–90.
194. Seo GJ, Chen CJ, Sullivan CS. Merkel cell polyomavirus encodes a microRNA with the ability to autoregulate viral gene expression. Virology. 2009;383:183–7.
195. Lee S et al. Identification and validation of a novel mature microRNA encoded by the Merkel cell polyomavirus in human Merkel cell carcinomas. J Clin Virol. 2011;52:272–5.
196. Umbach JL et al. MicroRNAs expressed by herpes simplex virus 1 during latent infection regulate viral mRNAs. Nature. 2008;454:780–3.

Epidemiology and Genetics (Including High Risk Patients, Polyomavirus, Prognostic Factors)

2

Garrett C. Lowe, Jerry D. Brewer, and Jeremy S. Bordeaux

Abbreviations

CLL	Chronic lymphocytic leukemia
HIV	Human immunodeficiency virus
LT	Large T
MCC	Merkel cell carcinoma
MCPyV	Merkel cell polyomavirus
NHL	Non-Hodgkin lymphoma
NMSC	Nonmelanoma skin cancer
PUVA	Psoralen-UV-A
RB	Retinoblastoma
SEER	Surveillance, Epidemiology, and End Results
SLNB	Sentinel lymph node biopsy

Overview and Incidence

Merkel cell carcinoma (MCC) is an uncommon, rapidly growing, and aggressive cutaneous malignancy of elderly persons, affecting mainly whites [1]. White-skinned individuals make up roughly 95 % of those affected; African Americans make up less than 1 % [2, 3]. Local recurrences, nodal involvement, metastases, and high mortality rates are more the rule than the exception in MCC. The most common region of the body affected by MCC is the head and neck, with roughly 50 % of MCCs occurring in this area [2, 4–6] and nearly one of every ten MCCs occurring on the eyelid and periocular areas [7, 8] (see Fig. 2.1). The incidence of MCC in the head and neck region increases substantially after the age of 65 years, especially in men [9]. The next most common sites are the upper and lower extremities, which are the more common sites of MCC involvement in individuals younger than 65 years [2, 5]. Upper-extremity MCC seems to carry a better prognosis and occurs in roughly 20 % of cases [4]. The lower extremities are affected in one of seven patients with MCC and seem to be associated with increased recurrence [10]. The trunk comprises 11 % of MCC development. In addition to these common sites of involvement, 5 % of MCCs occur in non-sun-exposed mucosal areas, the most common of which is the larynx [2]. Other less common locations for MCC include the breasts, buttocks, esophagus, penis, salivary glands, scrotum, and vulva [4, 11–14].

The majority (80 %) of MCCs measure less than 2 cm in diameter at diagnosis and present with localized disease clinically (50–70 %) [2, 5, 15]. The rest have regional node involvement or distant metastases, or both, at diagnosis [1, 16, 17]. Even with aggressive excision of localized MCC, the incidence of recurrence and metastasis is high, and these traits ultimately lead to death in

G.C. Lowe (✉) • J.D. Brewer
Department of Dermatology, Mayo Clinic, 200 1st Street SW, 55905 Rochester, MN, USA
e-mail: lowe.garrett@mayo.edu; brewer.jerry@mayo.edu

J.S. Bordeaux
Department of Dermatology, University Hospitals Case Medical Center, Case Western Reserve University, 11100 Euclid Avenue, Lakeside 3500, Cleveland, OH 44106-5000, USA
e-mail: Jeremy.Bordeaux@uhhospitals.org

M. Alam et al. (eds.), *Merkel Cell Carcinoma*, DOI 10.1007/978-1-4614-6608-6_2,

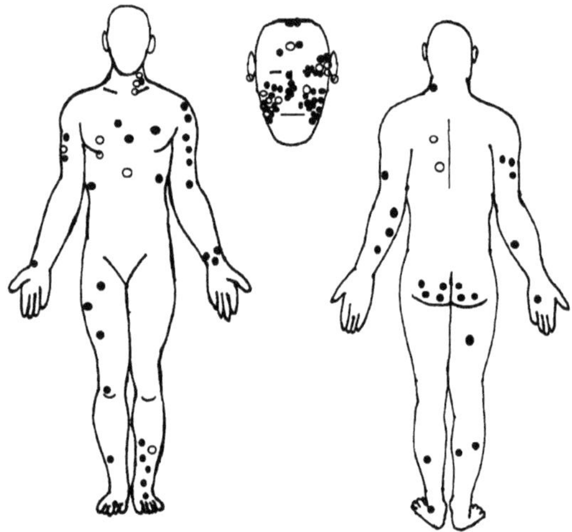

Fig. 2.1 Pictorial breakdown of Merkel cell carcinoma (MCC) distribution in a sample population from Finland. *Filled circles* represent MCC positive for Merkel cell polyomavirus; *open circles* represent MCC negative for the virus (Adapted from Sihto H, Kukko H, Koljonen V, Sankila R, Bohling T, Joensuu H. Clinical factors associated with Merkel cell polyomavirus infection in Merkel cell carcinoma. J Natl Cancer Inst. 2009;101:938–945. With permission Oxford University Press.)

approximately 30 % of individuals within 2 years of diagnosis [18] (median survival time, 33 months) [19].

The average age of persons affected with MCC is roughly 70 years (range, 7–104 years) [1, 5, 6, 20–22], with the male to female ratio believed to be 1.4:1.0 [1]. Of note, however, certain reports, such as one that evaluated MCC incidence in the Danish population, show a higher incidence in women than men [23]. In addition, this ratio moves closer to 1.0 in non-sun-exposed anatomical sites, and in these cases the average age is 60 years at diagnosis [2].

The estimated age-adjusted incidence of first primary MCC in the United States is currently 0.6 per 100,000 person-years (see Fig. 2.2), with the incidence rate of whites more than eight times that of African Americans and double the incidence of other ethnic groups [4]. From 1986 to 2001, the age-adjusted incidence of MCC increased 8 % per year, which was an alarming threefold increase [6]. The highest incidence rates of MCC were seen in Hawaii, Washington, and Utah [2, 6]. This increase surprisingly was more dramatic than the 3.03 % increase per year in melanoma incidence seen in that same period [6]. To date, the highest reported incidence rates of MCC in the medical literature come out of Western Australia, where age-adjusted incidence rates are 1.0 per 100,000 person-years in men and 0.63 per 100,000 person-years in women [24]. One of the first European epidemiologic studies of MCC came out of Spain and reported an age-adjusted incidence lower than that found in the United States: 0.13 per 100,000 person-years [25]. Similar incidence rates have been found in other European countries [26, 27].

The incidence of MCC has been increasing in different populations, having doubled since 1993 in the Netherlands by 2007 and tripled since 1983 in Finland by 2004 [26, 27]. The American Cancer Society recently estimated an increase of 1,500 new cases per year in the United States [18]. Several major risk factors are thought to contribute to this trend of increasing incidence: the increasing age of the general population, increased rates of immunosuppression, and increasing sun exposure habits over a lifetime [6]. Improved detection and reporting likely also contribute to the increasing incidence of MCC seen most prominently in the twenty-first century.

Ultraviolet Radiation

Strong clinical and epidemiologic evidence links ultraviolet (UV) radiation to the pathogenesis of MCC [1, 20, 28]. Higher incidence is found in geographic locations of higher ultraviolet radiation, in patients with fair skin, and in anatomic locations with sun exposure. In the United States, incidence of MCC increases with geographic regions of increasing sun exposure, as measured by the UV-B radiation index [29]. Review of the UV-B radiation index of different geographic areas designated in the Surveillance, Epidemiology, and End Results (SEER) Program shows a statistically significant linear correlation ($r=0.84$; $P=0.005$) existing between first primary MCC of the head and neck of white persons in the United States and the UV-B radiation index

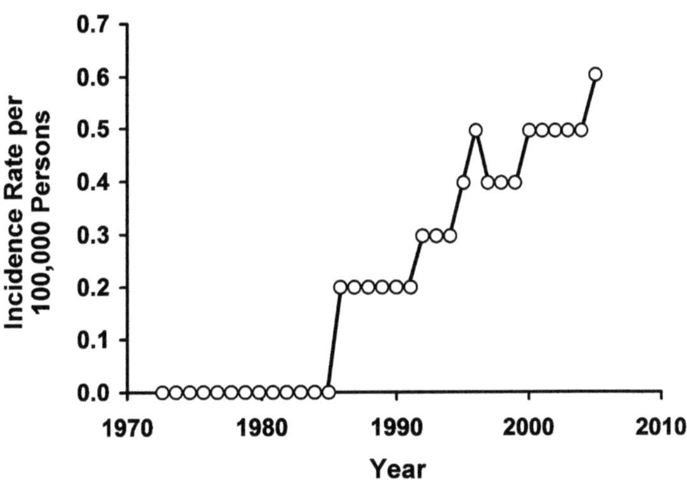

Fig. 2.2 Trends for Merkel cell carcinoma from 1973 to 2006 in the United States (Adapted from Albores-Saavedra J, Batich K, Chable-Montero F, Sagy N, Schwartz AM, Henson DE. Merkel cell carcinoma demographics, morphology, and survival based on 3870 cases: a population based study. J Cutan Pathol. 2010;37:20–27. With permission from John Wiley & Sons, Inc.)

of that SEER geographic area. The highest age-adjusted incidence rates of MCC were seen in Hawaii, a finding that correlates with the highest UV-B radiation index among the states [2]. In addition, the incidence of MCC is much greater in equatorial latitudes [6, 30] with highest incidence in Western Australia [24].

MCC is also most frequently found on sun-exposed skin. Interestingly, investigators in the United States found that MCC was much more likely to arise on the left side of the body than on the right, especially on the face and arms ($P<0.01$) [31]. This finding suggests that driver-side automobile UV light exposure, which is fivefold stronger on the left side of the body than on the right, is a strong contributing factor to the pathogenesis of MCC [31].

UV-A also appears to play a key role. The wavelengths in the UV-A light spectrum pass through window glass. Thus, UV-A most likely is strongly correlated with automobile UV exposure and the subsequent MCC development. Psoralen (methoxsalen) and UV-A used in combination (PUVA) for the treatment of psoriasis have also been correlated with MCC development [32]. In fact, a 100-fold increase in patients with psoriasis who were treated with PUVA was found when these patients were compared with the general population [33].

Recently, Merkel cell polyomavirus (MCPyV) mRNA transcript levels in patients with MCC proved to be UV light inducible, which may suggest an association between MCPyV, MCC development, and UV light [34].

Aging

The SEER National Database and all other cancer registries around the world confirm that MCC is a tumor of the elderly population. More than 70 % of primary MCCs occur in patients older than 70 years and the incidence rates of MCC increase dramatically with age [2, 6, 9] (see Fig. 2.3). For example, the annual incidence of MCC in people older than 85 years is 15.5 per 100,000 persons in Australia [24], and less than 5 % of all MCCs affect immunocompetent patients are younger than 50 years [2, 4, 5]. MCC development is exceedingly rare in children [21].

The immunological deterioration in both cell-mediated and humoral immunity that accompanies the aging process provides a possible explanation for the striking age-dependent trends of cutaneous carcinogenesis, including MCC development [35, 36]. Immunosenescence, or the gradual deterioration of the immune system brought on by the natural aging processes, results in decreasing numbers of functional immune cells, especially lymphocytes. The resulting decrease in immune function leads to a shift of

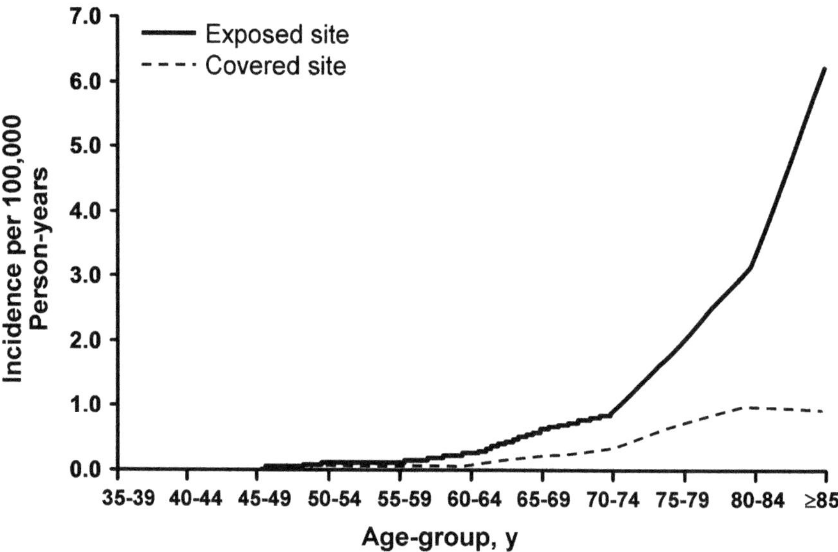

Fig. 2.3 Incidence trends for Merkel cell carcinoma by 5-year age-groups in Sweden between 1990 and 2005 for sun-exposed and non-sun-exposed tumor sites (Adapted from Hussain SK, Sundquist J, Hemminki K. Incidence trends of squamous cell and rare skin cancers in the Swedish national cancer registry point to calendar year and age-dependent increases. J Invest Dermatol. 2010;130:1323–1328. Nature Publishing Group.)

more T_H2 and fewer T_H1 cytokines, resulting in impaired immunity decreased tumor surveillance system [35].

Immunosuppression

Iatrogenic immunosuppression leads to decreased cell-mediated immunity and increased frequency of skin cancer, including MCC [37]. MCC is 15 times more likely to occur in individuals with long-term immunosuppression than in the general population [38]. Recent retrospective studies suggest that nearly 8 % of all MCC patients have immunosuppression [30]. Furthermore, the ratio of malignant melanoma to MCC is 6:1 in patients with long-term immunosuppression vs. the 65:1 ratio normally seen in the immunocompetent population[39].

Given that MCC is strongly correlated with aging, as well as UV radiation exposure, it is interesting to consider that both aging and UV radiation exposure result in decreased immune function and a blunted tumor surveillance system, which may lead to an accumulation of oncogenic events. Other specific forms of immunosuppression are discussed below.

Autoimmunity

Numerous autoimmune diseases have been associated with MCC [40–45]. Rheumatoid arthritis has been found to be the most prevalent autoimmune condition associated with skin cancer in a recent report and was associated specifically with an increased risk of MCC [46]. The incidence of MCC in patients with autoimmune disorders has been increasing over the past decade and may be secondary to the potent immunosuppressant medications used to treat these conditions [47–51]. In some cases, stopping the immunosuppressant medications has led to a regression of metastatic MCC [52, 53].

Organ Transplantation

The incidence of MCC is unusually high in organ transplant recipients compared with the general population, highlighting the importance of a functional immune system in prevention of MCC development [39, 54]. A tenfold increase of MCC in transplant recipients has been reported [29], with the incidence of MCC in these patients representing 0.9 % of all de novo cancers [39]. In addition, MCC arises at a much earlier age (mean, 53 years) [39], presents multifocally in 20 % of the cases [55], and is more often advanced at time of presentation and (stage II and III) in 70 % of cases involving transplant recipients [39, 54]. An estimated 60 % of organ transplant recipients with MCC die within 18 months of MCC diagnosis [39]. One recent report looking at renal transplant recipients with MCC in Finland showed that all patients died within 25 months of diagnosis. From this and other reports, it is strikingly apparent that organ transplant recipients are at much greater risk for skin cancer, including MCC. In addition, the clinical course of MCC in organ transplant recipients appears to be much more aggressive [56]. Aside from earlier age at MCC onset and seemingly more aggressive disease behavior, the other demographic characteristics and location of MCC appear similar, with a white male predominance and with the head and neck region being most commonly affected. MCC has been found to appear 6–8 years, on average, after organ transplantation, and the incidence of MCC increases remarkably 20 years after transplantation [57].

Acquired Immunodeficiency Syndrome

Human immunodeficiency virus (HIV) infection leads to an immunocompromised state with impaired cellular immunity, leaving patients highly susceptible to opportunistic, bacterial, and viral infections, as well as the development of certain cancers. The relative risk of MCC development in patients with HIV infection is 13.4, and HIV-infected individuals who undergo organ transplantation have an annual incidence of 12 per 100,000 persons [58]. Compared with the general population, HIV patients are diagnosed with MCC at a younger age (49 years) and tumors arise in anatomic sites other than the head and neck region in the majority of cases [59]. The average duration from HIV infection to MCC development is 9.5 years; the average CD4 count is 256 at the time of MCC diagnosis. Although the prognosis is poor in this population, treatment of AIDS with highly active antiretroviral therapy has led to remarkable improvements in patients with metastatic MCC [60].

Non-Hodgkin Lymphoma

Non-Hodgkin lymphoma (NHL) and chronic lymphocytic leukemia (CLL) are lymphoproliferative cancers. NHL ranks seventh among the most commonly diagnosed cancers in the world [61], and CLL is a member of the NHL family, representing 25 % of all leukemias [62]. A low-grade lymphoproliferative malignancy, CLL is characterized by clonal proliferation of B cells. The proliferation causes a marked decrease in the person's immune function. Investigators have shown that leukemic cells express immunosuppressive factors, as well as downregulate expression of CD40 ligand (CD154) on activated T cells, thus interfering with T-cell ability to interact with normal bystander B cells or other antigen-presenting cells [63]. Furthermore, CD154 has a role in the T-cell induction of immunoglobulin class switching and may result in a deficient IgG level of various IgG subclasses [64]. Other factors that affect the immunosuppression seen in patients with CLL include hypocomplementemia, altered expression of class 2 major histocompatibility complex antigens on leukemic cells, hypogammaglobulinemia, and impaired granulocyte function [65, 66].

A number of studies have reported an association between MCC and CLL [62, 67–73]. Individuals aged 50–69 years and those aged 70 years or older who have CLL have a striking 48- and 34-fold increase in age-adjusted incidence of MCC, respectively, compared with the incidence of the general population [74]. A small case series recently suggested that the course of MCC in the clinical setting of CLL is much more aggressive, with possible increased recurrence, metastasis, and MCC-related death [75]. A new subset of MCPyV was recently discovered in 25 % of CLL patients infected with MCPyV [76]. This discovery may argue for the potential role of MCPyV in the more aggressive nature of MCC in CLL patients. More research is needed to clarify the relationship of CLL and MCC and how one may influence the behavior of the other.

Association with Other Cancers

Patients with a diagnosis of MCC are at considerably increased risk of secondary malignancy, especially other skin cancers and hematologic cancers. The frequency of secondary malignancy in patients with MCC is as high as 25 % [32, 77, 78]. The risk of development of a secondary malignancy is estimated to be 2.1 % for each year after the diagnosis of a primary MCC [78]. The risk of a secondary malignancy is highest during the first year of follow-up [77, 78]. The cancer most commonly linked to MCC is squamous cell carcinoma, with reported associations as high as 40 % [79–81]. In Scandinavia, patients with NMSC and with melanoma had 8.35- and 4.29-fold increases for risk of second cancers compared with persons without primary MCC [82]. A population-based study from Denmark found that the overall cancer incidence more than 1 year after the diagnosis of MCC is twice that of the general population [23] and a national cohort study demonstrated similar findings [83]. Conversely, patients with other forms of cancer are at increased risk of MCC. A three- to seven-fold increase in MCC occurs after multiple myeloma, CLL, NHL, and malignant melanoma [77]. The MCC incidence rate at 12 months after the diagnosis of another cancer was 2.6 times higher than the expected incidence in the Danish population [23] and 1.7 times higher than in the United States [77].

Arsenic

Arsenic is a well-documented human carcinogen. NMSCs are the most common types of cancers that arise because of arsenic exposure. Contrary to the usual distribution of most NMSCs on sun-exposed sites, arsenic-related cancer typically occurs on sites not exposed to the sun [84]. MCC has been documented to be increased in geographic areas of high arsenic exposure. Data collected from two medical centers in Taiwan revealed that greater than 50 % of all MCCs occurred in residents with long-term arsenic exposure [85]. The exact mechanism by which arsenic influences the development of MCC has not been elucidated.

Merkel Cell Polyomavirus

In 2008, authors of published data theorized that a novel polyomavirus, termed Merkel cell polyomavirus (MCPyV), may influence MCC pathogenesis [86]. This virus was clonally integrated in the MCC tumor genome at various locations, strongly suggestive of viral infection and integration occurring in tumor cells before clonal expansion and tumor growth. In that study, the investigators detected viral levels in 80 % of MCC tumors and only 8 % of noncancerous tissue, with all but one MCC showing high viral loads. Since the report, efforts around the world have researched the possibility of human polyomavirus-associated tumorigenesis. Table 2.1 highlights the reproducible results published by independent researchers since 2008.

MCPyV belongs to a family of small nonenveloped, circular, double-stranded DNA viruses. Six of the polyomaviruses are known to infect humans, but for years these six viruses only produced tumor formation in animal models (hence, the term incorporates poly + oma) [87]. The link between this virus family and tumorigenesis has fueled research for decades, which in turn has led to the knowledge that all polyomaviruses encode T antigen oncoproteins and capsid proteins important for structural support, viral replication, virion assembly, host integration, and cellular transformation [88]. Feng et al. [86] described large T (LT) antigen mutations resulting in truncation in all MCPyV-positive tumor samples but not in MCPyV-positive control samples. The unique mutation found in MCPyV-positive tumor cells has been studied [89], and multiple distinct LT antigen mutations have been described in the MCPyV of MCC tumors. Normally, this antigen contains binding sites for the retinoblastoma (RB) tumor suppressor protein, cell-cycle regulatory heat shock proteins, and helicase domain.

Table 2.1 Summary of findings on Merkel cell polyomavirus

				Positivity	
Study authors	Year	Country	Positivity in MCC, % (*n*)	Noncancerous tissue (*n*)	Other cancers
Feng et al. [86]	2008	United States	80 [10]	8 % [59]	16 % of 25 skin and skin tumor tissue
Busam et al. [140]	2009	United States	88 [17]	–	–
Carter et al. [141]	2009	United States	77 [29]	–	–
Duncavage et al. [142]	2009	United States	76 [33]	–	–
Garneski et al. [92]	2009	United States/ Australia	43 [37]	0 % [15]	13 % of 15 SCC
Paulson et al. [102]	2009	United States	59 [22]	–	–
Ridd et al. [143]	2009	United States	54 [13]	3 % [37]	0 % of 119 other skin cancers
Bhatia et al. [106]	2010	United States	74 [23]	–	1 % of 52 non-MCC
Loyo et al. [144]	2010	United States	87 [7]	26 % [82]	11 % of 192 non-MCC
Sihto et al. [135]	2009	Finland	80 [88]	0 % [7]	0 % of 15 glioblastomas and melanomas
Sastre-Garau et al. [93]	2009	France	100 [10]	–	0 % of 1,241 non-MCC
Touze et al. [136]	2009	France	66 [31]	–	0 % of 9 other neuroendocrine tumors
Foulongne et al. [145]	2008	France	82 [11]	0 % [15]	–
Kassem et al. [90]	2008	Germany	77 [39]	0 % [45]	–
Becker et al. [94]	2009	Germany	85 [53]	–	13 % of 24 BCC
Helmbold et al. [146]	2009	Germany	92 [136]	9 % [44]	–
Wieland et al. [95]	2009	Germany	88 [34]	18 % [45]	16 % of other skin cancers
Andres et al. [147]	2010	Germany	64 [32]	17 % [12]	0 % of other skin cancers
Houben et al. [103]	2010	Germany	86 [50]	–	–
Varga et al. [148]	2009	Hungary	83 [6]	–	0 % of 29 other skin cancers
Wetzels et al. [149]	2009	Netherlands	40 [5]	–	0 % of 10 small-cell lung cancers
Mangana et al. [150]	2010	Switzerland	67 [28]	0 % [19]	–
Katano et al. [151]	2009	Japan	55 [11]	–	1 % of 241 of immune-compromised conditions and cancers
Nakajima et al. [152]	2009	Japan	79 [14]	–	–
Kuwamoto et al. [153]	2011	Japan	77 [26]	–	0 % of 4 mixed MCC and SCC; 0 % of 3 other skin cancers
Woo et al. [154]	2010	South Korea	100 [7]	–	–

BCC, basal cell carcinoma; *MCC*, Merkel cell carcinoma; *SCC*, squamous cell carcinoma; –, not available

The mutating events classic for MCPyV in MCC result in LT antigen truncation and loss of helicase function only, thus causing the virus to lose its ability to replicate epigenomically. This chain of events implies an integration before clonal expansion. In addition, recent reports of LT antigen mutations disrupting lysosome clustering and function and capsid mutations of VP1 altering viral integration have surfaced [90, 91]. These findings are in line with data supporting the monoclonal integration of the polyomavirus into Merkel cell tumors [90, 92–94]. Moreover, primary and metastatic specimens from the same patient have showed identical viral integration patterns, indicating that the integration process occurs before metastatic spread of tumor [86].

Since its discovery in 2008, MCPyV has been detected in normal tissue and in non-MCC cancerous tissue in small percentages (see Table 2.1). The only association reported between malignancy (other than MCC) and MCPyV is from a subset of patients who had CLL and tested positive for MCPyV, in whom rates were as high as 25 % [76]. Otherwise, no connection between MCPyV and other tumors has been seen [90, 95, 96]. MCPyV is ubiquitous in nature and infects nearly 90 % of healthy individuals by adulthood, as shown through seropositivity [97–99]. Some investigators have linked initial viral acquisition to respiratory tract infections [100] or to possible tonsillar persistence of the virus in childhood, or both [99]. Nevertheless, the exact mechanism through which this new human polyomavirus mediates carcinogenesis in MCC is still not clear. More than 1 pathway most likely exists for MCC tumorigenesis, however, because roughly 20 % of MCCs are negative for MCPyV (see Table 2.1). These MCPyV-negative MCCs have been theorized to arise from the accumulation of more complicated genetic aberrations [101] and develop together with MCPyV-positive MCC in the clinical setting of immunosuppression from long-term UV light exposure, aging, organ transplantation, concomitant cancers, and other factors.

In conclusion, the tight association of MCPyV with MCC; the clonal pattern of integration in tumor tissue, as well as in its metastasis; the expression of the mutant viral oncoproteins; and the striking incidence of this cancer in persons who have immunosuppression all strongly support a factor of causality for MCPyV in tumorigenesis [93]. However, it is abundantly clear is that other mechanisms are involved in the etiology and pathogenesis of MCC as well.

Genetics and Molecular Biology

The data presented in prior paragraphs show that the LT antigen of MCPyV-positive Merkel cell tumors interacts with RB protein for sustained tumor growth. Recently, Paulson et al. [102] analyzed chromosomal aberrations in 28 MCC tumors of 25 patients by using comparative genomic hybridization. They reported deletions from the long arm of chromosomes 5 and 13 and amplification of the short arm of chromosome 1. The *Rb1* tumor suppressor gene, which is encoded within 13q14-21, was deleted in 26 % of the tumors studied. Aberrant DNA methylation in promoter regions is now thought to be one of the most common molecular alterations in tumorigenesis [101]. Hypermethylation of promotor regions to the common locus gene for *p14ARF* and *p16INK4α(alpha)* has been reported in association with small percentages of Merkel cell tumors, which result in destabilization of p53 activity and improper signaling (phosphorylation) of the RB protein [38, 103]. The *p14ARF* gene works by inhibiting ubiquitin ligase necessary for p53 stability. One recent study suggests that p53 may be inactivated in about 50 % of Merkel cell tumors through hypermethylation of the promotor region [104]. Waltari et al. [105] reviewed 87 confirmed cases of MCC with DNA available in Finland. Among the tumors, 77 % were positive for MCPyV and only 22 % showed expression of tumor p53, with greater viral loads correlating with less p53 expression [106]. Tumor p53 expression was associated with absence of MCPyV DNA ($P=0.01$) and unfavorable MCC-specific survival ($P=0.02$) [105]. Increasing evidence suggests p53 and RB may have a role in one of the many pathways involved in MCC pathogenesis. Whether they are aberrantly expressed in MCPyV-positive or MCPyV-negative tumor cell lines, or both, is unclear.

Several studies have found recurrent chromosomal abnormalities in MCC through comparative genomic hybridization and fluorescence in situ hybridization techniques, in chromosomes 1, 3, 5, 6, 8, 10, 11, 13, 17, 19, and X [107–109]. The most common aberration is chromosomal 1p amplification in 39–63 % of MCC cases [102, 107]. L-*myc*, which is closely related to c-*myc*, is encoded within 1p34, suggesting involvement in tumor development in a subset of patients [102]. The proto-oncogene *myc* family is partially regulated by the E-cadherin /β(beta)-catenin complex. Interestingly, *p16INK4α (alpha)* is a target gene of β(beta)-catenin, and its overexpression has been linked to poor outcomes in other carcinomas, including colorectal tumors [110]. Recently, downregulation of the E-cadherin /β(beta)-catenin complex has been linked to MCC and is thought to possibly contribute to local invasion and metastasis [111].

Many studies have investigated the several oncogenic pathways involved in carcinogenesis, in attempts to find key genetic alterations in MCC (see Table 2.2). Unfortunately, the vast majority of studies show little involvement of such pathways. Bcl-2, an antiapoptotic protein, has been studied, and the results appear relevant. In 1996, two separate studies were conducted and found that 75 % of MCC expressed Bcl-2 [112, 113]. Furthermore, decreasing Bcl-2 in vivo in SCID mouse/human tumor xenograft model resulted in tumor shrinkage [114]. The antiapoptotic effect of Bcl-2 may be one of the mechanisms through which MCC avoids cell death, but it does little to explain the promitotic pathways seen in MCC [18]. Currently, hedgehog and kit signaling pathways are showing promise [105, 115] and investigations have led to speculation of their involvement in MCC. Research is ongoing to illuminate the molecular biology driving MCC.

Prognostic Factors

A fascinating and unusual form of skin cancer, MCC is defined with local and satellite recurrences, nodal involvement, metastases, high mortality rates, and overall poor prognosis. The initial tumor is typically small and fast growing with a high frequency of lymphovascular invasion. Investigators have suggested that the overall risk of lymphatic involvement or hematogenous metastasis, or both, is greater than 50 % at some point during the disease process [116]. MCC presents localized in 70–80 % of cases [32, 117–119], with the head and neck region most commonly affected. When relative rates of survival have been stratified in accordance with anatomical site, MCC of the upper and lower limbs is associated with the best prognosis and the worst prognosis, respectively [4, 10]. Not surprisingly, recurrent or second tumors are associated with a much dimmer prognosis [78]. When assessing prognostic indicators for MCC, conflicting studies pepper the literature because the natural history of MCC is not clear. Because of the relative rarity of this tumor, no prospective randomized trials have evaluated the prognostic factors in MCC. Further studies are needed.

The majority of studies suggest that tumors larger than 2 cm portend a worse prognosis, especially in elderly men [118–123]. For example, a review of all 251 cases of MCC in Memorial Sloan-Kettering Cancer Center's database between 1970 and 2002 found that tumor size and disease stage were the only independent predictors of survival [28]. However, published reports evaluating clinical tumor diameter as related to survival did not find that tumors smaller than 2 cm (stage I) were associated with better prognosis [124, 125].

Both melanoma and MCC are aggressive neoplasms of the skin. The paucity of data for MCC has led researchers to look to published data from large, randomized trials for malignant melanoma. Depth of invasion (Breslow depth) is well established as a prognostic indicator for melanoma. Unfortunately, depth of MCC as a reproducible histologic prognostic factor has not been elucidated [20]. Retrospective studies are drawn upon to make this connection. For instance, invasion into subcutaneous fat has been found to be significantly associated with poor outcomes, as defined by metastasis or death [126]. Skelton et al. [127] reviewed 132 cases and reported that depth of invasion was associated with worse survival, but without statistical significance. Tumor depth has been correlated with local recurrence [10, 124]. More recently, however, numerous authors have not been able to find a correlation between tumor thickness (depth of invasion) and overall survival [124, 125, 128].

Although diameter and thickness of primary tumors are inconsistent in prognostic value, stage of MCC at diagnosis is still considered a major determinant of survival [1, 4, 28, 119]. (Stages of disease are covered in full detail later in this book.) The 5-year disease-specific survival rate for MCC has been found to be roughly 65 % [28, 32], with stage I at 81 %, stage II at 67 %, stage III at 52 %, and stage IV at 11 %. Nodal involvement is a known prognostic indicator of many malignant neoplasms, including MCC. Clinically negative nodes in patients with MCC portend better prognosis than the presence of lymphadenopathy on physical examination. Furthermore, negative nodes confirmed by pathologic evaluation compared with clinically negative nodes are associated with significantly better prognosis [129]. Lemos et al. evaluated 5,823 cases from the National Cancer Data Base of MCC (median follow-up, 64 months) showing that patients with pathologically proven negative nodes had a survival rate of 76 % at 5 years whereas those with negative nodes by clinical evaluation alone had a survival rate of only 59 %. Evidence to date may support sentinel lymph node biopsy (SLNB) as the best staging tool for lymph node evaluation. Survival rates have reached 97 % at 5 years for patients with pathologically node-negative disease determined through SLNB [28]. The recurrence rate for patients with negative SLNB is three times less, at 20 %, than the 60 % recurrence in patients with a finding of node-positive disease through SLNB [130]. But, as with all prognostic indicators in MCC, authors from Memorial Sloan-Kettering Cancer Center published data in 2011 refuting whether sentinel lymph node status is associated with recurrence or survival [123].

Histologic growth patterns, cell types and size, mitotic activity, necrosis, lymphocytic infiltration, perineural invasion, and immunohistochemistry have all been evaluated in individual studies and have shown inconsistent associations with MCC prognosis [124, 126–128]. Diffuse growth patterns, lymphovascular invasion, and heavy lymphocytic infiltration have been associated with poor outcomes [122, 126]. Moreover, MCC tumors that are heavily infiltrated by CD8+ cells are dramatically less likely to recur or metastasize after treatment [131], as are tumors with large numbers of mast cells [122]. Mitotic index in MCC has not been shown to be related to patient survival [132].

In addition, *kit* mutations, but not c-*myc* oncogene activity, have been associated with a worse prognosis [132, 133].

Current evidence suggests that MCPyV is a causal factor that underlies the vast majority of MCC cases. There is no questioning the striking occurrence of the virus in Merkel cell tumors (see Table 2.1). However, whether it affects the prognosis is still unclear. Recently, no correlation between detection of MCPyV in the primary tumor and better survival was demonstrated by Handschel et al. [134]. However, the vast majority of studies show increased survival and less recurrence in patients in whom MCPyV positivity was found compared with control subjects [135–138]. Moreover, patients with high levels of serum antibodies against MCPyV have been found to have better progression-free survival [139]. High titers of MCPyV, coupled with better disease-free survival, in patients with CD8+ infiltrated MCC tumors [131] suggest that stronger immune function correlates with better clinical outcomes.

Table 2.2 Cancer-associated pathways and genes studied in MCC oncogenesis

Cancer-associated pathway/gene	Likely relevant	Summary of findings	Reference
p53	–	No mutations found in 12 of 15 samples	Van Gele, et al. [155]
Ras	–	No activating mutations in *H-ras*, *K-ras*, or *N-ras* found in 6 MCC cell lines	Popp et al. [80]
B-RAF^{V600E}	–	No mutations in 46 MCCs	Houben et al. [156]
MAP kinase activity	–	MAP kinase silenced in 42/44 MCCs	Houben et al. [156]
WNT	–	No mutations in β(beta)-catenin, APC, AXIN1, or AXIN2 in 12 MCC tumors	Liu et al. [157]
c-kit	–	No activating mutations in 9 MCC tumors	Swick et al. [158]
PTEN	?	No mutations in 20 of 21 samples but loss of heterozygosity for region in 43 %	Van Gele et al. [159]
bcl-2	+	High expression in 15 of 20 MCC tumors; *bcl-2* antisense decreases tumor size in xenograft model	Kennedy et al. [112]; Plettenberg et al. [113]; Schlagbauer-Wadl et al. [114]

MCC, Merkel cell carcinoma; –, negative; +, positive; ?, not known
Source: Adapted from Lemos B, Nghiem P. Merkel cell carcinoma: more deaths but still no pathway to blame. J Invest Dermatol. 2007;127:2100–2103. With permission from Nature Publishing Group

References

1. Medina-Franco H, Urist MM, Fiveash J, Heslin MJ, Bland KI, Beenken SW. Multimodality treatment of Merkel cell carcinoma: case series and literature review of 1024 cases. Ann Surg Oncol. 2001;8: 204–8.
2. Agelli M, Clegg LX, Becker JC, Rollison DE. The etiology and epidemiology of Merkel cell carcinoma. Curr Probl Cancer. 2010;34:14–37.
3. Anderson LL, Phipps TJ, McCollough ML. Neuroendocrine carcinoma of the skin (Merkel cell carcinoma) in a black. J Dermatol Surg Oncol. 1992;18:375–80.
4. Albores-Saavedra J, Batich K, Chable-Montero F, Sagy N, Schwartz AM, Henson DE. Merkel cell carcinoma demographics, morphology, and survival based on 3870 cases: a population based study. J Cutan Pathol. 2010;37:20–7.
5. Agelli M, Clegg LX. Epidemiology of primary Merkel cell carcinoma in the United States. J Am Acad Dermatol. 2003;49:832–41.
6. Hodgson NC. Merkel cell carcinoma: changing incidence trends. J Surg Oncol. 2005;89:1–4.
7. Kivela T, Tarkkanen A. The Merkel cell and associated neoplasms in the eyelids and periocular region. Surv Ophthalmol. 1990;35:171–87.
8. Soltau JB, Smith ME, Custer PL. Merkel cell carcinoma of the eyelid. Am J Ophthalmol. 1996;121: 331–2.
9. Hussain SK, Sundquist J, Hemminki K. Incidence trends of squamous cell and rare skin cancers in the Swedish national cancer registry point to calendar year and age-dependent increases. J Invest Dermatol. 2010;130:1323–8.
10. Poulsen M, Round C, Keller J, Tripcony L, Veness M. Factors influencing relapse-free survival in Merkel cell carcinoma of the lower limb: a review of 60 cases. Int J Radiat Oncol Biol Phys. 2010;76: 393–7.
11. Alzaraa A, Thomas GD, Vodovnik A, Modgill VK. Merkel cell carcinoma in a male breast: a case report. Breast J. 2007;13:517–9.
12. Best TJ, Metcalfe JB, Moore RB, Nguyen GK. Merkel cell carcinoma of the scrotum. Ann Plast Surg. 1994;33:83–5.
13. Daghistani W, Younan R, Brutus JP. Merkel cell carcinoma of the hand: case report and literature review. Chir Main. 2010;29:128–31.
14. Tomic S, Warner TF, Messing E, Wilding G. Penile Merkel cell carcinoma. Urology. 1995;45:1062–5.
15. Hitchcock CL, Bland KI, Laney III RG, Franzini D, Harris B, Copeland III EM. Neuroendocrine (Merkel cell) carcinoma of the skin: its natural history, diagnosis, and treatment. Ann Surg. 1988;207:201–7.
16. Eng TY, Boersma MG, Fuller CD, et al. A comprehensive review of the treatment of Merkel cell carcinoma. Am J Clin Oncol. 2007;30:624–36.
17. Veness MJ, Perera L, McCourt J, et al. Merkel cell carcinoma: improved outcome with adjuvant radiotherapy. ANZ J Surg. 2005;75:275–81.
18. Lemos B, Nghiem P. Merkel cell carcinoma: more deaths but still no pathway to blame. J Invest Dermatol. 2007;127:2100–3.
19. Eftekhari F, Wallace S, Silva EG, Lenzi R. Merkel cell carcinoma of the skin: imaging and clinical features in 93 cases. Br J Radiol. 1996;69:226–33.
20. Heath ML, Nghiem P. Merkel cell carcinoma: if no breslow, then what? J Surg Oncol. 2007;95:614–5.
21. Schmid C, Beham A, Feichtinger J, Aubock L, Dietze O. Recurrent and subsequently metastasizing Merkel cell carcinoma in a 7-year-old girl. Histopathology. 1992;20:437–9.
22. Sonak RA, Trede K, Gerharz CD. [Merkel cell tumor of the hand in a 104-year-old patient: case report with review of the literature]. Handchir Mikrochir Plast Chir. 1996;28:43–5. German.
23. Kaae J, Hansen AV, Biggar RJ, et al. Merkel cell carcinoma: incidence, mortality, and risk of other cancers. J Natl Cancer Inst. 2010;102:793–801.
24. Girschik J, Thorn K, Beer TW, Heenan PJ, Fritschi L. Merkel Cell carcinoma in Western Australia: a population-based study of incidence and survival. Br J Dermatol. 2011;165(5):1051–7.
25. Vilar-Coromina N, Perez Bueno F, Alsina Maqueda M, Vilardell Gil L, Izquierdo Font A, Marcos-Gragera R. [Merkel cell cancer of the skin: population-based incidence and survival 1995–2005]. Med Clin (Barc). 2009;132:701–3.
26. Kukko H, Bohling T, Koljonen V, et al. Merkel cell carcinoma: a population-based epidemiological study in Finland with a clinical series of 181 cases. Eur J Cancer. 2011;48(5):737–42.
27. Reichgelt BA, Visser O. Epidemiology and survival of Merkel cell carcinoma in the Netherlands: a population-based study of 808 cases in 1993–2007. Eur J Cancer. 2011;47:579–85.
28. Allen PJ, Bowne WB, Jaques DP, Brennan MF, Busam K, Coit DG. Merkel cell carcinoma: prognosis and treatment of patients from a single institution. J Clin Oncol. 2005;23:2300–9.
29. Miller RW, Rabkin CS. Merkel cell carcinoma and melanoma: etiological similarities and differences. Cancer Epidemiol Biomarkers Prev. 1999;8:153–8.
30. Heath M, Jaimes N, Lemos B, et al. Clinical characteristics of Merkel cell carcinoma at diagnosis in 195 patients: the AEIOU features. J Am Acad Dermatol. 2008;58:375–81.
31. Paulson KG, Iyer JG, Nghiem P. Asymmetric lateral distribution of melanoma and Merkel cell carcinoma in the United States. J Am Acad Dermatol. 2011;65: 35–9.
32. Goessling W, McKee PH, Mayer RJ. Merkel cell carcinoma. J Clin Oncol. 2002;20:588–98.
33. Lunder EJ, Stern RS. Merkel-cell carcinomas in patients treated with methoxsalen and ultraviolet A radiation. N Engl J Med. 1998;339:1247–8.

34. Mogha A, Fautrel A, Mouchet N, et al. Merkel cell polyomavirus small T antigen mRNA level is increased following in vivo UV-radiation. PLoS One. 2010;5:e11423.
35. Castle SC, Uyemura K, Fulop T, Makinodan T. Host resistance and immune responses in advanced age. Clin Geriatr Med. 2007;23:463–79, v.
36. O'Connor WJ, Brodland DG. Merkel cell carcinoma. Dermatol Surg. 1996;22:262–7.
37. Rangwala S, Tsai KY. Roles of the immune system in skin cancer. Br J Dermatol. 2011;165(5):953–65.
38. Becker JC, Schrama D, Houben R. Merkel cell carcinoma. Cell Mol Life Sci. 2009;66:1–8.
39. Penn I, First MR. Merkel's cell carcinoma in organ recipients: report of 41 cases. Transplantation. 1999;68:1717–21.
40. Gianfreda M, Caiffi S, De Franceschi T, et al. [Merkel cell carcinoma of the skin in a patient with myasthenia gravis]. Minerva Med. 2002;93:219–22.
41. Lentz SR, Krewson L, Zutter MM. Recurrent neuroendocrine (Merkel cell) carcinoma of the skin presenting as marrow failure in a man with systemic lupus erythematosus. Med Pediatr Oncol. 1993;21: 137–41.
42. Lillis J, Ceilley RI, Nelson P. Merkel cell carcinoma in a patient with autoimmune hepatitis. J Drugs Dermatol. 2005;4:357–9.
43. McLoone NM, McKenna K, Edgar D, Walsh M, Bingham A. Merkel cell carcinoma in a patient with chronic sarcoidosis. Clin Exp Dermatol. 2005;30: 580–2.
44. Nemoto I, Sato-Matsumura KC, Fujita Y, et al. Leukaemic dissemination of Merkel cell carcinoma in a patient with systemic lupus erythematosus. Clin Exp Dermatol. 2008;33:270–2.
45. Satolli F, Venturi C, Vescovi V, Morrone P, De Panfilis G. Merkel-cell carcinoma in Behçet's disease. Acta Derm Venereol. 2005;85:79.
46. Lanoy E, Engels EA. Skin cancers associated with autoimmune conditions among elderly adults. Br J Cancer. 2010;103:112–4.
47. Cohen Y, Amir G, Polliack A. Development and rapid dissemination of Merkel-cell carcinomatosis following therapy with fludarabine and rituximab for relapsing follicular lymphoma. Eur J Haematol. 2002;68:117–9.
48. Gooptu C, Woollons A, Ross J, et al. Merkel cell carcinoma arising after therapeutic immunosuppression. Br J Dermatol. 1997;137:637–41.
49. Krishna SM, Kim CN. Merkel cell carcinoma in a patient treated with adalimumab: case report. Cutis. 2011;87:81–4.
50. Stone JH, Holbrook JT, Marriott MA, et al. Solid malignancies among patients in the Wegener's Granulomatosis Etanercept Trial. Arthritis Rheum. 2006;54:1608–18.
51. Wirges ML, Saporito F, Smith J. Rapid growth of Merkel cell carcinoma after treatment with rituximab. J Drugs Dermatol. 2006;5:180–1.
52. Friedlaender MM, Rubinger D, Rosenbaum E, Amir G, Siguencia E. Temporary regression of Merkel cell carcinoma metastases after cessation of cyclosporine. Transplantation. 2002;73:1849–50.
53. Muirhead R, Ritchie DM. Partial regression of Merkel cell carcinoma in response to withdrawal of azathioprine in an immunosuppression-induced case of metastatic Merkel cell carcinoma. Clin Oncol (R Coll Radiol). 2007;19:96.
54. Buell JF, Trofe J, Hanaway MJ, et al. Immunosuppression and Merkel cell cancer. Transplant Proc. 2002;34:1780–1.
55. Rubel JR, Milford EL, Abdi R. Cutaneous neoplasms in renal transplant recipients. Eur J Dermatol. 2002;12:532–5.
56. Koljonen V, Kukko H, Tukiainen E, et al. Incidence of Merkel cell carcinoma in renal transplant recipients. Nephrol Dial Transplant. 2009;24:3231–5.
57. Bordea C, Wojnarowska F, Millard PR, Doll H, Welsh K, Morris PJ. Skin cancers in renal-transplant recipients occur more frequently than previously recognized in a temperate climate. Transplantation. 2004;77:574–9.
58. Engels EA, Frisch M, Goedert JJ, Biggar RJ, Miller RW. Merkel cell carcinoma and HIV infection. Lancet. 2002;359:497–8.
59. Izikson L, Nornhold E, Iyer JG, Nghiem P, Zeitouni NC. Merkel cell carcinoma associated with HIV: review of 14 patients. AIDS. 2011;25:119–21.
60. Burack J, Altschuler EL. Sustained remission of metastatic Merkel cell carcinoma with treatment of HIV infection. J R Soc Med. 2003;96:238–9.
61. Adami J, Frisch M, Yuen J, Glimelius B, Melbye M. Evidence of an association between non-Hodgkin's lymphoma and skin cancer. BMJ. 1995;310:1491–5.
62. Agnew KL, Ruchlemer R, Catovsky D, Matutes E, Bunker CB. Cutaneous findings in chronic lymphocytic leukaemia. Br J Dermatol. 2004;150:1129–35.
63. Cantwell M, Hua T, Pappas J, Kipps TJ. Acquired CD40-ligand deficiency in chronic lymphocytic leukemia. Nat Med. 1997;3:984–9.
64. Lacombe C, Gombert J, Dreyfus B, Brizard A, Preud'Homme JL. Heterogeneity of serum IgG subclass deficiencies in B chronic lymphocytic leukemia. Clin Immunol. 1999;90:128–32.
65. Kipps TJ. Genetics of chronic lymphocytic leukaemia. Hematol Cell Ther. 2000;42:5–14.
66. Kipps TJ. Chronic lymphocytic leukemia. Curr Opin Hematol. 2000;7:223–34.
67. Barroeta JE, Farkas T. Merkel cell carcinoma and chronic lymphocytic leukemia (collision tumor) of the arm: a diagnosis by fine-needle aspiration biopsy. Diagn Cytopathol. 2007;35:293–5.
68. Cervigon I, Gargallo AB, Bahillo C, et al. [Merkel cell carcinoma in a patient with chronic lymphocytic leukemia]. Actas Dermosifiliogr. 2006;97:264–6.
69. Papageorgiou KI, Kaniorou-Larai MG. A case report of Merkel cell carcinoma on chronic lymphocytic leukemia: differential diagnosis of coexisting lymphadenopathy and indications for early aggressive treatment. BMC Cancer. 2005;5:106.
70. Quaglino D, Di Leonardo G, Lalli G, et al. Association between chronic lymphocytic leukae-

mia and secondary tumours: unusual occurrence of a neuroendocrine (Merkel cell) carcinoma. Eur Rev Med Pharmacol Sci. 1997;1:11–6.

71. Robak E, Biernat W, Krykowski E, Jeziorski A, Robak T. Merkel cell carcinoma in a patient with B-cell chronic lymphocytic leukemia treated with cladribine and rituximab. Leuk Lymphoma. 2005;46:909–14.
72. Vlad R, Woodlock TJ. Merkel cell carcinoma after chronic lymphocytic leukemia: case report and literature review. Am J Clin Oncol. 2003;26:531–4.
73. Ziprin P, Smith S, Salerno G, Rosin RD. Two cases of Merkel cell tumour arising in patients with chronic lymphocytic leukaemia. Br J Dermatol. 2000;142: 525–8.
74. Tadmor T, Aviv A, Polliack A. Merkel cell carcinoma, chronic lymphocytic leukemia and other lymphoproliferative disorders: an old bond with possible new viral ties. Ann Oncol. 2011;22:250–6.
75. Khezri F, Brewer JD, Weaver AL. Merkel cell carcinoma in the setting of chronic lymphocytic leukemia. Dermatol Surg. 2011;37:1100–5.
76. Pantulu ND, Pallasch CP, Kurz AK, et al. Detection of a novel truncating Merkel cell polyomavirus large T antigen deletion in chronic lymphocytic leukemia cells. Blood. 2010;116:5280–4.
77. Howard RA, Dores GM, Curtis RE, Anderson WF, Travis LB. Merkel cell carcinoma and multiple primary cancers. Cancer Epidemiol Biomarkers Prev. 2006;15:1545–9.
78. Brenner B, Sulkes A, Rakowsky E, et al. Second neoplasms in patients with Merkel cell carcinoma. Cancer. 2001;91:1358–62.
79. Euvrard S, Kanitakis J, Pouteil-Noble C, Claudy A, Touraine JL. Skin cancers in organ transplant recipients. Ann Transplant. 1997;2:28–32.
80. Popp S, Waltering S, Herbst C, Moll I, Boukamp P. UV-B-type mutations and chromosomal imbalances indicate common pathways for the development of Merkel and skin squamous cell carcinomas. Int J Cancer. 2002;99:352–60.
81. Walsh NM. Primary neuroendocrine (Merkel cell) carcinoma of the skin: morphologic diversity and implications thereof. Hum Pathol. 2001;32:680–9.
82. Bzhalava D, Bray F, Storm H, Dillner J. Risk of second cancers after the diagnosis of Merkel cell carcinoma in Scandinavia. Br J Cancer. 2011;104:178–80.
83. Koljonen V, Kukko H, Tukiainen E, et al. Second cancers following the diagnosis of Merkel cell carcinoma: a nationwide cohort study. Cancer Epidemiol. 2010;34:62–5.
84. Boonchai W, Green A, Ng J, Dicker A, Chenevix-Trench G. Basal cell carcinoma in chronic arsenicism occurring in Queensland, Australia, after ingestion of an asthma medication. J Am Acad Dermatol. 2000;43:664–9.
85. Lien HC, Tsai TF, Lee YY, Hsiao CH. Merkel cell carcinoma and chronic arsenicism. J Am Acad Dermatol. 1999;41:641–3.
86. Feng H, Shuda M, Chang Y, Moore PS. Clonal integration of a polyomavirus in human Merkel cell carcinoma. Science. 2008;319:1096–100.
87. Poulin DL, DeCaprio JA. Is there a role for SV40 in human cancer? J Clin Oncol. 2006;24:4356–65.
88. Rollison DE, Giuliano AR, Becker JC. New virus associated with Merkel cell carcinoma development. J Natl Compr Canc Netw. 2010;8:874–80.
89. Shuda M, Feng H, Kwun HJ, et al. T antigen mutations are a human tumor-specific signature for Merkel cell polyomavirus. Proc Natl Acad Sci USA. 2008;105:16272–7.
90. Kassem A, Schopflin A, Diaz C, et al. Frequent detection of Merkel cell polyomavirus in human Merkel cell carcinomas and identification of a unique deletion in the VP1 gene. Cancer Res. 2008;68:5009–13.
91. Liu X, Hein J, Richardson SC, et al. Merkel cell polyomavirus large T antigen disrupts lysosome clustering by translocating human Vam6p from the cytoplasm to the nucleus. J Biol Chem. 2011;286:17079–90.
92. Garneski KM, Warcola AH, Feng Q, Kiviat NB, Leonard JH, Nghiem P. Merkel cell polyomavirus is more frequently present in North American than Australian Merkel cell carcinoma tumors. J Invest Dermatol. 2009;129:246–8.
93. Sastre-Garau X, Peter M, Avril MF, et al. Merkel cell carcinoma of the skin: pathological and molecular evidence for a causative role of MCV in oncogenesis. J Pathol. 2009;218:48–56.
94. Becker JC, Houben R, Ugurel S, Trefzer U, Pfohler C, Schrama D. MC polyomavirus is frequently present in Merkel cell carcinoma of European patients. J Invest Dermatol. 2009;129:248–50.
95. Wieland U, Mauch C, Kreuter A, Krieg T, Pfister H. Merkel cell polyomavirus DNA in persons without Merkel cell carcinoma. Emerg Infect Dis. 2009;15: 1496–8.
96. Dworkin AM, Tseng SY, Allain DC, Iwenofu OH, Peters SB, Toland AE. Merkel cell polyomavirus in cutaneous squamous cell carcinoma of immunocompetent individuals. J Invest Dermatol. 2009;129: 2868–74.
97. Pastrana DV, Tolstov YL, Becker JC, Moore PS, Chang Y, Buck CB. Quantitation of human seroresponsiveness to Merkel cell polyomavirus. PLoS Pathog. 2009;5:e1000578.
98. Kean JM, Rao S, Wang M, Garcea RL. Seroepidemiology of human polyomaviruses. PLoS Pathog. 2009;5:e1000363.
99. Chen T, Hedman L, Mattila PS, et al. Serological evidence of Merkel cell polyomavirus primary infections in childhood. J Clin Virol. 2011;50:125–9.
100. Goh S, Lindau C, Tiveljung-Lindell A, Allander T. Merkel cell polyomavirus in respiratory tract secretions. Emerg Infect Dis. 2009;15:489–91.
101. Kuwamoto S. Recent advances in the biology of Merkel cell carcinoma. Hum Pathol. 2011;42:1063–77.
102. Paulson KG, Lemos BD, Feng B, et al. Array-CGH reveals recurrent genomic changes in Merkel cell carcinoma including amplification of L-Myc. J Invest Dermatol. 2009;129:1547–55.
103. Houben R, Schrama D, Alb M, et al. Comparable expression and phosphorylation of the retinoblas-

toma protein in Merkel cell polyoma virus-positive and negative Merkel cell carcinoma. Int J Cancer. 2010;126:796–8.
104. Lassacher A, Heitzer E, Kerl H, Wolf P. p14ARF hypermethylation is common but INK4a-ARF locus or p53 mutations are rare in Merkel cell carcinoma. J Invest Dermatol. 2008;128:1788–96.
105. Waltari M, Sihto H, Kukko H, et al. Association of Merkel cell polyomavirus infection with tumor p53, KIT, stem cell factor, PDGFR-alpha and survival in Merkel cell carcinoma. Int J Cancer. 2011;129: 619–28.
106. Bhatia K, Goedert JJ, Modali R, Preiss L, Ayers LW. Merkel cell carcinoma subgroups by Merkel cell polyomavirus DNA relative abundance and oncogene expression. Int J Cancer. 2010;126:2240–6.
107. Van Gele M, Speleman F, Vandesompele J, Van Roy N, Leonard JH. Characteristic pattern of chromosomal gains and losses in Merkel cell carcinoma detected by comparative genomic hybridization. Cancer Res. 1998;58:1503–8.
108. Gancberg D, Feoli F, Hamels J, et al. Trisomy 6 in Merkel cell carcinoma: a recurrent chromosomal aberration. Histopathology. 2000;37:445–51.
109. Larramendy ML, Koljonen V, Bohling T, Tukiainen E, Knuutila S. Recurrent DNA copy number changes revealed by comparative genomic hybridization in primary Merkel cell carcinomas. Mod Pathol. 2004;17:561–7.
110. Wassermann S, Scheel SK, Hiendlmeyer E, et al. p16INK4a is a beta-catenin target gene and indicates low survival in human colorectal tumors. Gastroenterology. 2009;136:196–205 e192.
111. Panelos J, Batistatou A, Paglierani M, et al. Expression of Notch-1 and alteration of the E-cadherin/beta-catenin cell adhesion complex are observed in primary cutaneous neuroendocrine carcinoma (Merkel cell carcinoma). Mod Pathol. 2009;22:959–68.
112. Kennedy MM, Blessing K, King G, Kerr KM. Expression of bcl-2 and p53 in Merkel cell carcinoma: an immunohistochemical study. Am J Dermatopathol. 1996;18:273–7.
113. Plettenberg A, Pammer J, Tschachler E. Merkel cells and Merkel cell carcinoma express the BCL-2 protooncogene. Exp Dermatol. 1996;5:102–7.
114. Schlagbauer-Wadl H, Klosner G, Heere-Ress E, et al. Bcl-2 antisense oligonucleotides (G3139) inhibit Merkel cell carcinoma growth in SCID mice. J Invest Dermatol. 2000;114:725–30.
115. Brunner M, Thurnher D, Pammer J, et al. Expression of hedgehog signaling molecules in Merkel cell carcinoma. Head Neck. 2010;32:333–40.
116. Kukko HM, Koljonen VS, Tukiainen EJ, Haglund CH, Bohling TO. Vascular invasion is an early event in pathogenesis of Merkel cell carcinoma. Mod Pathol. 2010;23:1151–6.
117. Morrison WH, Peters LJ, Silva EG, Wendt CD, Ang KK, Goepfert H. The essential role of radiation therapy in securing locoregional control of Merkel cell carcinoma. Int J Radiat Oncol Biol Phys. 1990;19:583–91.
118. Meeuwissen JA, Bourne RG, Kearsley JH. The importance of postoperative radiation therapy in the treatment of Merkel cell carcinoma. Int J Radiat Oncol Biol Phys. 1995;31:325–31.
119. Guler-Nizam E, Leiter U, Metzler G, Breuninger H, Garbe C, Eigentler TK. Clinical course and prognostic factors of Merkel cell carcinoma of the skin. Br J Dermatol. 2009;161:90–4.
120. Boyle F, Pendlebury S, Bell D. Further insights into the natural history and management of primary cutaneous neuroendocrine (Merkel cell) carcinoma. Int J Radiat Oncol Biol Phys. 1995;31:315–23.
121. Koljonen V, Bohling T, Granhroth G, Tukiainen E. Merkel cell carcinoma: a clinicopathological study of 34 patients. Eur J Surg Oncol. 2003;29:607–10.
122. Beer TW, Ng LB, Murray K. Mast cells have prognostic value in Merkel cell carcinoma. Am J Dermatopathol. 2008;30:27–30.
123. Fields RC, Busam KJ, Chou JF, et al. Recurrence and survival in patients undergoing sentinel lymph node biopsy for Merkel cell carcinoma: analysis of 153 patients from a single institution. Ann Surg Oncol. 2011;18:2529–37.
124. Sandel IV HD, Day T, Richardson MS, Scarlett M, Gutman KA. Merkel cell carcinoma: does tumor size or depth of invasion correlate with recurrence, metastasis, or patient survival? Laryngoscope. 2006; 116:791–5.
125. Goldberg SR, Neifeld JP, Frable WJ. Prognostic value of tumor thickness in patients with Merkel cell carcinoma. J Surg Oncol. 2007;95:618–22.
126. Mott RT, Smoller BR, Morgan MB. Merkel cell carcinoma: a clinicopathologic study with prognostic implications. J Cutan Pathol. 2004;31:217–23.
127. Skelton HG, Smith KJ, Hitchcock CL, McCarthy WF, Lupton GP, Graham JH. Merkel cell carcinoma: analysis of clinical, histologic, and immunohistologic features of 132 cases with relation to survival. J Am Acad Dermatol. 1997;37:734–9.
128. Llombart B, Monteagudo C, Lopez-Guerrero JA, et al. Clinicopathological and immunohistochemical analysis of 20 cases of Merkel cell carcinoma in search of prognostic markers. Histopathology. 2005;46:622–34.
129. Lemos BD, Storer BE, Iyer JG, et al. Pathologic nodal evaluation improves prognostic accuracy in Merkel cell carcinoma: analysis of 5823 cases as the basis of the first consensus staging system. J Am Acad Dermatol. 2010;63:751–61.
130. Gupta SG, Wang LC, Penas PF, Gellenthin M, Lee SJ, Nghiem P. Sentinel lymph node biopsy for evaluation and treatment of patients with Merkel cell carcinoma: The Dana-Farber experience and meta-analysis of the literature. Arch Dermatol. 2006;142:685–90.
131. Paulson KG, Carter JJ, Johnson LG, et al. Antibodies to Merkel cell polyomavirus T antigen oncoproteins

reflect tumor burden in Merkel cell carcinoma patients. Cancer Res. 2010;70:8388–97.

132. Jemec B, Chana J, Grover R, Grobbelaar AO. The Merkel cell carcinoma: survival and oncogene markers. J Eur Acad Dermatol Venereol. 2000;14:400–4.
133. Andea AA, Patel R, Ponnazhagan S, et al. Merkel cell carcinoma: correlation of KIT expression with survival and evaluation of KIT gene mutational status. Hum Pathol. 2010;41:1405–12.
134. Handschel J, Muller D, Depprich RA, et al. The new polyomavirus (MCPyV) does not affect the clinical course in MCCs. Int J Oral Maxillofac Surg. 2010;39:1086–90.
135. Sihto H, Kukko H, Koljonen V, Sankila R, Bohling T, Joensuu H. Clinical factors associated with Merkel cell polyomavirus infection in Merkel cell carcinoma. J Natl Cancer Inst. 2009;101:938–45.
136. Touze A, Gaitan J, Maruani A, et al. Merkel cell polyomavirus strains in patients with Merkel cell carcinoma. Emerg Infect Dis. 2009;15:960–2.
137. Bhatia K, Goedert JJ, Modali R, Preiss L, Ayers LW. Immunological detection of viral large T antigen identifies a subset of Merkel cell carcinoma tumors with higher viral abundance and better clinical outcome. Int J Cancer. 2010;127:1493–6.
138. Laude HC, Jonchere B, Maubec E, et al. Distinct Merkel cell polyomavirus molecular features in tumour and non tumour specimens from patients with Merkel cell carcinoma. PLoS Pathog. 2010;6: e1001076.
139. Touze A, Le Bidre E, Laude H, et al. High levels of antibodies against Merkel cell polyomavirus identify a subset of patients with Merkel cell carcinoma with better clinical outcome. J Clin Oncol. 2011;29:1612–9.
140. Busam KJ, Jungbluth AA, Rekthman N, et al. Merkel cell polyomavirus expression in Merkel cell carcinomas and its absence in combined tumors and pulmonary neuroendocrine carcinomas. Am J Surg Pathol. 2009;33:1378–85.
141. Carter JJ, Paulson KG, Wipf GC, et al. Association of Merkel cell polyomavirus-specific antibodies with Merkel cell carcinoma. J Natl Cancer Inst. 2009;101: 1510–22.
142. Duncavage EJ, Zehnbauer BA, Pfeifer JD. Prevalence of Merkel cell polyomavirus in Merkel cell carcinoma. Mod Pathol. 2009;22:516–21.
143. Ridd K, Yu S, Bastian BC. The presence of polyomavirus in non-melanoma skin cancer in organ transplant recipients is rare. J Invest Dermatol. 2009;129:250–2.
144. Loyo M, Guerrero-Preston R, Brait M, et al. Quantitative detection of Merkel cell virus in human tissues and possible mode of transmission. Int J Cancer. 2010;126:2991–6.
145. Foulongne V, Kluger N, Dereure O, Brieu N, Guillot B, Segondy M. Merkel cell polyomavirus and Merkel cell carcinoma. France Emerg Infect Dis. 2008;14:1491–3.
146. Helmbold P, Lahtz C, Enk A, et al. Frequent occurrence of RASSF1A promoter hypermethylation and Merkel cell polyomavirus in Merkel cell carcinoma. Mol Carcinog. 2009;48:903–9.
147. Andres C, Belloni B, Puchta U, Sander CA, Flaig MJ. Prevalence of MCPyV in Merkel cell carcinoma and non-MCC tumors. J Cutan Pathol. 2010;37:28–34.
148. Varga E, Kiss M, Szabo K, Kemeny L. Detection of Merkel cell polyomavirus DNA in Merkel cell carcinomas. Br J Dermatol. 2009;161:930–2.
149. Wetzels CT, Hoefnagel JG, Bakkers JM, Dijkman HB, Blokx WA, Melchers WJ. Ultrastructural proof of polyomavirus in Merkel cell carcinoma tumour cells and its absence in small cell carcinoma of the lung. PLoS One. 2009;4:e4958.
150. Mangana J, Dziunycz P, Kerl K, Dummer R, Cozzio A. Prevalence of Merkel cell polyomavirus among Swiss Merkel cell carcinoma patients. Dermatology. 2010;221:184–8.
151. Katano H, Ito H, Suzuki Y, et al. Detection of Merkel cell polyomavirus in Merkel cell carcinoma and Kaposi's sarcoma. J Med Virol. 2009;81:1951–8.
152. Nakajima H, Takaishi M, Yamamoto M, et al. Screening of the specific polyoma virus as diagnostic and prognostic tools for Merkel cell carcinoma. J Dermatol Sci. 2009;56:211–3.
153. Kuwamoto S, Higaki H, Kanai K, et al. Association of Merkel cell polyomavirus infection with morphologic differences in Merkel cell carcinoma. Hum Pathol. 2011;42:632–40.
154. Woo KJ, Choi YL, Jung HS, et al. Merkel cell carcinoma: our experience with seven patients in Korea and a literature review. J Plast Reconstr Aesthet Surg. 2010;63:2064–70.
155. Van Gele M, Kaghad M, Leonard JH, et al. Mutation analysis of P73 and TP53 in Merkel cell carcinoma. Br J Cancer. 2000;82:823–6.
156. Houben R, Michel B, Vetter-Kauczok CS, et al. Absence of classical MAP kinase pathway signalling in Merkel cell carcinoma. J Invest Dermatol. 2006;126:1135–42.
157. Liu S, Daa T, Kashima K, Kondoh Y, Yokoyama S. The Wnt-signaling pathway is not implicated in tumorigenesis of Merkel cell carcinoma. J Cutan Pathol. 2007;34:22–6.
158. Swick BL, Ravdel L, Fitzpatrick JE, Robinson WA. Merkel cell carcinoma: evaluation of KIT (CD117) expression and failure to demonstrate activating mutations in the C-KIT proto-oncogene: implications for treatment with imatinib mesylate. J Cutan Pathol. 2007;34:324–9.
159. Van Gele M, Leonard JH, Van Roy N, Cook AL, De Paepe A, Speleman F. Frequent allelic loss at 10q23 but low incidence of PTEN mutations in Merkel cell carcinoma. Int J Cancer. 2001;92:409–13.
160. Agraharkar ML, Cinclair RD, Kuo YF, Daller JA, Shahinian VB. Risk of malignancy with long-term immunosuppression in renal transplant recipients. Kidney Int. 2004;66:383–9.

Part II

Diagnosis

3 Clinical Diagnosis

Nancy Kim, Sandra Y. Han, and Siegrid S. Yu

Introduction and History

MCC was first described by Cyril Toker in 1972. He named it trabecular carcinoma of the skin because of its histological appearance of trabecular or column-like growth [1]. Toker initially believed MCC to be a tumor of sweat gland origin. In 1978, Tang and Toker performed ultrastructural studies of MCC which showed dense core neurosecretory granules in the cytoplasm of tumor cells [2]. As Merkel cells were known to be the only cells in the skin containing these granules, they hypothesized that trabecular carcinoma of the skin originated from Merkel cells [3, 4]. This continues to be debated in the literature with most current authors believing that MCC is related to Merkel cells and that the cells are of neuroendocrine origin [4, 5]. Other authors postulate that a pluripotent stem cell is responsible for MCC [6, 7].

N. Kim • S.S. Yu (✉)
Department of Dermatology, UCSF Dermatologic Surgery & Laser Center, 1701 Divisadero Street, Third Floor, San Francisco, CA 94115-0316, USA
e-mail: KimN@derm.ucsf.edu; nkimmd@gmail.com; Yus@derm.ucsf.edu

S.Y. Han
Department of Dermatology, University of California, San Francisco, 1701 Divisadero Street, Third Floor, San Francisco, CA 94115, USA
e-mail: sandrayhan@yahoo.com

With all the different hypotheses about the origin of MCC, it is not surprising that there have been a plethora of different names used to describe it in the literature such as trabecular carcinoma of the skin, cutaneous apudoma, primary small cell carcinoma of the skin, primary undifferentiated carcinoma of the skin, anaplastic carcinoma of the skin, cutaneous neuroendocrine carcinoma, and MCC [8]. The term Merkel cell carcinoma was first introduced in 1980 and has since become the most commonly used term to describe the tumor [9].

Merkel cell carcinoma is so rare that it was previously difficult to assess the true incidence of this disease. More recently, epidemiologic information has been gleaned through mining large cancer registries, which pool data across large regions. Agnelli and Clegg analyzed the population covered by the Surveillance Epidemiology and End Results (SEER) program of the National Cancer Institute [10, 11]. The year 1986 was chosen as the starting year for analysis because this was the inaugural year for the histologic code for MCC with the advent of the International Statistical Classification of Diseases and Related Health Problems (ICD) in the form of ICD-0, rendering it more easily trackable. Through this research it has become apparent that although rare, incidence of Merkel cell carcinoma is increasing. Reported incidence in the Surveillance, Epidemiology, and End Results (SEER) database has quadrupled from 1986 to 2006 likely because of new pathologic techniques that reduce the

M. Alam et al. (eds.), *Merkel Cell Carcinoma*, DOI 10.1007/978-1-4614-6608-6_3,

number of missed diagnoses. In 1986 the incidence of Merkel cell carcinoma in the United States was estimated at 0.15 cases per 100,000 people [12]. In 2001, the incidence rose to 0.44 cases per 100,000 [12]. By 2006, the incidence had increased to 0.6 per 100,000 [13]. In 2006, there were 1,630 cases of Merkel cell carcinoma in the United States [13].

The incidence of Merkel cell carcinoma will only continue to increase as diagnostic techniques for detecting MCC, such as cytokeratin-20 immunohistochemistry, become more widely used. The importance of cytokeratin-20 immunostains in diagnosing Merkel cell carcinomas histologically was first published in 1992 [14]. Prior to the advent of cytokeratin-20 immunostains, the diagnosis of Merkel cell carcinoma had to be verified with cumbersome electron microscopy techniques.

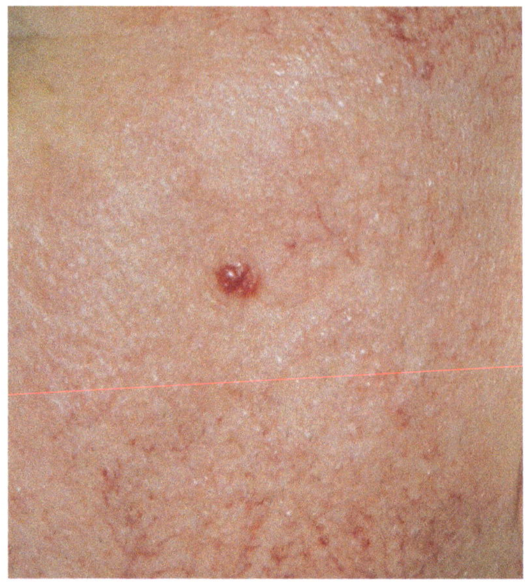

Fig. 3.1 This new asymptomatic, firm, *red* papule on the cheek of an elderly patient was diagnosed as a Merkel cell carcinoma. This is a typical presentation for MCC

Key Features

MCC can be a difficult tumor to clinically diagnose, as it tends to be asymptomatic, and does not have pathognomonic clinical features. Ultimately, the diagnosis is made by biopsy and histopathologic examination. To facilitate diagnosis of MCC, the pneumonic "AEIOU" was coined to summarize the five most common clinical findings of Merkel cell carcinoma (Asymptomatic, Expanding rapidly, Immunosuppression [15, 16], Older than 50 years, and Ultraviolet exposure) [17]. In one study, 89 % of patients met 3 or more criteria, 52 % met 4 or more criteria, and 7 % met all criteria [17].

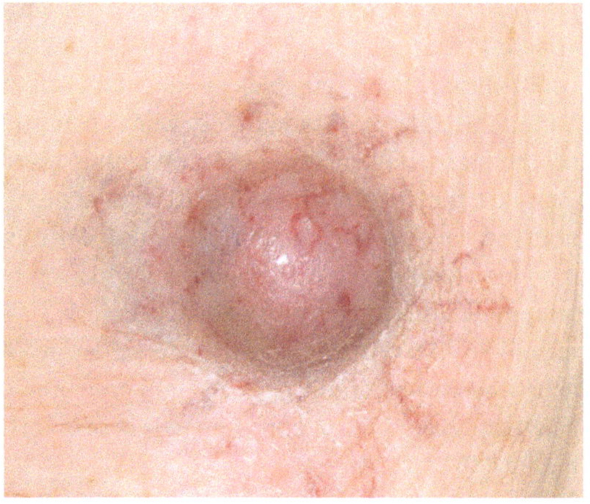

Fig. 3.2 This Merkel cell carcinoma presented as a dull *pink* tumor with overlying telangiectasias. The majority of MCCs exhibit *pink* or *red* color

MCC presented as an asymptomatic lesion in 88 % of patients in one large study [17]. Ulceration or epidermal disruption is rarely reported. Typically, lesions present as a firm, red-to-purple, non-tender papules or nodules [17] (see Fig. 3.1). MCCs present in a number of colors, though red/pink primary lesions predominate (see Figs. 3.2 and 3.3) and are seen in 56 % of patients [17]. Blue/violaceous lesions were noted in 26 % (see Fig. 3.4).

Sixty-three percent of patients reported rapid growth in the size of their tumor over a period of 3 months [17]. Only 11 % of patients did not notice any changes in size of primary lesions. Sizes of primary lesions at time of diagnosis vary widely. In a study of 191 patients, the diameter of the primary tumor was highly variable, with a median tumor size of 1.8 cm [17]. 21.3 % of patients presented with a diameter of less than 1 cm for the primary tumor, 43.3 % of patients

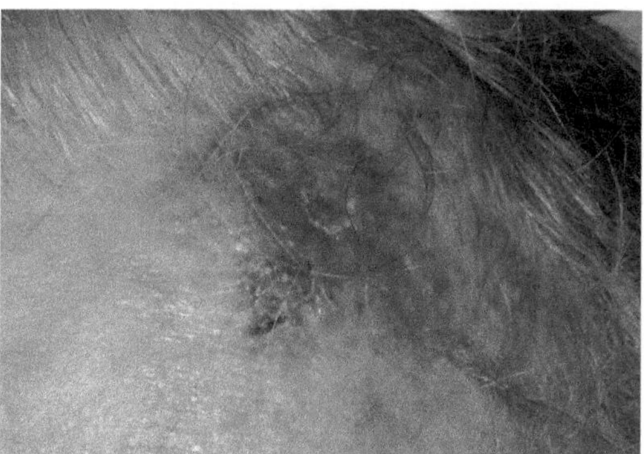

Fig. 3.3 Merkel cell carcinomas may be poorly circumscribed, presenting here as an ill-defined, erythematous plaque with central scale

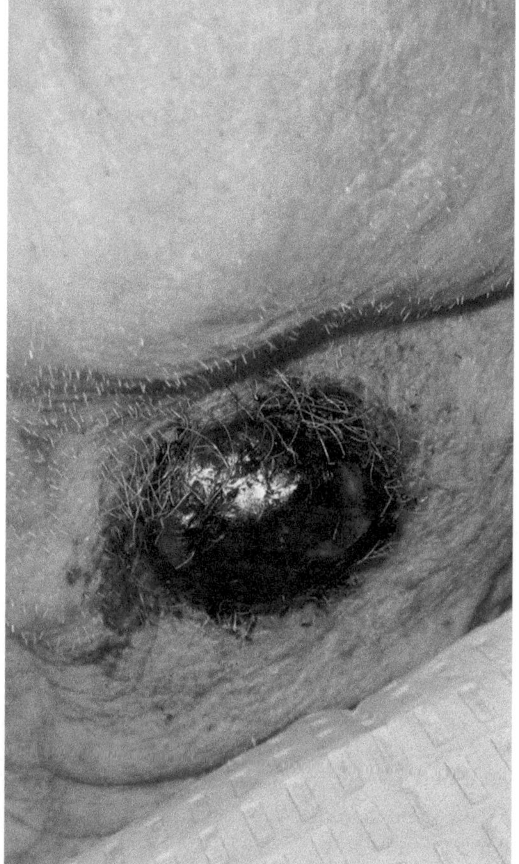

Fig. 3.4 Note the violaceous hue of this Merkel cell cancer that grew 4 cm over the course of 1 month

with a diameter between 1 and 2 cm, and 35.3 % of patients with a diameter greater than 2 cm (see Figs. 3.5 and 3.6).

Patients with immunosuppression are at higher risk for the development of MCC. MCC has been

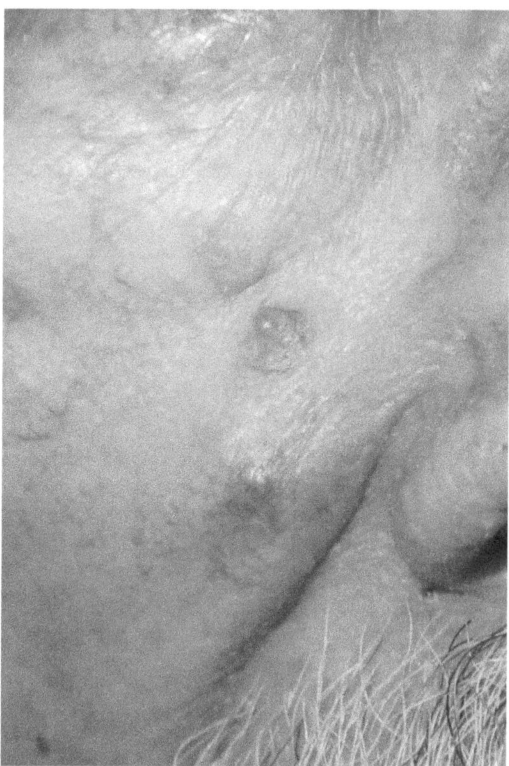

Fig. 3.5 The superior lesion was the site of a biopsy of a primary Merkel cell carcinoma. The original lesion was approximately 0.6 cm. There is tumor growth at the periphery of the biopsy scar. The papule directly inferior was an in-transit metastasis that measured 0.8 cm and developed within 1 month of the primary diagnosis

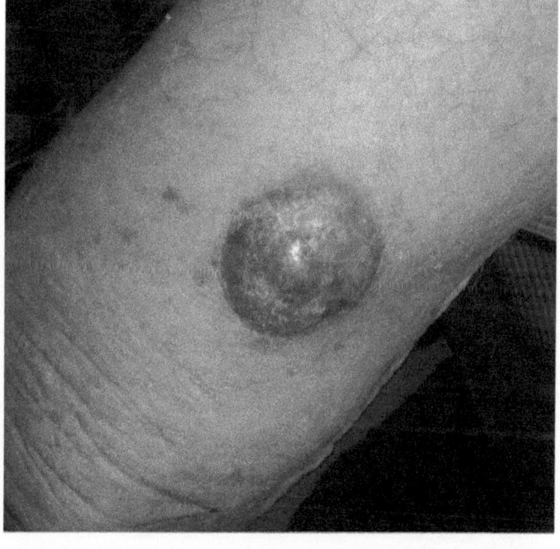

Fig. 3.6 This rapidly enlarging Merkel cell measured 3.5 cm at initial presentation. Approximately one-third of Merkel cells tumors are >2 cm at the time of diagnosis

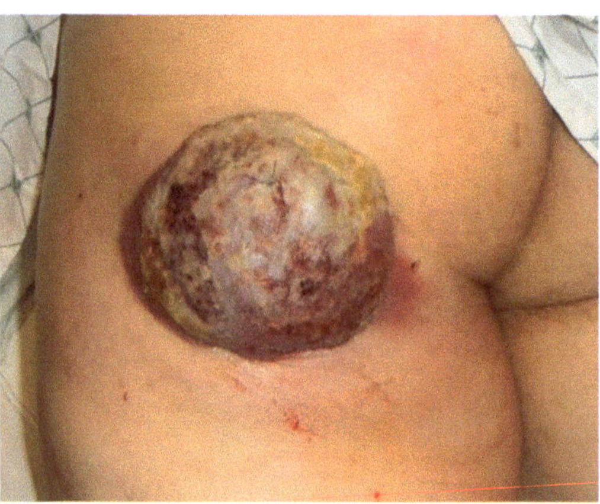

Fig. 3.7 This patient developed Merkel cell carcinoma on the left buttock with associated bulky inguinal lymphadenopathy 9 years after receiving a liver transplant. Immune suppression is a risk factor for developing MCC, and these patients usually present with advanced disease

associated with a diverse number of autoimmune diseases as well as with organ transplants [18–24]. In one study, 7.8 % of MCC patients were found to have some form of immunosuppression including HIV, CLL, and solid organ transplants [17]. Among transplant patients, renal transplant patients acquire MCC most commonly, with the average time span between organ transplantation and development of MCC being 7 years [25]. The discovery of a novel human polyomavirus integrated in the genome of a majority of Merkel cell carcinomas may explain the increased incidence of MCC in immunosuppressed patients [26]. Not surprisingly, organ transplant and immune suppressed patients present with MCC at younger ages than nonimmune suppressed patients. The mean age of presentation in organ transplant patients is 53 years [25]. In these patients the disease is typically well-advanced at the time of presentation (see Fig. 3.7).

In immunocompetent patients, MCC tends to affect older patients over the age of 65. In one large study, the median age at diagnosis was 69 years [17]. Ninety percent of patients with MCC were older than 50 years. A male predominance has also been noted in patients who develop the disease. In the SEER (Surveillance, Epidemiology and End Results) data, the incidence of first primary MCC is 2:1, men to women in Caucasian and African American patients [10]. In all other ethnic groups, the ratio of men to women affected by the disease is 1.5:1. Furthermore, when men are affected by MCC, they typically present at a younger age at the time of diagnosis than women. The mean age for the diagnosis of MCC is 71 years in men and 76 years in women. It is also primarily a disease of fair-skinned people. In one large study, Caucasians had an overall age-adjusted incidence of 0.36 per 100,000 person years [10]. In comparison, African Americans had an incidence rate of 0.045 and all other ethnic groups had an incidence rate of 0.4 [10]. Ninety-eight percent of patients were white, only 4 of 191 patients were nonwhite (3 Asian and 1 black) [17].

Ultraviolet exposure (both UVA and UVB) and both ionizing [27, 28] and infrared radiation [7, 29, 30] are all linked with an increase in the incidence of MCC. MCC is much more prevalent in areas with a high UVB radiation index [10]. When the SEER database was examined in relation to the incidence of first Merkel cell carcinoma and the UVB radiation index, it was found that the overall age-adjusted incidence of first primary MCC in Caucasians is highest in Hawaii, the geographic location with the highest UVB radiation index [10]. MCC is also most commonly located on UV-exposed areas such as the head and neck (see Fig. 3.8). There is a positive correlation between incidence of head and neck MCC and increased UVB radiation index. Not only does UVB induce MCC, but UVA and ionizing radiation and infrared radiation have also been found to be linked to an increased incidence of MCC. UVA radiation is a more powerful mutagen then UVB radiation [31]. Patients with psoriasis who underwent oral methoxsalen (psoralen) and UVA photo-chemotherapy have an MCC incidence 100× greater than the general population [32].

The most common sites for MCC include the head and neck; these two sites account for 48 % of all MCC diagnoses. Incidence of MCC of the upper limb is 19 %, followed by a 16 % incidence of MCC of the lower limb (see Fig. 3.9), and 11 % incidence of MCC of the trunk [10] (see Fig. 3.10). Ultraviolet-protected locations such

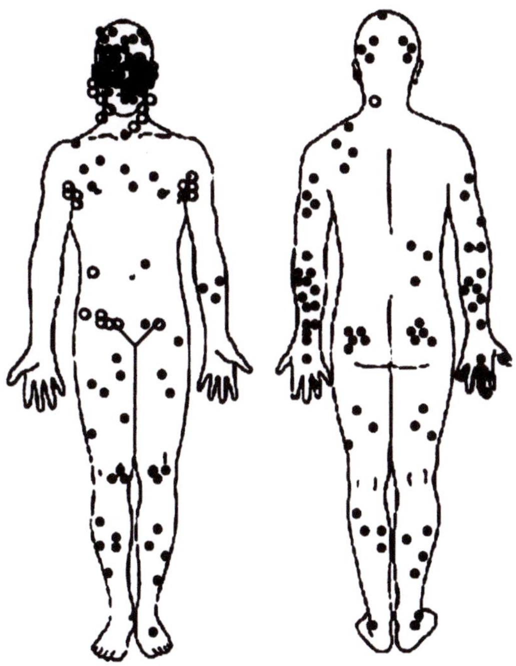

Fig. 3.8 Distribution of Merkel cell carcinoma at presentation in 195 patients. Primary skin lesion (*solid circle*) was seen in 168 patients (86 %). In all, 27 (14 %) presented with nodal involvement and no known primary (*open circles*) (reprinted from Heath M, Jaimes N, Lemos B, Mostaghimi A, Wang LC, Penas PF, Nghiem P. Clinical Characteristics of Merkel cell carcinoma at diagnosis in 195 patients: the AEIOU features. J Am Acad Dermatol 2008;58:375–81. With permission from Elsevier)

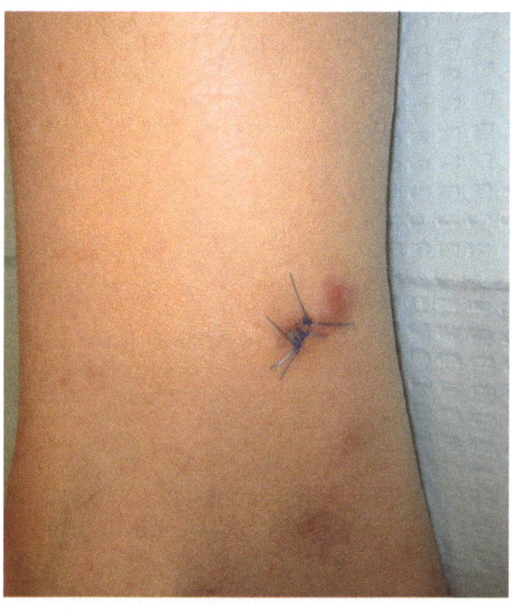

Fig. 3.9 Merkel cell carcinomas may present on the extremities. This MCC (with sutures at the biopsy site) developed on the medial lower leg. Primary MCCs of the limbs have the best prognosis

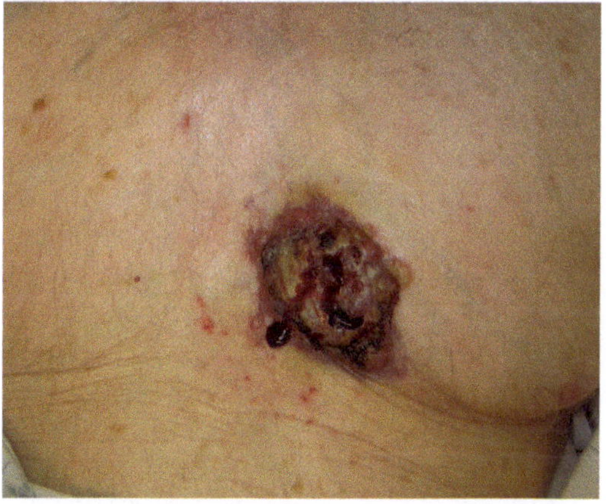

Fig. 3.10 This friable, rapidly growing Merkel cell carcinoma presented on the chest of an elderly male. Primary presentation on the trunk is associated with a worse prognosis

as the trunk, back, and buttocks are less commonly affected than ultraviolet-exposed sites. In men, it has been found that the site of first primary MCC varies by age [10]. Head and neck MCC accounts for 30 % of first primary MCC in men under 65 years of age. In men younger than 65 years of age, the largest proportion of cases occurs on the trunk and limbs. By the time men reach 75 years or older, the percentage of cases which are head and neck increases to 55 %.

Some unusual primary sites for MCC to occur include mucosal sites [10], the lacrimal gland [33], and the parotid gland [34]. Approximately 5 % of all cases of first primary MCC present in mucosal sites. From 1992 to 2001, the total number of cases of first primary MCC was 1,027 and of these cases, 50 had an initial presentation in a mucosal anatomic site [10]. The most typical sites affected by mucosal MCC are the larynx, followed by the nasal cavity, pharynx, mouth, and tongue. There have also been rare reports of vulvar [35] and penile MCC [36]. Similar to MCC in other sites, there is a slight male predominance for mucosal MCC of 1.3:1. Mucosal

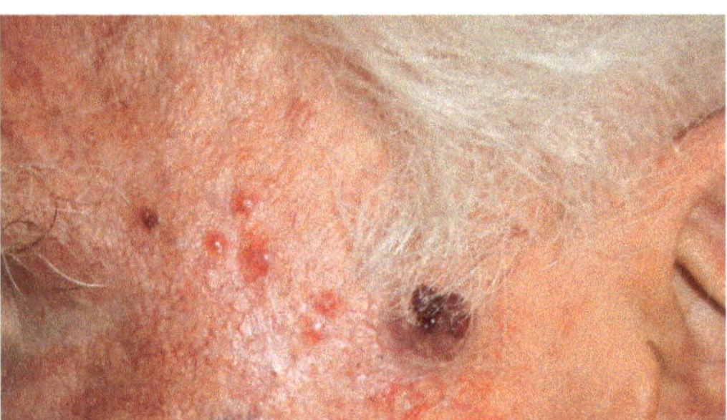

Fig. 3.11 This patient developed rapidly in-transit metastatic lesions within 3 weeks of developing a primary lesion of Merkel cell carcinoma. The primary tumor is the lateral violaceous, ulcerated nodule

MCC typically presents in younger patients than MCC in other sites with mean age is 62 years vs. 74 years in other MCC patients.

The location of the MCC presentation is statistically significant for staging [10]. The MCC site with the best prognosis is presentation on the limbs, which generally correlates with less advanced disease. MCC presentation on the trunk is associated with distant metastasis at the time of diagnosis. Mucosal MCC is also associated with worse prognosis than primary cutaneous MCC at other anatomic sites. Mucosal MCC is difficult to detect and therefore typically is more advanced at the time of diagnosis. The relative survival of individuals with first primary MCC of the mucosa is poorer than that of individuals with first primary MCC in other cutaneous sites. The 2-year relative survival rate is 49 % for first primary MCC of the mucosa compared with a 76 % relative survival rate for first primary MCC of the skin. Case reports for mucosal MCC describe high rates of local recurrence, regional and distant metastases, and even fulminating courses [37].

MCC is a therapeutic challenge because of its high rate of locoregional recurrence as well as its tendency to spread to distant sites. In-transit metastases for MCC are not uncommon (see Fig. 3.11). These in-transit metastases most commonly have the appearance of other similar cutaneous metastases and present as firm papules or nodules with or without epidermal change (see Fig. 3.12). Distantly metastatic MCC has been reported almost everywhere in the body, including but not limited to the retroperitoneum, pancreas, kidney, brain, and gastrointestional tract [38–44]. These distant metastases are typically found with imaging.

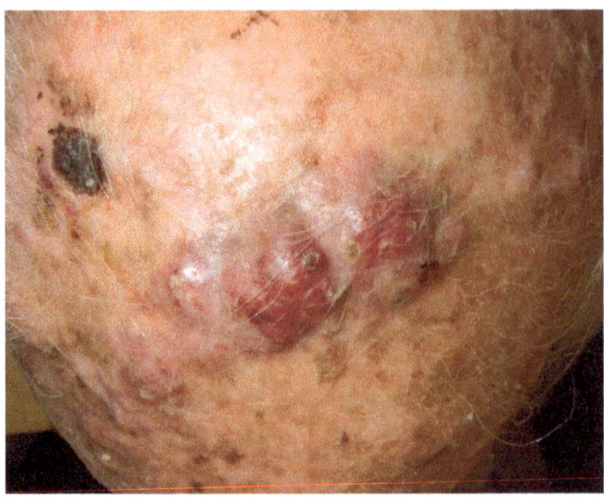

Fig. 3.12 This patient had a known history of renal cell carcinoma, and initial clinical suspicion of these firm nodules on the scalp was that of metastatic renal cell carcinoma. Biopsy, however, revealed Merkel cell carcinoma, presenting as in-transit disease. In-transit MCCs may mimic other cutaneous metastases

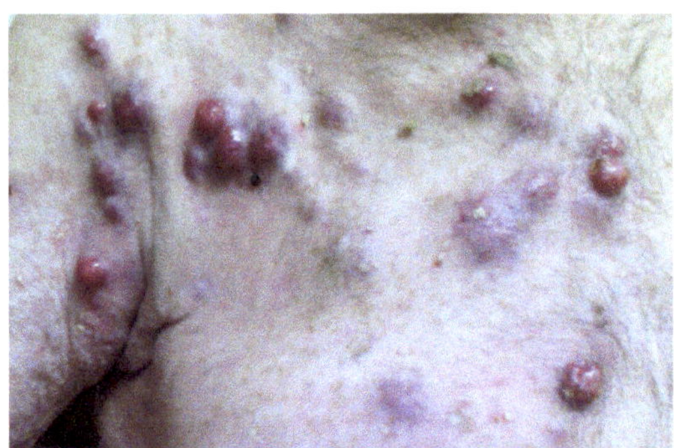

Fig. 3.13 This patient had numerous distantly metastatic cutaneous and visceral lesions at the time of initial diagnosis. Prognosis of such advanced disease is uniformly very poor

The most important prognostic feature is the stage of MCC at time of initial presentation. The extent of disease at the time of diagnosis varies widely. In the SEER database, 50 % of cases present with localized disease (stage I) and 50 % with disease that has spread beyond the local site (see Fig. 3.13). While patients presenting with cutaneous MCC distant from the primary site have been thought to have two separate primary

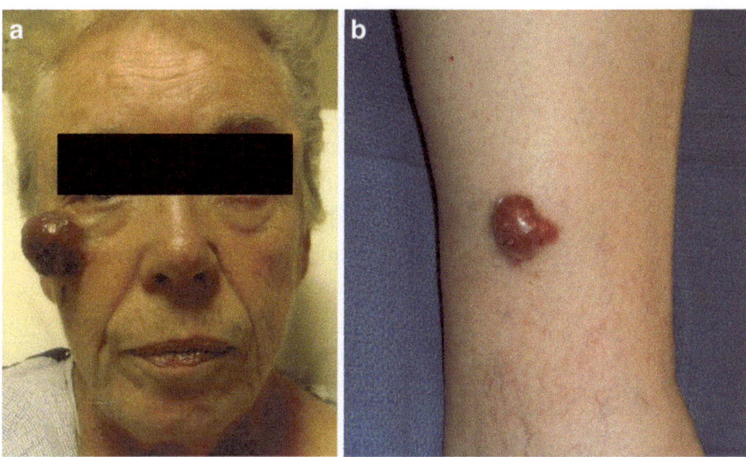

Fig. 3.14 (**a**) This patient had a primary Merkel cell carcinoma of her right cheek. (**b**) She subsequently developed a tumor on the contralateral lower leg that also proved to be MCC. Comparative genomic hybridization demonstrated this leg lesion to be a metastatic lesion, likely spread hematogenously from the cheek, rather than a second primary MCC of the leg

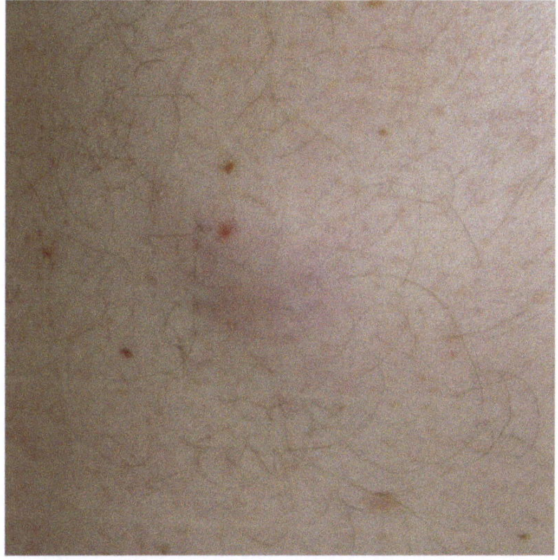

Fig. 3.15 This patient developed a firm, subcutaneous nodule initially thought to be a lipoma. Fine needle aspiration demonstrated Merkel cell carcinoma, confirmed on histopathologic evaluation of the excised specimen

MCCs, this notion has recently been challenged. A recent report used array comparative genomic hybridization to demonstrate hematogenous spread of a primary MCC to a distant cutaneous site (see Fig. 3.14) [45].

Subcutaneous primary tumor is an unusual presentation of MCC (see Fig. 3.15). Reports in the literature describe a subcutaneous nodule or mass with minimal to no overlying epidermal change as the initial presentation [46–50]. The sites of these nodules have varied from the cheek [46] to the arm [47] to the inguinal region 6 [48–50]. Interestingly, the groin is overrepresented as the site of these subcutaneous nodules in the few reported cases of subcutaneous presentation. Differential diagnoses for these nodules and masses have included lipoma, carcinoid, and cutaneous metastases until pathological examination rendered the diagnosis of MCC.

Another less common presentation of MCC is an enlarged lymph node without any findings of primary cutaneous disease [51–61] In one series, nodal MCC with an unknown primary was reported to be the initial presentation of 14 % of MCCs [17] (see Fig. 3.16). Of reported cases, the most common site of MCC presenting in the lymph node has been inguinal, though axillary [51, 53], submandibular [51, 52, 58], and retroperitoneal [59] sites have also been noted. The prognosis of these nodal presentations of MCC with unknown primary has been demonstrated to be better than those of primary cutaneous MCC with nodal metastasis [61]. The general prevailing viewpoint is that these nodal MCCs represent nodal metastasis from a regressed primary cutaneous MCC. An alternative theory is that these lymph nodal MCCs are primary sites of tumor formation [51], but given that Merkel cells have never been localized as primary cells of lymph

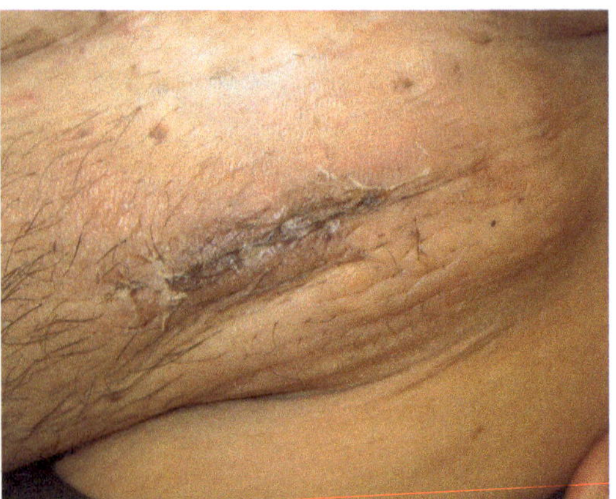

Fig. 3.16 A less common presentation of Merkel cell carcinoma is disease of the lymph nodes without an identifiable primary cutaneous tumor. This patient presented with enlarged inguinal lymph nodes. The photo shows postsurgical changes following an excisional biopsy, which revealed MCC

nodes, this theory is less favorable. As distinction from other poorly differentiated small cell or neuroendocrine tumors may be difficult, stringent pathologic techniques must be employed to diagnose MCC presenting in a lymph node without a known corresponding cutaneous lesion.

Additional Features

Patients with MCC often have an associated (i.e. preceding, concurrent or following the diagnosis of MCC) malignancy, especially cutaneous or lymphoproliferative disorders [62–65]. The tumor most commonly found in association with MCC is squamous cell carcinoma, which has been reported in approximately 40 % of cases [7, 66]. In the SEER registry, all cases of first primary cancers ($N=2{,}048{,}739$) were examined and found to have a statistically significant risk of developing MCC as a second primary cancer ($N=221$) and relatively quickly. Eighty nine percent of the second primary MCCs ($N=197$) developed within 1 year of the diagnosis of the first primary cancer [Howard]. The non-cutaneous cancers that correlated with a statistically significant increased risk of MCC as a second primary cancer were non-Hodgkin lymphoma ($N=16$), chronic lymphocytic leukemia ($N=14$), and multiple myeloma ($N=4$) [67].

Being diagnosed with MCC is also associated with an increased risk (estimated actuarial risk is 2.1 % per year of follow-up) of developing a second primary cancer based on data from the Israel Tumor Registry [68]. On average, the second primary tumor is found 3.6 years after the diagnosis of MCC.

Differential Diagnosis

The differential diagnosis of MCC is diverse. The most common presumed diagnosis for a Merkel cell carcinoma is a cyst (see Fig. 3.17) or acneiform lesion (see Fig. 3.18) in 32 % of cases [17]. The most common malignant differential diagnoses included nonmelanoma skin cancer (19 %) (see Figs. 3.19 and 3.20), lymphoma (6 %), metastatic carcinoma (2 %), and sarcoma (2 %). In a study reviewing the providers' clinical impression at the time of biopsy, clinicians misdiagnosed MCC as a benign lesion in 57 % of cases and correctly diagnosed it as a malignant lesion in 34 % of cases. In 8 % of cases, they felt it was indeterminate. Of those lesions thought to be malignant by the clinician, the most common clinical diagnosis was nonmelanoma skin cancer. Only 1 % of the time did the clinicians correctly suspect MCC as the correct diagnosis [17].

Clues for the clinician that might suggest MCC as a diagnosis should include patient's elderly age, location of the lesion in a sun-exposed location, lack of symptomatology of the lesion, rapid growth, and immunosuppression. In elderly patients, the threshold for biopsy should be lowered, particularly if the lesion is rapidly growing, even if it is not symptomatic. Clinicians should be alert for lesions arising in chronically sun-exposed regions. It is well known that immunosuppressed patients have a greatly increased incidence of cutaneous non-melanoma skin cancers such as basal cell and squamous cell

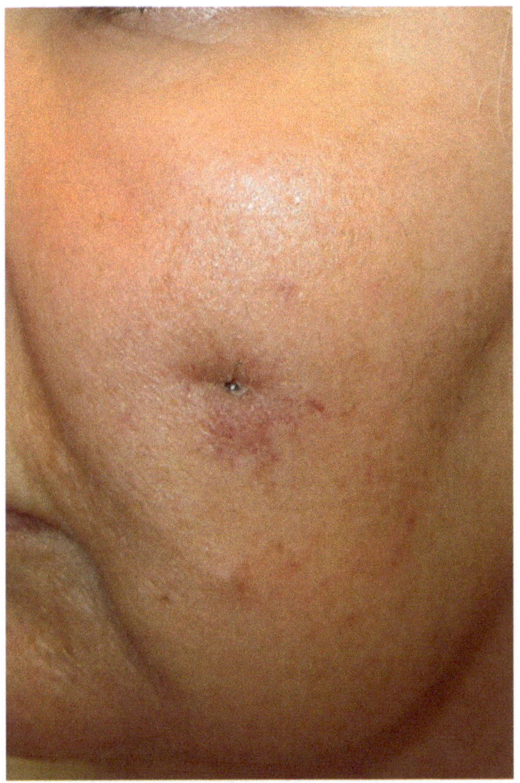

Fig. 3.17 This patient developed a tender, erythematous nodule on her cheek. The lesion was thought to be an infected cyst and treated with incision and drainage and systemic antibiotics. Due to persistence of the lesion, a biopsy was conducted, and Merkel cell carcinoma was diagnosed

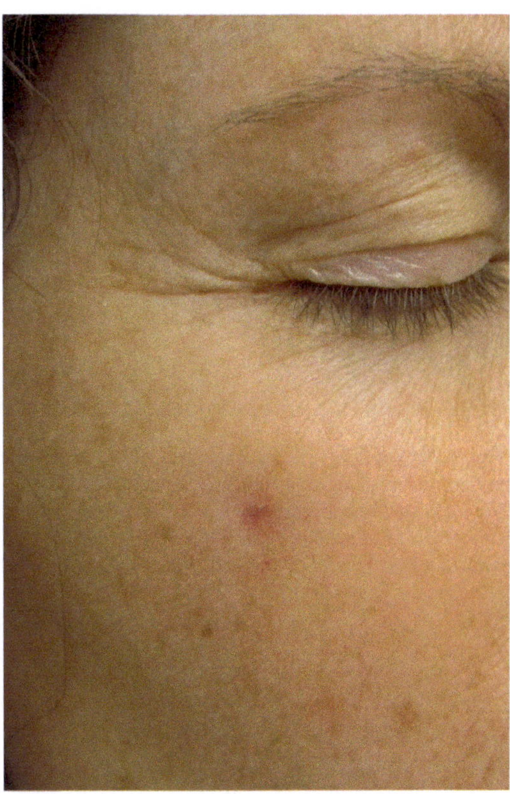

Fig. 3.18 The acneiform papule on the cheek of this woman was diagnosed as Merkel cell carcinoma following biopsy. Clinicians should be prompted to further evaluate any lesions that fail to resolve, even in those patients who are several decades younger than the average age of those diagnosed with MCC

carcinomas but clinicians should be thinking of MCC in the differential for any rapidly growing lesion on an immunosuppressed patient.

MCC may be distinguished from acneiform and cystic lesions by the fact that MCCs tend to enlarge rapidly and are most often asymptomatic. Acneiform and cystic lesions can enlarge rapidly when inflamed, however, inflamed acneiform and cystic lesions tend to be painful and symptomatic. Cysts are often characterized by the presence of a punctum as well as occasional expression of keratinocytic debris. Acneiform lesions often are comedonal and may also express keratinocytic debris. These are findings that would not be found in an MCC.

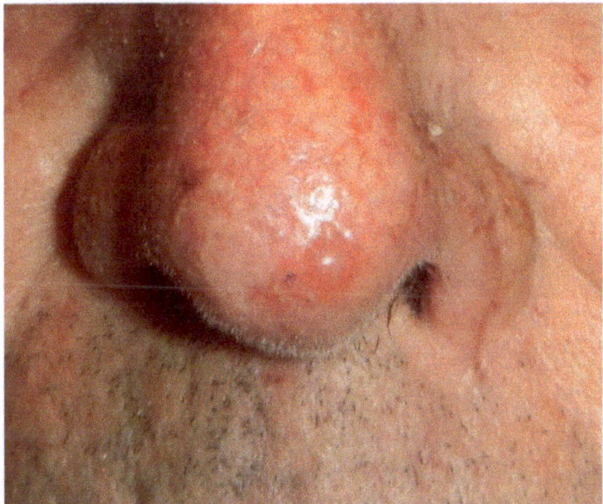

Fig. 3.19 The pearly nature of the Merkel cell carcinoma on the nasal tip mimics that of a basal cell carcinoma

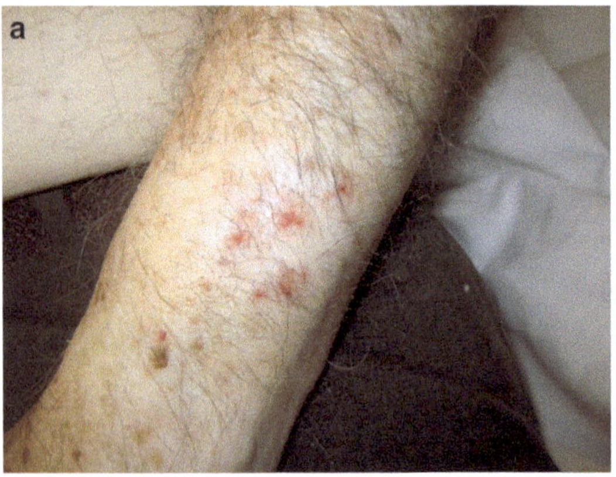

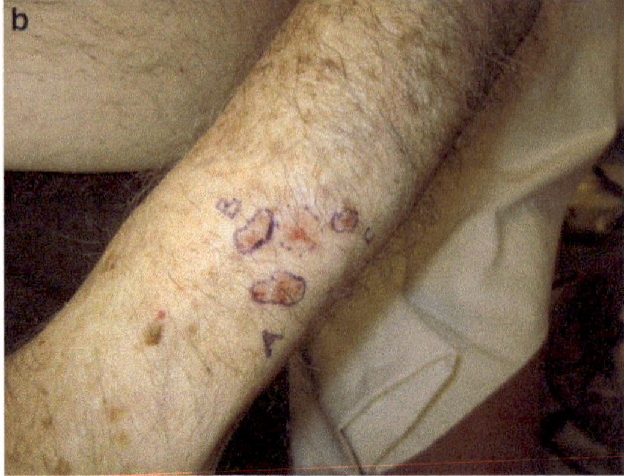

Fig. 3.20 (**a**) Merkel cell carcinomas may clinically mimic cutaneous squamous cell carcinoma. MCC has also been reported to arise in association with squamous cell carcinoma in situ. This patient presented with four ill-defined, erythematous papules of the forearm, which all appeared morphologically similar. The central lesion was biopsied first, revealing MCC. (**b**) Biopsies of lesions *A*, *B*, and *C* revealed squamous cell carcinoma in situ. The post-biopsy MCC is highlighted with *dotted* markings

Similarly, if the differential diagnosis was lipoma, lipomas are typically stable in size and do not grow rapidly. Lipomas are usually non-tender and asymptomatic unless they are angiolipomas, which can be painful. MCC would be differentiated by rapid growth from most typical lipomas. MCCs typically have some overlying red-violaceous hue, whereas lipomas are skin-colored as they are subcutaneous lesions that do not exhibit any epidermal change.

Non-melanoma skin cancers are typically slowly growing in immunocompetent patients in comparison with MCC. It would be unusual to find a basal cell carcinoma or squamous cell carcinoma that rapidly grew over a period of 1–3 months. The exception to this would be keratoacanthoma which is a rapidly growing subtype of squamous cell carcinoma with a typically crateriform appearance. MCCs tend to grow rapidly, but are typically not ulcerated and this would differentiate MCC from keratoacanthoma.

Lymphoma, sarcoma, and metastatic carcinoma are rapidly growing lesions which are dome-shaped and can show color variation from red to pink to blue to violaceous. They can be relatively asymptomatic. These are diagnoses that would require a biopsy to definitively diagnose and differentiate from MCC.

Diagnostic Tools Under Development

A unique polyomavirus, Merkel cell polyomavirus (MCV), has been isolated and described using digital transcriptome subtraction and two cDNA libraries generated from four MCC tissues [69]. This MCV appears to have a role in the pathogenesis of MCC. A member of the polyomavirus family, MCV is a small double-stranded DNA virus (between 40 and 50 nm in diameter). Other polyomaviruses (JC virus and BK virus) have demonstrated an ability to induce tumor formation [70–72]. Polyomaviruses replicate by encoding large and small T-antigens, nonstructural proteins which bind to the host cell proteins and lock the host cell into the S phase of DNA replication [73, 74]. Tumor suppressor proteins, p53 and pocket retinoblastoma (pRb), can be inactivated by the large T-antigen of polyomavirus [71].

One study demonstrated the presence of MCV in tissues obtained from 8 to 10 MCC patients (80 %) with monoclonal viral integration in 5 of these 10 tumors (50 %) [69]. In patients with primary and metastatic MCC tissues, the viral integration pattern was studied and it was found that the patterns were identical between the primary and metastatic lesions, indicating that MCV integrated prior to the metastasis of the tumor. Subsequent studies have demonstrated a range of MCV DNA in MCC tumors ranging from 40 to 100 % [75, 76]. Differences in methodology may account for this discrepancy in findings.

As MCV has only been recently described, much remains to be learned about its mode of transmission, natural life cycle, presence or absence of a latent phase, and tumor induction. Serological studies show a high prevalence of seropositivity with an increasing prevalence of MCV seropositivity with increasing age. By age 15, school children are 40–50 % likely to be seropositive for MCV. By the time patients reach 50 or above, 80 % of screened patients are seropositive for MCV [77]. The significance of this virus in MCC pathogenesis will have to be elucidated. Clinical diagnosis will be aided by a greater understanding of the role of MCV in the pathogenesis of MCC as clinicians will have a better understanding of which patients are most at risk and what risk factors may lead to the development of MCC.

Conclusions

MCC is a rare and potentially lethal neuroendocrine carcinoma whose pathogenesis remains unclear. It appears to have multifactorial contributing factors including advanced age, immunosuppression, ultraviolet exposure, and fair skin. This tumor presents a diagnostic challenge for clinicians as it does not have a typical or predictable morphologic appearance and often mimics a benign lesion. However, features such as rapid growth within 3 months concurrently with lack of symptomatology in a Caucasian patient over the age of 65 should alert clinicians to have a lower threshold to perform a skin biopsy. The suspicion should be even greater should the patient be immune suppressed.

Data regarding epidemiology of MCC and the presentation of MCC is obtained through culling large cancer registries, as the disease is exceedingly rare. With greater access to information and better diagnostic techniques, more data will become available to clinicians. Earlier diagnosis will lead to better prognosis for patients as this disease has a high rate of local and regional metastasis and has a higher mortality rate than melanoma.

References

1. Toker C. Trabecular carcinoma of the skin. Arch Dermatol. 1972;105:107–10.
2. Tang CK, Toker C. Trabecular carcinoma of the skin: an ultrastructural study. Cancer. 1978;42:2311–21.
3. Merkel F. Tastzellen and Taskoerperchen bei Den Hausthieren and bei Menschchen. Arch Mikrosk J Anat. 1875;11:636–52.
4. Halata Z, Grim M, Bauman KI. Friedrich Sigmund Merkel and his "Merkel cell", morphology, development, and physiology: a review and new results. Anat Rec A Discov Mol Cell Evol Biol. 2003;271:225–39.
5. Szeder V, Grim M, Halata Z, Sieber-Blum M. Neural crest origin of mammalian Merkel cells. Dev Biol. 2003;253:258–63.
6. Yoker SR. Merkel cell carcinoma. Adv Dermatol. 2003;19:185–205.
7. Hewitt JB, Sherif A, Kerr KM, Stankler L. Merkel cell and squamous cell carcinomas arising in erythema ab igne. Br J Dermatol. 1993;128:591–2.
8. Haag ML, Glass LF, Fense NA. Merkel cell carcinoma. Diagnosis and treatment. Dermatol Surg. 1995;21:669–83.
9. De Wolff-Peeters C, Marien K, Mebis J, Desmet V. A cutaneous APUDoma or Merkel cell tumor? A morphologically recognizable tumor with a biological and histological malignant aspect in contrast with its clinical behavior. Cancer. 1980;46:1810–6.
10. Agnelli M, Clegg LX. Epidemiology of primary Merkel cell carcinoma in the United States. J Am Acad Dermatol. 2003;49:832–41.
11. Hankey BF, Ries LA, Edwards BK. The surveillance, epidemiology, and end results program: a national resource. Cancer Epidemiol Biomarkers Prev. 1999;8: 117–21.
12. Hodgson NC. Merkel cell carcinoma: changing incidence trends. J Surg Oncol. 2005;89:1–4.
13. Albores-Saavedra J, Batich K, Chable-Montero F, Sagy N, Schwartz AM, Henson DE. Merkel cell carcinoma demographics, morphology, and survival based on 3870 cases: a population based study. J Cutan Pathol. 2010;37:20–7.
14. Moll R, Lowe A, Laufer J, Franke WW. Cytokeratin 20 in human carcinomas. A new histodiagnostic marker detected by monoclonal antibodies. Am J Pathol. 1992;140:427–47.

15. Lanoy E, Costagliola D, Engels EA. Skin cancers associated with HIV infection and solid-organ transplantation among elderly adults. Int J Cancer. 2010;126:1724–31.
16. Engels EA. Epidemiology of nonkeratinocytic skin cancers among persons with AIDS in the United States. AIDS. 2009;23:385–93.
17. Heath M, Jaimes N, Lemos B, Mostaghimi A, Wang LC, Penas PF, et al. Clinical characteristics of Merkel cell carcinoma at diagnosis in 195 patients: the AEIOU features. J Am Acad Dermatol. 2008;58:375–81.
18. Gooptu C, Woollons A, Ross J, Price M, Wojnarowska F, Morris PJ, et al. Merkel cell carcinoma arising after therapeutic immunosuppression. Br J Dermatol. 1997;137:637–41.
19. Lentz SR, Krewson L, Zutter MM. Recurrent neuroendocrine (Merkel cell) carcinoma of the skin presenting as marrow failure in a man with systemic lupus erythematosus. Med Pediatr Oncol. 1993;21: 137–41.
20. Nemoto I, Sato-Matsumura KC, Fujita Y, Natsuga K, Ujiie H, Tomita Y, et al. Leukaemic dissemination of Merkel cell carcinoma in a patient with systemic lupus erythematosus. Clin Exp Dermatol. 2008;33:270–2.
21. McCloone NM, McKenna K, Edgar D, Walsh M, Binham A. Merkel cell carcinoma in a patient with chronic sarcoidosis. Clin Exp Dermatol. 2005;30: 580–2.
22. Lillis J, Ceilley RI, Nelson P. Merkel cell carcinoma in a patient with autoimmune hepatitis. J Drugs Dermatol. 2005;4:357–9.
23. Satolli F, Venturi C, Vescovi V, Morrone P, De Panfilis G. Merkel cell carcinoma in Behcet's disease. Acta Derm Venereol. 2005;85:79.
24. Gianfreda M, Caiffi S, De Franceschi T, Dodero C, Durante R, Faletti P, et al. Merkel cell carcinoma of the skin in a patient with myasthenia gravis. Minerva Med. 2002;93:219–22.
25. Buell JF, Trofe J, Hanaway MJ, Beebe TM, Gross TG, Alloway RR, et al. Immunosuppression and Merkel cell carcinoma. Transplant Proc. 2002;34:1780–1.
26. Engels EA, Frisch M, Goedert JJ, Biggar RJ, Miller RW. Merkel cell carcinoma and HIV infection. Lancet. 2002;359:497–8.
27. Lardy F, Gautier C, Etesse-Pichon S, Martin JC, Demeaux H, Geniaux M, et al. [Post radiotherapy cutaneous neuro-endocrine carcinoma]. Ann Dermatol Venereol. 1996;123:464–7.
28. Tuneu A, Pujol RM, Moreno A, Barnadas MA, de Moragas JM. Postirradiation Merkel cell carcinoma. J Am Acad Dermatol. 1989;20:505–7.
29. Iacocca MV, Abernethy JL, Stefanato CM, Allan AE, Bhawan J. Mixed Merkel cell carcinoma and squamous cell carcinoma of the skin. J Am Acad Dermatol. 1998;39(5 Pt 2):882–7.
30. Jones CS, Tyring SK, Lee PC, Fine JD. Development of neuroendocrine (Merkel cell) carcinoma mixed with squamous cell carcinoma in erythema ab igne. Arch Dermatol. 1988;124:110–3.
31. Brash DE. Sunlight and the onset of skin cancer. Trends Genet. 1997;13:410–4.
32. Lunder EJ, Stern RS. Merkel cell carcinomas in patients treated with methoxsalen and ultraviolet A radiation. N Engl J Med. 1998;339:1247–8.
33. Gess AJ, Silkiss RZ. A Merkel cell carcinoma of the lactrimal gland. Ophthal Plast Reconstr Surg. 2012;28(1):e11–3.
34. Ghaderi M, Coury J, Oxenberg J, Spector H. Primary Merkel cell carcinoma of the parotid gland. Ear Nose Throat J. 2010;89:E24–7.
35. Iavazzo C, Terzi M, Arapantoni-Dadioti P, Dertimas V, Vorgias G. Vulvar merkel carcinoma: a case report. Case Rep Med. 2011;2011:546972.
36. Tomic S, Warner TF, Messing E, Wilding G. Penile Merkel cell carcinoma. Urology. 1995;45:1062–5.
37. Yom SS, Rosenthal DI, El Naggar AK, Kies MS, Hessel AC. Merkel cell carcinoma of the tongue and head and neck oral mucosal sites. Oral Surg Oral Med Oral Pathol Oral Radiol Endod. 2006;101:761–8.
38. Kim EJ, Kim HS, Kim HO, Jung CK, KO YH, Kim TH Park Ym. Merkel cell carcinoma of the inguinal lymph node with an unknown primary site. J Dermatol 2009;36:170–3.
39. Matkowskyj KA, Hosseini A, Linn JG, Yang GY, Kuzel TM, Wayne JD. Merkel cell carcinoma metastatic to the small bowel mesentery. Rare Tumors. 2011;3:e2.
40. Kirwan C, Carney D, O'Keefe M. Merkel cell carcinoma metastasis to the iris in a 23 year old female. Ir Med J. 2009;102:53–4.
41. Noto R, Giaquinta A, Alessandria I, Soma P, Latteri S, Grasso G, et al. Right leg swelling as primary presentation of metastatic Merkel cell carcinoma. Minerva Med. 2008;99(3):341–5.
42. Chang DT, Mancuso AA, Riggs Jr CE, Mendenhall WM. Merkel cell carcinoma of the skin with leptomeningeal metastases. Am J Otolaryngol. 2005;26: 210–3.
43. Dim DC, Nugent SL, Darwin P, Peng HQ. Metastatic merkel cell carcinoma of the pancreas mimicking primary pancreatic endocrine tumor diagnosed by endoscopic ultrasound-guided fine needle aspiration cytology: a case report. Acta Cytol. 2009;53:223–8.
44. Medhi S, Purandare NC, Dua SG, Gujral S. Bilateral renal metastases in a case of Merkel cell carcinoma. J Cancer Res Ther. 2010;6:353–5.
45. Ahronowitz IZ, Daud AI, Leong SP, Shue EH, Bastian BC, McCalmont TH, et al. An isolated Merkel cell metastasis at a distant cutaneous site presenting as a second 'primary' tumor. J Cutan Pathol. 2011;38:801–7.
46. Sarma DP, Heagley DE, Chalupa J, Cox M, Shehan JM. An unusual clinical presentation of Merkel cell carcinoma: a case report. Case Report Med. 2010; 905414.
47. Huang G, Chang W, Lee H, Taylor JAM, Cheng T, Chen C. Merkel cell carcinoma arising from the subcutaneous fat of the arm with intact skin. Dermatol Surg. 2005;31:717–9.
48. Balaton AJ, Capron F, Baviera EE, Meyrignac P, Vaury P, Vuong PN. Neuroendocrine carcinoma (Merkel cell tumor?) presenting as a subcutaneous tumor. An ultrastructural and immunohistochemical

study of three cases. Pathol Res Pract. 1989;184: 211–6.
49. Tsai YY, Hsiao CH, Chiu HC, Chen M, Tsai TF. CK7+/CK20- Merkel cell carcinoma presenting as inguinal subcutaneous nodules with subsequent epidermotropic metastasis. Acta Derm Venereol. 2010;90: 438–9.
50. Gambichler T, Kobus S, Kreuter A, Wieland U, Stücker M. Primary Merkel cell carcinoma clinically presenting as a deep oedematous mass of the groin. Eur J Med Res. 2010;15:274–6.
51. Eusebi V, Capellar C, Coss A, Rosai J. Neuroendocrine carcinoma within lymph nodes in the absence of a primary tumor, with special reference to Merkel cell carcinoma. Am J Surg Pathol. 1992;16:658–66.
52. Straka JA, Straka MB. A review of Merkel cell carcinoma with emphasis on lymph node disease in the absence of a primary site. Am J Otolaryngol. 1997;18: 55–65.
53. Ferrara G, Ianniello GP, Di Vizio D, Nappi O. Lymph node Merkel cell carcinoma with no evidence of cutaneous tumor—report of two cases. Tumori. 1997; 83:868–72.
54. Samarendra P, Berkovtiz L, Kumari S, Alexis R. Primary nodal neuroendocrine (Merkel cell) tumor in a patient with HIV infection. South Med J. 2000;93: 920–2.
55. Fotia G, Barni R, Bellan C, Neri A. Lymph nodal Merkel cell carcinoma: primary or metastatic disease? A clinical case. Tumori. 2002;88:424–6.
56. Silberstein E, Korets M, Cagnano E, Katchko L, Rosenberg L. Neuroendocrine (Merkel cell) carcinoma in regional lymph nodes without primary site. Isr Med Assoc J. 2003;5:450–1.
57. Kuwabara H, Mori H, Uda H, Takei K, Ishibashi Y, Takatani N. Nodal neuroendocrine (Merkel cell) carcinoma without an identifiable primary tumor. Acta Cytol. 2003;47:515–7.
58. Nazarian Y, Shalmon B, Horowitz Z, Bedrin L, Pfeffer MR, Talmi YP. Merkel cell carcinoma of unknown primary site. J Laryngol Otol. 2007;121e1.
59. Boghossian V, Owen ID, Nuli B, Xiao PQ. Neuroendocrine (Merkel cell) carcinoma of the retroperitoneum with no identifiable primary site. World J Surg Oncol. 2007;5:117.
60. Kim EJ, Kim HS, Kim HO, Jung CK, KO YH, Kim TH, et al. Merkel cell carcinoma of the inguinal lymph node with an unknown primary site. J Dermatol. 2009;36:170–3.
61. Tarantola TT, Vallow LA, Halyard MY, Weenig RH, Warschaw KE, Weaver AL, Roenigk RK, Brewer JD, Otley CC. Unknown primary Merkel cell carcinoma. 23 New cases and a Review. J Am Acad Dermatol. 2013;68(3):433–40.
62. Goessling W, McKee PH, Mayer RJ. Merkel cell carcinoma. J Clin Oncol. 2002;20:588–98.
63. Cohen Y, Amir G, Polliack A. Development and rapid dissemination of Merkel cell carcinomatosis following therapy with fludarabine and rituximab for relapsing follicular lymphoma. Eur J Haematol. 2002;68:117–9.
64. Silva EG, Mackay B, Goepfert H, Burgess MA, Fields RS. Endocrine carcinoma of the skin (Merkel cell carcinoma). Pathol Annu. 1984;19(Pt 2):1–30.
65. Ziprin P, Smith S, Salerno G, Rosin RD. Two cases of Merkel cell tumour arising in patients with chronic lymphocytic leukaemia. Br J Dermatol. 2000;142: 525–8.
66. Cerroni L, Kerl H. Primary cutaneous neuroendocrine (Merkel cell) carcinoma in association with squamous- and basal-cell carcinoma. Am J Dermatopathol. 1997; 19:610–3.
67. Howard RA, Dores GM, Curtis RE, Anderson WF, Travis LB. Merkel cell carcinoma and multiple primary cancers. Cancer Epidemiol Biomarkers Prev. 2006;15:1545–9.
68. Brenner B, Sulkes A, Rakowsky E, Feinmesser M, Yukelson A, Bar-Haim E, et al. Second neoplasms in patients with Merkel cell carcinoma. Cancer. 2001;91: 1358–62.
69. Feng H, Shuda M, Chang Y, Moore PS. Clonal integration of a polyomavirus in human Merkel cell carcinoma. Science. 2008;319:1096–100.
70. Major EO, Mourrain P, Cummins C. JC virus-induced owl monkey glioblastoma cells in culture: biological properties associated with viral early gene product. Virology. 1984;136:359–67.
71. Shah KV, Daniel RW, Strandberg JD. Sarcoma in a hamster inoculated with BK virus, a human papovavirus. J Natl Cancer Inst. 1975;54:945–50.
72. Zur HH. Novel human polyomaviruses-re-emergence of a well known virus family as possible human carcinogens. Int J Cancer. 2008;123:247–50.
73. Caracciolo V, Reiss K, Khalili K, De Falco G, Giordano A. Role of the interaction between large T antigen and Rb family members in the oncogenicity of JC virus. Oncogene. 2006;25:5294–301.
74. Moens U, Van Ghelue M, Johannessen M. Oncogenic potentials of the human polyomavirus regulatory proteins. Cell Mol Life Sci. 2007;64:1656–78.
75. Sastre-Garau X, Peter M, Avril MF, Laude H, Couturier J, Rozenberg F, et al. Merkel cell carcinoma of the skin: pathological and molecular evidence of a causative role of MCV in oncogenesis. J Pathol. 2009;218:48–56.
76. Wetzels CT, Hoefnagel JG, Bakkers JM, Dijkman HB, Blokx WA, Melchers WJ. Ultrastructural proof of polyomavirus in Merkel cell carcinoma tumour cells and its absence in small cell carcinoma of the lung. PLoS One. 2009;4:4958.
77. Kean JM, Rao S, Wang M, Garcea RL. Seroepidemiology of human polyomaviruses. PLoS Pathog. 2009;5:e1000363.
78. Allen PJ, Bowne WB, Jaques DP, Brennan MF, Busam K, Coit DG. Merkel cell carcinoma: prognosis and treatment of patients from a single institution. J Clin Oncol. 2005;23:2300–9.

4 Staging

Sherrif F. Ibrahim and Siegrid S. Yu

Introduction

The American Joint Committee on Cancer (AJCC) defines staging as *the process of determining how much cancer there is in the body and where it is located* [1].

The philosophy of cancer classification and staging draws from the premise that cancers of the same anatomic site and histology share similar patterns of growth and clinical outcomes. The staging of various human malignancies is of critical importance for several reasons. Tumor staging can be a clinically useful tool for therapeutic decision-making, estimation of prognosis, and evaluation of treatment results. Standardized staging is also critical as a means of communication and collaborative scientific investigation.

Accurate staging provides the practitioner with the best road map for treatment. If certain workups or therapies have been shown to be more beneficial for certain stages, then consistent staging allows a physician to make optimal management decisions that are rooted in the collective experiences of similar cases around the world. Stage at presentation often provides the best prognostic factor for survival, determines course of treatment, and allows for consistent and systematic reporting of data, as it is a standardized means by which to describe the extent of involvement and severity of a given cancer. When a patient is newly diagnosed with cancer, his or her first response is commonly, "how long do I have?" Without accurate staging, this question becomes impossible to answer. Consensus staging methods allow the practitioner to reply with a response based upon the best available knowledge, which is determined from the collective reported literature and expected course of a given type of cancer.

Furthermore, a uniform and reproducible staging system provides practitioners with a common language by which to discuss specific details of a given patient's tumor both with the patient and with other health care professionals. In the case of Merkel cell carcinoma (MCC) and other rare tumors, cases are so few in number that studies in the literature tend to be retrospective in nature. Without a comprehensive, uniformly adopted staging system based upon factors that provide proven useful prognostic information, evaluations that compare various studies and meta-analyses that group data from multiple studies are difficult, if not impossible. The evolution of MCC staging is outlined below.

S.F. Ibrahim (✉)
Department of Dermatology, University of Rochester Medical Center, 400 Red Creek Drive, Suite 200, Rochester, NY 14623, USA
e-mail: sherrif_ibrahm@urmc.rochester.edu

S.S. Yu
Department of Clinical Dermatology, UCSF Dermatologic Surgery & Laser Center, 1701 Divisadero Street, Third Floor, San Francisco, CA 94115-0316, USA
e-mail: YuS@derm.ucsf.edu

M. Alam et al. (eds.), *Merkel Cell Carcinoma*, DOI 10.1007/978-1-4614-6608-6_4,

Staging of Merkel Cell Carcinoma

To date, six staging systems for MCC have been published, the first in 1991 and the most recent in 2010 (Table 4.1) [2–7]. Four of the first five staging systems were based on data from 1 to 3 institutions and from 70 to 251 patients. One system published by the AJCC in 2006 was based upon no MCC-specific data and included information from 82 other types of non-melanoma skin cancer [3]. As these systems were conflicting with one another, the goals of staging, such as prognosis assessment, communication with other health care professionals, and scientific study of MCC, were impossible to achieve. For example, disparities among the prior systems included: three-tier vs. four-tier systems, either stage II or stage III defining regional nodal disease, and varying primary tumor sizes for determining the tumor (T) categories. "Stage III MCC" could refer to invasive local disease, regional nodal disease, or distant metastatic disease depending on which staging system was used. The most recent staging system, reported by Lemos and colleagues, is the first consensus system and is by far the most comprehensive, incorporating data from almost 6,000 patients from institutions around the United States [7]. Collectively, the various staging systems for MCC have evolved over the past 20 years and were largely predicated on patient and disease characteristics shown by epidemiological analyses to be predictive of patient outcomes and overall survival. As the incidence of MCC continues to increase, there has been heightened awareness, improved diagnostic approaches, and more intensive efforts to better record these cases globally. This is reflected in the progression of staging systems outlined below.

Yiengpruksawan et al. 1991

Yiengpruksawan and colleagues were the first to report a staging system for use in the workup and management of MCC [2]. This data was based on the retrospective study of 70 patients treated at Memorial Sloan-Kettering Cancer Center between 1969 and 1989, with a median follow-up of 28 months. Sixty-six of the 70

Table 4.1 Summary of reported staging systems for Merkel cell carcinoma

Staging system	Subjects	Stage I	Stage II	Stage III	Stage IV
Yiengpruksawan et al. [2]	70, single institution	Local	Regional nodal	Distant metastatic	–
Allen et al. [4]	190, single institution	IA: local <2 cm IB: local ≥2 cm	Regional nodal	Distant metastatic	–
AJCC sixth edition [3]	No specific data used	Local ≤2 cm	Local >2 cm	Regional nodal or local with deep invasion	Distant metastatic
Allen et al. [5]	251, single institution	Local <2 cm	Local ≥2 cm	Regional nodal	Distant metastatic
Clark et al. [6]	110, three institutions	Local ≤1 cm	IIA: local ≤1 cm with ≤2 positive regional nodes IIB: local ≥2 cm	More than two positive regional nodes	Distant metastatic
Lemos et al. [7]	5,823, nationwide	IA: local, histologically node negative IB: local, clinically node negative	IIA: local >2 cm, histologically node negative IIB: local >2 cm, clinically node negative IIC: deeply invasive tumors	IIIA: any tumor with nodal micrometastases IIIB: any tumor with macrometastases or in-transit metastases	Distant metastatic

patients were recorded between 1980 and 1989. The authors proposed a three-tiered clinical system based on local (stage I), regional (stage II), or distant metastatic (stage III) disease at time of presentation. Stage I patients were shown to have an improved 5-year survival rate over stage II (64 % vs. 47 %, $P=0.04$), and tumors occurring on the head and neck had an improved survival compared with non-head and neck sites (91 % vs. 48 %, $P=0.02$). When tumors were stratified by anatomic location (head/neck, buttock/trunk, extremities), stage at presentation was a significant predictor of survival for the head/neck and buttock/trunk cohorts, but not for MCC of the extremities ($P<0.01$). Sex, age, tumor size (≤2 vs. >2 cm), local recurrence, surgical margin, and proximity of the tumor to the draining lymph node basin for MCC located on an extremity were not shown to affect outcome or course. While this report was the first to propose a staging system for MCC, there were several limitations. A three-tiered system was incongruent with the common four-tiered systems used by the AJCC, by which stage I and II define low- and high-risk local disease, respectively, stage III typically refers to local metastatic disease and stage IV is reserved for distant metastatic disease. Furthermore, because staging was based upon clinical examination alone, (i.e., no imaging was used), there was no inclusion of stage III patients, as no evidence of distant metastatic disease was found upon initial presentation of any of the subjects, thus no conclusions could be determined for the subset of patients who might present with advanced disease. Lastly, it drew data from a relatively small number of subjects from a single institution, thus potentially including selection biases and incorporating information not consistent among all cases of MCC.

Allen et al. 1999

The Yiengpruksawan staging system served as a foundation for the second MCC staging system, which differed from the first by incorporating more detailed information regarding tumor size. Specifically, the authors reported that stratification by primary tumor size more accurately predicted survival in patients presenting with local disease [4]. Also accrued from data collected retrospectively from Memorial Sloan-Kettering Cancer Center, this report studied patients diagnosed with MCC between 1969 and 1996. Of the 109 patients, adequate follow-up data was available for 102 (94 %) with a median follow-up time of 35 months. Fifty-three percent were treated during the last 6 years of the study period, and all but 6 (94 %) since 1980. Interestingly, at the time of publication, the authors noted only 425 cases of MCC reported in the literature since 1972.

By multivariate analysis, the only independent predictor of survival was disease stage at time of presentation ($P\leq0.0001$). When multivariate analysis was stratified by stage, the only independent predictor of survival in patients who presented with local disease was size of the primary lesion ($P=0.04$). Patients with local disease who had tumors ≥2 cm in diameter had survival rates similar to patients with regional disease ($P=0.48$). By univariate analysis, location on the head and neck was associated with a significantly improved survival, but only when tumors were <2 cm ($P=0.03$). Tumors located on the head and neck were statistically smaller at presentation than tumors located elsewhere. Given the apparent significance of primary tumor size in patients with local disease, tumors were therefore staged according to status at initial presentation in a similar three-tiered fashion as previously reported; however, those patients with local (stage I) disease were further subclassified based on primary tumor size. Stage I patients with tumors <2 cm in maximum diameter were subcategorized as stage IA and those patients with tumors ≥2 cm as stage IB. Primary tumor size did not impact predictive value for patients with regional or distantly metastatic disease When size was removed from the multivariate analysis and incorporated into a staging system (stage IA/IB), then stage at time of presentation was highly significant in predicting disease-specific and relapse-free survival ($P=0.008$). Seventy-six percent of patients initially presented with stage I disease, and overall survival for these patients was 81 %. With respect to nodal disease, elective lymph node dissection (ELND) was an independent predictor of relapse-free survival, and none of the patients who underwent ELND died of disease. However, this was a limited number of patients with local disease, which carries a favorable prognosis. This relapse-free survival did not translate into an overall survival advantage.

This staging system was an improvement over the previous system in that it called attention to the importance of primary tumor size in the stratification of survival statistics. As it was drawn from data prior to the wide use of sentinel lymph node biopsy (SLNB), data relating to pathologic nodal staging was briefly mentioned, but did not carry sufficient statistical power to lead to an overall survival advantage. Despite the observation that primary tumor size should be incorporated into staging, the authors chose to subdivide stage I disease into stage IA and IB as opposed to expansion to a four-tiered system, which would be more consistent with staging systems for other human malignancies.

American Joint Commission on Cancer (AJCC)

The AJCC sixth edition published in 2002 listed MCC along with over 80 other types of non-melanoma skin cancer in a single staging system referred to as "Carcinoma of the Skin" [3]. Included among these cancers are both squamous cell carcinoma and basal carcinoma. With over 2,000,000 cases of non-melanoma skin cancers being treated annually in the United States [8], the use of a single staging system incorporating tumors with an enormously diverse range of biological behaviors and clinical prognoses was of minimal utility. To maintain consistency with other staging systems, the proposed AJCC guidelines moved skin cancer staging to a four-tiered system. Both stage I and stage II included patients with local disease, with those patients having tumors >2 cm being categorized as stage II. A patient was classified as having stage III disease if the primary tumor extended beyond the dermis into underlying tissue OR if regional nodal disease was present. Stage IV referred to patients with distant metastases.

While the transition to a four-tiered staging system was an attempt to gain consistency among established staging systems for other malignancies, grouping of MCC with other, much more common and less aggressive non-melanoma skin cancers was quickly determined to not reflect the seriousness of MCC and provided little useable staging information. These concerns were addressed in a subsequent AJCC staging system, which removed MCC from staging of other non-melanoma skin cancer and has provided independent staging and treatment guidelines based upon the study of Lemos et al., discussed below [9].

Allen et al. 2005

In 2005, the group from Memorial Sloan-Kettering proposed a fourth staging system, also based on retrospective data accumulated from their institution, this time with 251 patients treated between 1970 and 2002 [5]. The series of reports from this single institution reflects the investigators' dedication to the study of this disease, the increased incidence of MCC, and better efforts to accumulate and analyze data, as 65 % of the patients in the most recent report were treated in the last 7 years of the study. The staging system in the 2005 report was developed to incorporate data from previous studies, again reflecting that size was of prognostic value for localized disease as well as to maintain consistency with the most recent AJCC staging system for skin and other cancers that was available at the time [3]; stage I and II represent low- and high-risk local disease, respectively, stage III regional metastatic disease, and stage IV is reserved for distant metastatic disease. The result is a four-tiered MCC system that separates local disease based on low- and high-risk primary tumors, with tumors <2 cm categorized as stage I, and tumors ≥2 cm categorized as stage II tumors. Stage III disease refers to regional nodal involvement, and stage IV is when distant metastases are present. The overall 5-year disease-specific survival in this study was 64 %, and the stage at presentation was the only patient, tumor, or treatment-related factor shown to predict survival. The authors further subdivided those patients with localized disease into those who were clinically node negative and those were shown to be pathologically node negative either by SLNB or ELND, and found that those patients who were confirmed to be pathologically node negative had a 5-year survival rate of 97 % while those patients who were noted to be node negative based on clinical exam alone had a lowered 75 % survival ($P=0.009$). Those patients that were clinically negative for nodal disease but subsequently shown to be pathologically node positive had a 5-year survival rate of 62 %. Furthermore, those patients who had only a single positive lymph node were shown to have a 5-year survival rate of 65 %, while those patients who had more than four proven nodes with disease involvement had only a 30 % 5-year survival rate ($P<0.001$), indicating that not only did the presence or absence of nodal disease affect stage-specific outcomes but that the extent of nodal disease burden was also of prognostic value. Although pathologic nodal staging was not incorporated in their staging system, the authors did recommend that all patients diagnosed with MCC undergo SLNB, as approximately 25 % of the patients included in the study with clinically negative lymph nodes, were shown to have nodal involvement by histologic evaluation. Numerous additional authors have confirmed this relatively high rate of SLNB positivity at time of disease presentation [10, 11]. Thus, by moving patients after pathologic evaluation from stage I or II (node negative) to stage III (node positive), staging was more accurate and survival for both stages improved. The authors stressed the importance of pathologic nodal staging, as they felt it provided a more accurate estimate of stage-specific survival and identifies a subgroup of patients with excellent long-term survival. In their study, those patients who had negative nodes confirmed histologically had a nodal recurrence rate of 11 %, while those that were shown to be only clinically node negative had a nodal recurrence rate of 44 %.

This report by Allen and colleagues was seminal in many ways. It was among the first papers to draw direct attention to the need for consistent staging across different institutions, particularly when comparing survival rates. The timing of the study was also important, as it was published after SLNB and immunohistochemistry techniques had been validated for cancers such as melanoma and breast cancer; thus pathologic assessment of nodal status could be achieved with greatly reduced morbidity to the patient. With increased sensitivity for detecting even microscopic nodal disease, a population of low-risk patients with excellent prognosis was identified. This staging system is widely used in reports today and served as a foundation for the development of downstream staging methods.

Clark et al. 2007

In 2007, Clark and colleagues retrospectively studied 110 patients diagnosed with MCC of the head and neck from three tertiary care hospitals in Australia and Canada, with a specific goal of determining if adjuvant radiation therapy improved survival [6]. The secondary aim of the study was to determine by stage which patients might derive greater benefit from combined surgery and radiation and to identify independent predictors for survival based on multivariate regression analyses. This report used two staging systems, the system proposed by Allen et al. [5], and the second, revised system that took into account primary tumor size, number of positive regional lymph nodes, and distant metastases in a TNM (Tumor, Node, Metastases) staging system similar to that used for other malignancies [12, 13]. In this revised system, stage I disease is defined as tumors ≤1 cm without nodal involvement; stage IIA as small tumors with ≤2 positive regional lymph nodes; stage IIB as large tumors (>1 cm) without lymph node involvement; stage III disease as any sized tumor with greater than two positive regional nodes; and stage IV as any patient with metastatic involvement. By categorizing patients in both staging systems, they were able to perform a direct comparison and remark on the differences between the two. By their analyses, both staging systems were able to significantly predict overall and disease-specific survival ($P<0.0001$ for both systems). They

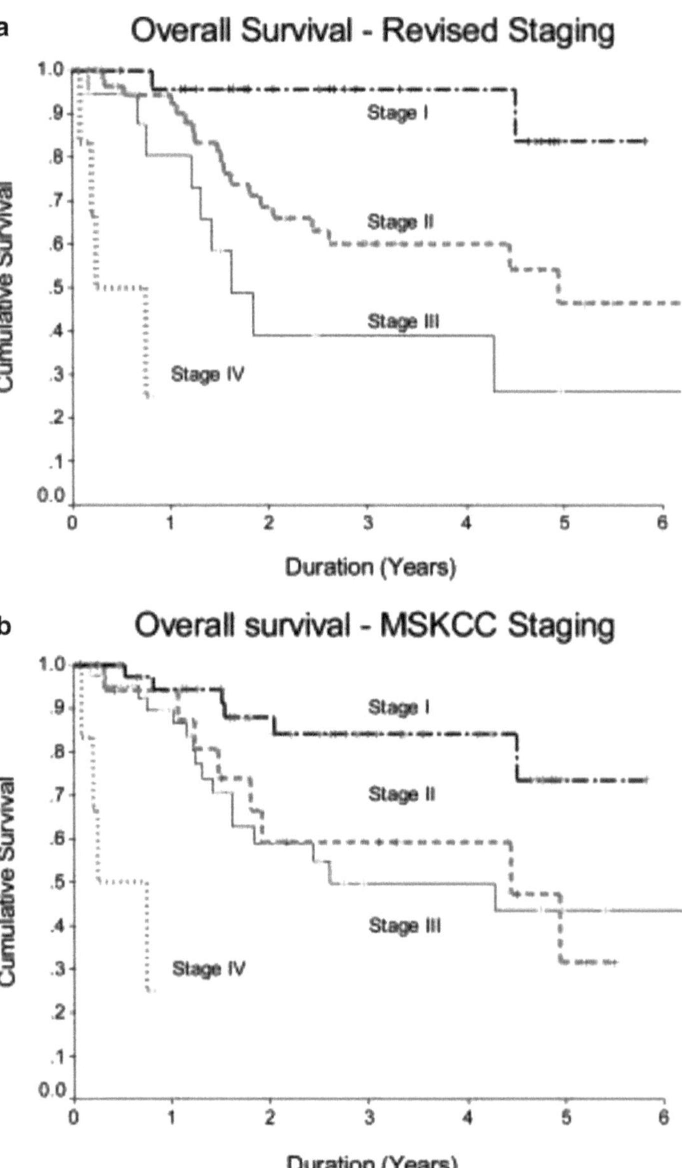

Fig. 4.1 The revised staging system was superior to the Memorial Sloan-Kettering Cancer Center (MSKCC) staging in terms of stratification of survival by stage [Reprinted from Clark, J.R., Veness, M.J., Gilbert, R., O'Brien, C.J. & Gullane, P.J. Merkel cell carcinoma of the head and neck: is adjuvant radiotherapy necessary? Head Neck 2007; 29: 249–257. With permission from John Wiley & Sons, Inc.]

concluded that the revised system was superior in stratifying cumulative survival based on stage, as the Allen et al. system clustered stage II and stage III patients (Fig. 4.1). Furthermore, the authors commented that they were better able to identify a cohort at very low risk of dying from MCC.

With regard to treatment, analyses were unable to show an overall disease-specific survival for patients treated with combined modalities than those treated with a single therapeutic modality. To determine if a subset of patients derived maximal benefit from combination treatment, disease-specific survival was stratified according to stage, and only stage II patients in both staging systems had a significant difference in survival ($P=0.015$ for the Allen et al. system, $P=0.002$ for the revised system), implying that patients with advanced local disease fared better with combination therapy as compared to those with nodal involvement. This was particularly true for those patients who presented as stage IIB (advanced local disease, no evidence of nodal involvement). On multivariate analysis, age >70 years, tumor size >1 cm, and the number of nodal metastases were all shown to significantly impact overall and disease-specific survival. When size and metastases were replaced with tumor stage on regression analysis, stage was the most powerful predictor of survival.

This report was critical in the development of MCC staging in several ways. It was the first report to directly include pathologic nodal involvement in staging, a concept that was drawn from the previous staging system and one that is included as a main feature in subsequent systems. Secondly, the authors sought not only to better stratify patients as to survival rates but also identified subsets of patients that might benefit from specific therapeutic intervention. In this staging system, those patients who are classified as stage II derived a significant survival advantage from adjuvant radiation therapy, with stage IIB patients having the greatest benefit. Therefore patients that may have been previously categorized as having low-risk tumors, who may have not been referred for adjuvant radiation therapy, may indeed benefit most from this intervention. Because there were relatively few patients who presented with stage III disease, the authors recommend combination therapy for all stage II and III patients, while suggesting a "watch-and-wait" approach for those patients who present with stage I disease who are shown to be pathologically node negative. Thus, dedicated efforts were made to better define treatment recommendations for patients based upon disease parameters with the goals of defining standard treatment approaches.

American Joint Commission on Cancer (AJCC) 2010

The AJCC recognized the unique characteristics of MCC and the need to create a separate staging system specific for this tumor. The authors of the most recent MCC staging system, published by Lemos and colleagues in 2010 [7], created the first consensus staging system, specifically developed from the best available data to address the disparities in the existing staging systems for the disease. Important information about the behavior and prognosis of MCC is presented in the previous reports and components of these prior staging systems are incorporated in subsequent staging methodologies. Most notably, primary tumor size clearly surfaced as an important prognostic factor in the estimation of various survival statistics and remained incorporated into all subsequent staging systems since its first use. Allen et al. [5] drew attention to the use of SLNB and made an early recommendation that pathologic nodal evaluation should be considered in all MCC patients. As the use of the SLNB technique gained more widespread use, numerous large studies have shown that nearly one in three patients have microscopic nodal disease despite having no clinical evidence of regional disease [5, 10, 11, 14, 15]. Building on these reports, the central contribution of this new staging system is the review of how nodal status is determined and inclusion of this into staging. The authors discuss pathologic vs. clinical nodal staging, and furthermore, when nodal disease is present, whether it is macroscopic or microscopic only. Additionally, deeply invasive primary tumors have separate category, as does in-transit disease. While previous systems were derived from 251 or fewer cases and from 3 or fewer institutions, this system was based on data from the National Cancer Data Base (NCDB), a national tumor registry maintained by the Commission on Cancer, and included 10,020 patients with MCC from 1986 to 2004 as well as from meetings of an MCC multidisciplinary board that included many of the authors from previous studies. Of the subjects drawn from the NCDB, only those patients with 5-year follow-up data (5,823 patients) were included in the study with a median follow-up time of 64.1 months for patients who were alive at time of analysis. Because the NCDB does not record disease-specific survival, all calculations are based on relative survival. Like its most recent predecessor, the consensus system was designed along the TNM staging systems well known in oncology, but resulted from data from more than ten times as many patients than in prior staging systems for MCC (Table 4.2). While it is similar

Table 4.2 TNM criteria and stage groupings of new American Joint Committee on Cancer staging system for Merkel cell carcinoma

T	N	M	
Tx, primary tumor cannot be assessed	Nx, regional nodes cannot be assessed N0, no regional node metastasis[a]	Mx, distant metastasis cannot be assessed	
T0, no primary tumor	cN0, nodes not clinically detectable[a]	M0, no distant metastasis	
Tis, in situ primary tumor	cN1, nodes clinically detectable[a]	M1, distant metastasis[b]	
T1, primary tumor ≤2 cm T2, primary tumor >2 but ≤5 cm	pN0, nodes negative by pathologic examination	M1a, distant skin, distant subcutaneous tissues, or distant lymph nodes	
T3, primary tumor >5 cm	pNx, nodes not examined pathologically	distant lymph nodes	
T4, primary tumor invades bone, muscle, fascia, or cartilage	N1a, micrometastasis[c] N1b, macrometastasis[d] N2, in-transit metastasis[e]	M1b, lung M1c, all other visceral sites	
Stage		Stage grouping	
0	Tis	N0	M0
IA	T1	pN0	M0
IB	T1	cN0	M0
IIA	T2/T3	pN0	M0
IIB	T2/T3	cN0	M0
IIC	T4	N0	M0
IIIA	Any T	N1a	M0
IIIB	Any T	N1b/N2	M0
IV	Any T	Any N	M1

[a]"N0" denotes negative nodes by clinical, pathologic, or both types of examination. Clinical detection of nodal disease may be via inspection, palpation, and/or imaging; cN0 is used only for patients who did not undergo pathologic node staging

[b]Because there are no data to suggest significant effect of M categories on survival in Merkel cell carcinoma, M1a–c are included in same stage grouping

[c]Micrometastases are diagnosed after sentinel or elective lymphadenectomy

[d]Macrometastases are defined as clinically detectable nodal metastases confirmed pathologically by biopsy or therapeutic lymphadenectomy

[e]In-transit metastasis is tumor distinct from primary lesion and located either: (1) between primary lesion and draining regional lymph nodes; or (2) distal to primary lesion

to that of Clark and colleagues by stratifying patients into four main tiers (I and II for local disease, III for nodal disease, IV for distant metastatic disease), this system subdivides local disease stages into "A" and "B" groups based on the method of nodal evaluation. For local disease, those patients who are shown clinically to be node negative are designated as the less favorable "B" subgroup (i.e., IB or IIB), while those that are shown to be node negative by pathologic examination are designated as the "A" subgroup (i.e., IA or IIB). These substages were created based on the differences in 5-year survival if a patient was shown to be node negative by pathologic staging (76 %) or by clinical staging (59 %) (Fig. 4.2). Stage II disease is further divided into a "C" subgroup in the case of node-negative disease with a tumor that invades bone, muscle,

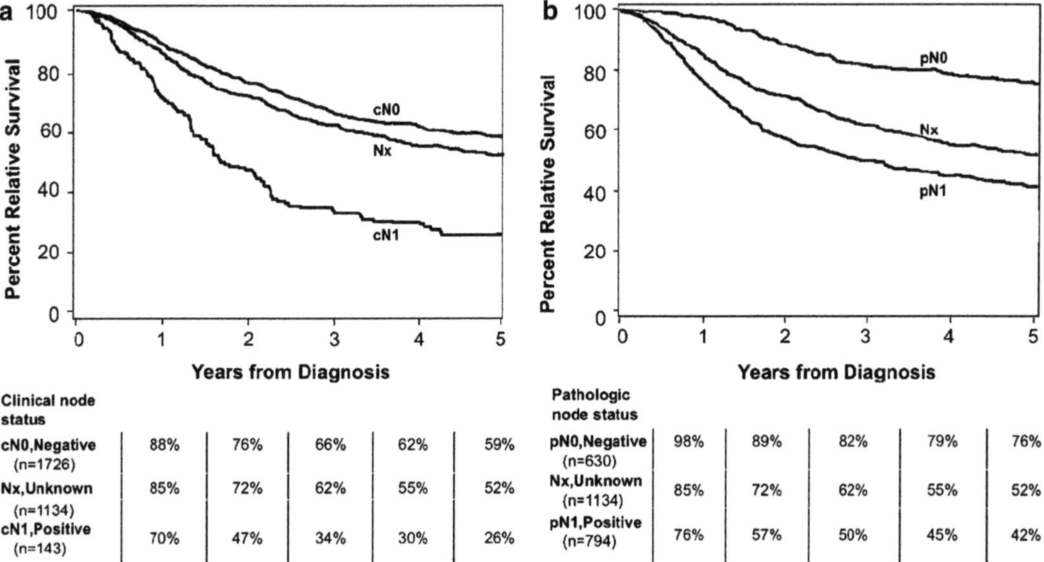

Clinical node status					
cN0,Negative (n=1726)	88%	76%	66%	62%	59%
Nx,Unknown (n=1134)	85%	72%	62%	55%	52%
cN1,Positive (n=143)	70%	47%	34%	30%	26%

Pathologic node status					
pN0,Negative (n=630)	98%	89%	82%	79%	76%
Nx,Unknown (n=1134)	85%	72%	62%	55%	52%
pN1,Positive (n=794)	76%	57%	50%	45%	42%

Fig. 4.2 Relative survival by nodal status: clinical vs. pathologic evaluation. Age- and sex-adjusted percent relative survival curves are shown for all patients with Merkel cell carcinoma who had follow-up data and did not have distant metastatic disease ($n=4{,}427$). Patients for whom no regional nodal data were available (1,134 cases) are represented by same curve (Nx). Pathologic node-negative status (pN0) was established either by elective lymphadenectomy or by sentinel lymph node biopsy (SLNB). Pathologic node-positive status (pN1) was established by elective or therapeutic lymphadenectomy, fine needle aspirate, SLNB, or other biopsy technique. Age- and sex-adjusted excess hazard ratio comparing clinical node-negative with pathologic node-negative (*top lines*) is 1.80 (95 % confidence interval 1.4–2.4; $P<0.0001$). The age- and sex-adjusted excess hazard ratio comparing clinical node positive with pathologic node positive (*bottom lines*) is 1.48 (95 % confidence interval 1.1–1.9; $P=0.004$). There was very little overlap in data in this cohort for method of nodal evaluation because patients had only clinical or pathologic nodal data recorded in majority of cases. Specifically, 240 (5 %) of 4,427 cases included in this analysis had both pathologic and clinical nodal data recorded. These cases are included in pathologic category (**b**) and excluded from clinical nodal analysis (**a**) because pathologic data were considered to be more accurate [Reprinted from Lemos, B.D. et al. Pathologic nodal evaluation improves prognostic accuracy in Merkel cell carcinoma: analysis of 5823 cases as the basis of the first consensus staging system. J. Am. Acad. Dermatol 2010; 63:751–761. With permission from Elsevier]

fascia, or cartilage. Stage III disease refers to node-positive disease, with stage IIIA reserved for micrometastatic involvement (diagnosed histologically after SLNB or nodal dissection), and stage IIIB referring to macrometastases (clinically detectable lymph node involvement confirmed by histology, or in-transit metastases) (5-year relative survival, 42 % for stage IIIA vs. 26 % for stage IIIB, $P=0.004$). Drawing on previous studies which concluded that tumor size is prognostic for survival in local disease, this staging system uses a 2 cm cutoff to differentiate between stage I (≤2 cm) and stage II (>2 cm) disease, with stage I having a 5-year survival of 66 %, while stage II drops to 51 % ($P<0.0001$). Further stratification of patients with tumors ≤1 and 2 cm resulted in the same survival rate (81 % for ≤1 cm vs. 79 % for all stage IA tumors) (Fig. 4.3). In the discussion of this report, the authors call attention to the fact that approximately 1/3 of patients with MCC who present with a negative clinical nodal evaluation will be shown to be node positive by SLNB [10]. Although not all patients will undergo pathologic nodal evaluation, this staging system does not group patients who are shown by pathologic evaluation to be node negative with those who were only evaluated clinically. Thus, it may provide more accurate prognostic information for each individual patient by optimal utilization of the

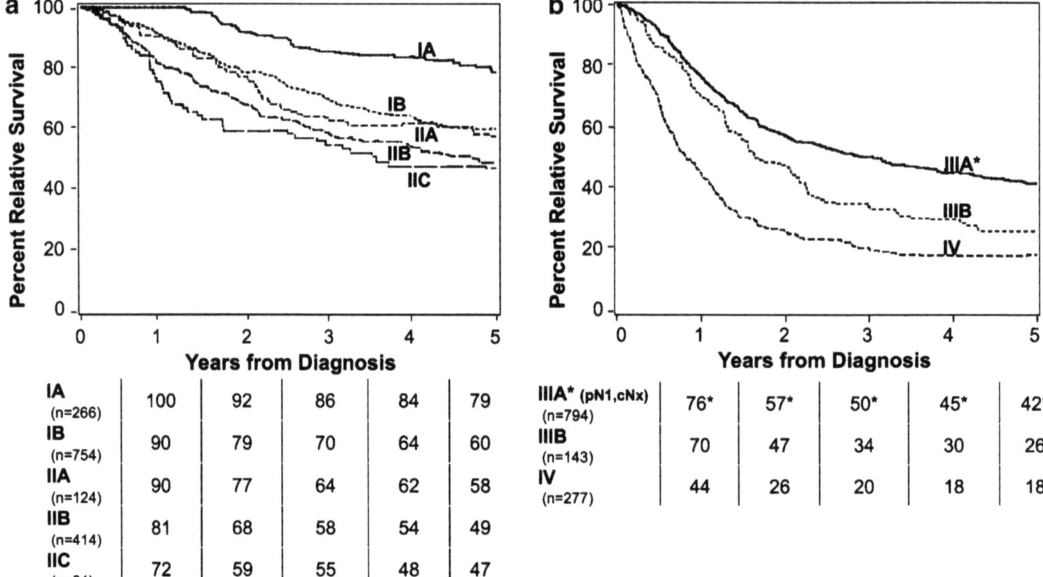

IA (n=266)	100	92	86	84	79
IB (n=754)	90	79	70	64	60
IIA (n=124)	90	77	64	62	58
IIB (n=414)	81	68	58	54	49
IIC (n=84)	72	59	55	48	47

IIIA* (pN1,cNx) (n=794)	76*	57*	50*	45*	42*
IIIB (n=143)	70	47	34	30	26
IV (n=277)	44	26	20	18	18

Fig. 4.3 Relative survival by nodal status: clinical vs. pathologic evaluation. Age- and sex-adjusted percent relative survival curves are shown for all patients with Merkel cell carcinoma who had follow-up data and did not have distant metastatic disease (n=4,427). Patients for whom no regional nodal data were available (1,134 cases) are represented by same curve (Nx). Pathologic node-negative status (pN0) was established either by elective lymphadenectomy or by SLNB. Pathologic node-positive status (pN1) was established by elective or therapeutic lymphadenectomy, fine needle aspirate, SLNB, or other biopsy technique. Age- and sex-adjusted excess hazard ratio comparing clinical node-negative with pathologic node-negative (*top lines*) is 1.80 (95 % confidence interval 1.4–2.4; P<0.0001). The age- and sex-adjusted excess hazard ratio comparing clinical node positive with pathologic node positive (*bottom lines*) is 1.48 (95 % confidence interval 1.1–1.9; P=0.004). There was very little overlap in data in this cohort for method of nodal evaluation because patients had only clinical or pathologic nodal data recorded in majority of cases. Specifically, 240 (5 %) of 4,427 cases included in this analysis had both pathologic and clinical nodal data recorded. These cases are included in pathologic category (**b**) and excluded from clinical nodal analysis (**a**) because pathologic data were considered to be more accurate [Reprinted from Lemos, B.D. et al. Pathologic nodal evaluation improves prognostic accuracy in Merkel cell carcinoma: analysis of 5823 cases as the basis of the first consensus staging system. J. Am. Acad. Dermatol 2010; 63:751–761. With permission from Elsevier]

available information. Stage IV disease refers to patients with any type of primary tumor or lymph node status with distant metastatic disease and carries an 18 % 5-year survival.

In summary, the consensus staging system takes into account the best available data from a large number of patients from multiple institutions. It builds upon prior staging systems that were able to demonstrate statistically significant differences in survival statistics based upon primary tumor size and is the first to incorporate nodal status based on both clinical and pathologic data. Thus, the system takes into account the best available data for each patient and provides the most accurate prognostic information by separating patients with clinically negative nodal disease from those who are shown by pathology to be free of nodal disease in a system that is in line with traditional TNM staging systems used for other forms of cancer. The authors call attention to the limitations of their staging system including the lack of the NCDB to record disease-specific survival, and therefore only relative survival was collected. This would result in an overestimation of mortality associated with MCC if patients had other coexisting conditions that might impact mortality. Along these lines, information on tumor recurrence was not available, precluding the determination of disease-free survival.

Conclusions and Future Directions

As standardized clinical and histopathologic staging of MCC becomes better integrated into the protocols of major cancer centers, improved methods of patient and tumor evaluation will ultimately lead to more uniform staging for this disease. It is clear from the above discussion that staging for MCC has been an evolutionary process as more high-quality data is recorded and reported. Regardless of the system used, it is clear that MCC is an aggressive tumor with high proclivity for regional and distant spread, but excellent survival rates if disease is shown by pathologic as well as clinical measures to be confined to the primary site. Further refinements in staging will require more detailed acquisition of parameters for patients and tumors. New checklists for pathologists have been published [16] to standardize the histologic analyses of MCC tumors in an effort to determine if one or more of these features may reliably impact prognosis. Collectively, these efforts will lead to better management of this aggressive disease and identification of those patients who would benefit from various interventions.

References

1. What is Cancer Staging? American Joint Committee on Cancer. 5 May 2010. http://www.cancerstaging.org/mission/whatis.html. Accessed 9 Oct 2012.
2. Yiengpruksawan A, Coit DG, Thaler HT, Urmacher C, Knapper WK. Merkel cell carcinoma. Prognosis and management. Arch Surg. 1991;126:1514–9.
3. Greene FL, Page DL, Fleming ID, et al (Eds). AJCC cancer staging manual. 6th ed. New York: Springer; 2002.
4. Allen PJ, Zhang ZF, Coit DG. Surgical management of Merkel cell carcinoma. Ann Surg. 1999;229:97–105.
5. Allen PJ et al. Merkel cell carcinoma: prognosis and treatment of patients from a single institution. J Clin Oncol. 2005;23:2300–9.
6. Clark JR, Veness MJ, Gilbert R, O'Brien CJ, Gullane PJ. Merkel cell carcinoma of the head and neck: is adjuvant radiotherapy necessary? Head Neck. 2007;29:249–57.
7. Lemos BD et al. Pathologic nodal evaluation improves prognostic accuracy in Merkel cell carcinoma: analysis of 5823 cases as the basis of the first consensus staging system. J Am Acad Dermatol. 2010;63:751–61.
8. Rogers HW et al. Incidence estimate of nonmelanoma skin cancer in the United States, 2006. Arch Dermatol. 2010;146:283–7.
9. Edge SB, Byrd DR, Compto CC, et al (Eds). AJCC cancer staging manual. 7th ed. New York: Springer; 2010.
10. Gupta SG et al. Sentinel lymph node biopsy for evaluation and treatment of patients with Merkel cell carcinoma: the Dana-Farber experience and meta-analysis of the literature. Arch Dermatol. 2006;142:685–90.
11. Schwartz JL et al. Features predicting sentinel lymph node positivity in Merkel cell carcinoma. J Clin Oncol. 2011;29:1036–41.
12. Sobin LH, Greene FL. TNM classification: clarification of number of regional lymph nodes for pNo. Cancer. 2001;92:452.
13. Greene FL, Sobin LH. A worldwide approach to the TNM staging system: collaborative efforts of the AJCC and UICC. J Surg Oncol. 2009;99:269–72.
14. Howle JR, Hughes TM, Gebski V, Veness MJ. Merkel cell carcinoma: an Australian perspective and the importance of addressing the regional lymph nodes in clinically node-negative patients. J Am Acad Dermatol. 2012;67(1):33–40.
15. Fields RC et al. Five hundred patients with Merkel cell carcinoma evaluated at a single institution. Ann Surg. 2011;254:465–73; discussion 473–5.
16. Rao P et al. Protocol for the examination of specimens from patients with Merkel cell carcinoma of the skin. Arch Pathol Lab Med. 2010;134:341–4.

Histopathologic Diagnosis

5

Jeffrey North and Timothy H. McCalmont

Neuroendocrine tumors, including Merkel cell carcinoma (MCC), belong to the small cell carcinoma category and are characterized histopathologically by monomorphous, small- to medium-sized cells with scant cytoplasm. Their nuclei have granular chromatin with inconspicuous or small nucleoli. In MCC, mitotic figures and single necrotic (apoptotic) cells are frequent, but nuclear pleomorphism is modest. The tumors typically have a center of gravity in the dermis, but epidermal, follicular, or subcutaneous involvement is occasionally present. In the dermis, the tumor is distributed as nodular aggregations, sheets, or interanastomosing cords in a trabecular pattern. The latter pattern prompted Toker's designation of "trabecular carcinoma" in the initial description of MCC in 1972. MCC can often exhibit divergent differentiation or may be seen in association with other neoplasms. Up to 28 % of MCCs occur as a composite with squamous cell carcinoma (SCC).

Due to undifferentiated histopathologic features, confirmatory immunostaining is necessary in most cases. Labeling with Cam5.2, cytokeratin 20 (CK20), or neurofilament in a paranuclear dot pattern is relatively sensitive and quite specific for MCC. Cytokeratin 7 (CK7) and thyroid transcription factor-1 (TTF-1) are typically negative, but rare examples of MCC with a CK7-positive/CK20-negative immunophenotype have been described.

Tumor size, tumor thickness, and the presence of lymphovascular invasion have prognostic significance in MCC. Several studies have investigated different immunostains for potential prognostic ability. Immunopositivity for p63 and lack of CD8+ intratumoral lymphocytes, both associated with a poor prognosis, look particularly promising. However, small sample sizes and lack of independent confirmatory studies are critical limiting factors in these and other studies of prognostic immunomarkers in MCC.

On the genetic level, chromosomal gains and losses are detectable by comparative genomic hybridization (CGH) in most MCCs. Gains involving chromosome 1 and losses on chromosome 3p are the most frequent aberrations. Greater genomic instability, i.e., greater numbers of chromosomal gains or losses, has been associated with a poor prognosis. CGH analysis has also been used as an ancillary test in some diagnostically challenging cases.

J. North (✉)
Department of Dermatology, University of Missouri, One Hospital Dr., MA111, Columbus, MO 65212, USA
e-mail: jeffreypaulnorth@gmail.com

T.H. McCalmont
Department of Pathology (Dermatopathology), University of California, San Francisco, 1701 Divisadero Street, Suite 280, San Francisco, CA 94115, USA
e-mail: tim.mccalmont@ucsf.edu

Introduction and History

MCC is a neuroendocrine tumor. Neuroendocrine cells are intermediary cells between the nervous and endocrine systems capable of receiving signals from neurons that trigger the release of

M. Alam et al. (eds.), *Merkel Cell Carcinoma*, DOI 10.1007/978-1-4614-6608-6_5,

hormones from the neuroendocrine cell. Such cells are found throughout the body in various organs, and thus neuroendocrine tumors can be found at many sites, including carcinoid tumors resembling the serotonin-secreting enterochromaffin cells of the small intestine, small (oat) cell carcinoma of the lung, and pheochromocytoma of the adrenal gland. Due to varying names in the medical literature, the terminology regarding neuroendocrine tumors can be confusing, with a semantic spectrum including small cell carcinoma, carcinoid tumor, and APUDoma. The latter term refers to the tumor cells' ability to utilize *a*mine *p*recursor *u*ptake and *d*ecarboxylation to produce bioactive amines (e.g., serotonin and catecholamines).

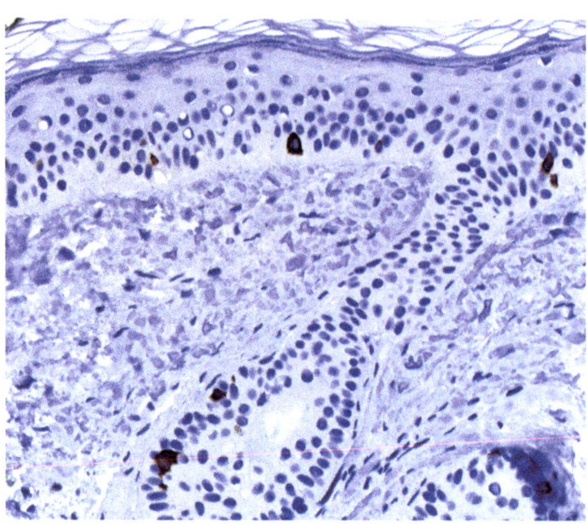

Fig. 5.1 Normal distribution of Merkel cells. A cytokeratin 20 (CK20) stain highlights individual Merkel cells in the basal epidermis and follicular epithelium. CK20 ×400

Merkel Cells

In 1875, Friedrich Merkel described pale basal epidermal cells, associated with nerve fibers, which he believed functioned as cutaneous mechanoreceptors. He designated these cells "Tastzellen" (touch cells), and they were later named Merkel cells in his honor. Merkel cells have round nuclei with little cytoplasm and can be difficult to delineate from neighboring keratinocytes in conventional sections. However, they are readily identifiable with immunohistochemical stains (Fig. 5.1) or by their neurosecretory granules seen with electron microscopy.

Merkel cells are believed to be of ectodermal derivation and are found primarily in the epidermis, follicular epithelium, and mucosa. Occasionally, Merkel cells can be present in the papillary dermis as well. Merkel cells are most abundant in the glabrous skin of the hands and feet, where they sometimes cluster at the tips of rete ridges. They transduce action potentials, synthesize neuropeptides, and express proneural transcription factors, which initially led to the belief that Merkel cells derive from the neural crest. However, increasing evidence, including the presence of cytoplasmic keratin, desmosomal attachments, and the frequent association of SCC and MCC, has led to an alternate hypothesis that Merkel cells derive from an ectodermal stem cell. While some lineage-tracing experiments have supported the neural crest hypothesis [1], there are recent compelling studies with lineage-tracing experiments in mice demonstrating that epidermal stems cell give rise to Merkel cells [2].

Merkel Cell Carcinoma

In 1972, Cyril Toker described five cases of a cutaneous carcinoma of uncertain derivation with a trabecular growth pattern occurring in older patients [3]. He proposed the term "trabecular carcinoma" and hypothesized eccrine or apocrine lineage, as some showed primitive tubule and rosette formation. Six years later, he noted the presence of neurosecretory granules in three of these tumors via electron microscopy and postulated that this carcinoma derived from Merkel cells [4].The name Merkel cell tumor was first used in 1980 [5]. Other designations that have been employed include Toker tumor, cutaneous APUDoma, primary small cell carcinoma of the skin, neuroendocrine tumor of the skin, "murky cell" carcinoma, and anaplastic carcinoma of the skin.

While the term MCC has now gained wide acceptance, some doubts persist as to whether this type of carcinoma truly derives from Merkel cells or simply phenotypically resembles Merkel cells. MCC is typically found in the dermis of sun-exposed skin of the head and neck. In contrast, Merkel cells are located primarily in the epidermis and adnexal epithelium and are concentrated within acral skin, which is an infrequent site for MCC. Some differences in the neurosecretory profiles of Merkel cells and MCC have also raised doubts about their relationship [6]. However, as more reports have emerged of epidermal involvement of MCC, including purely intraepidermal forms [7], as well as studies showing that MCCs express VIP, much like Merkel cells [8], the hypothesis that MCC derives from Merkel cells or Merkel cell precursors has gained strength. The discrepancy in anatomic distribution reflects the importance of ultraviolet light exposure in the pathogenesis of this malignancy.

Key Features

Histopathologically, MCCs have monomorphous, small- to medium-sized, ovoid cells with scant amphophilic cytoplasm. Nuclei are typically round with granular or stippled chromatin and variable hyperchromasia and have been described as having a smudged appearance (Fig. 5.2a). Some cases of MCC have a more irregular nuclear contour with vesicular chromatin and more abundant cytoplasm (Fig. 5.2b). The latter features were associated with a lack of detectable Merkel cell polyoma virus infection in one small study [9].While nuclear pleomorphism is usually mild, mitotic figures abound (75 % of cases with 4–9 per high power field) and sometimes exceed ten mitosis per high power field. Apoptotic cells are also frequent (Fig. 5.2b).

Architecturally, MCC is typically centered in the dermis with a thin "Grenz" zone of dermal collagen separating it from the epidermis. Tumor cells form sheets (Fig. 5.3), cluster in nodular aggregations (Fig. 5.4), or form partially interanastomosing cords in a trabecular pattern (Fig. 5.5). Some tumor cells are crowded closely together and exhibit a "ball-in-mitt" pattern in which a round cell is partially encompassed by one or two adjacent crescentic cells (Fig. 5.6). Sometimes less cohesive aggregations are present with gaps between tumor cells. Poor circumscription is present in the majority of cases, with small nodular aggregations or infiltrative cords of cells among dermal collagen bundles at the periphery or extending into the subcutis (Fig. 5.7). Lymphovascular invasion is common in MCC,

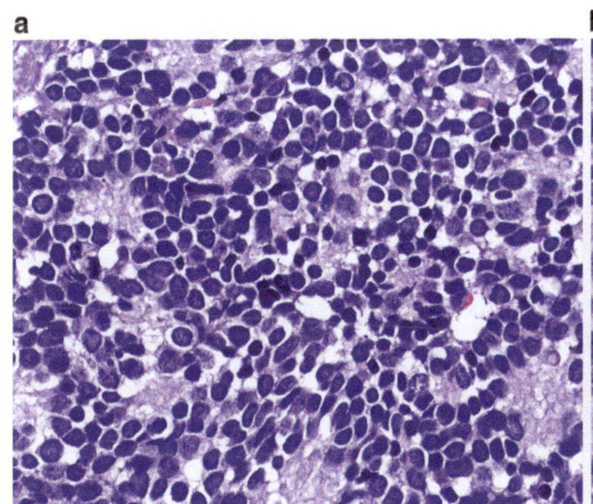

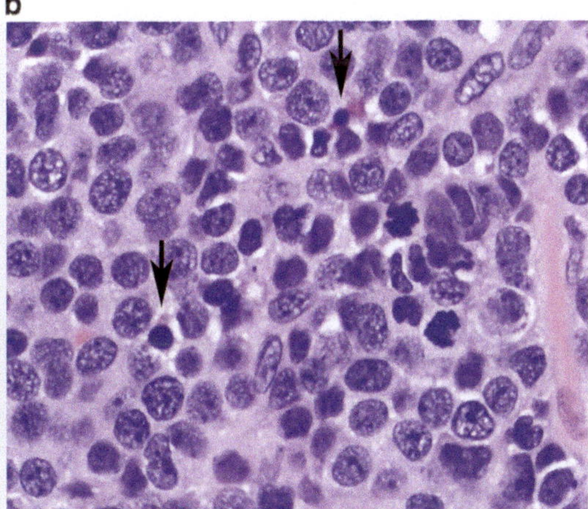

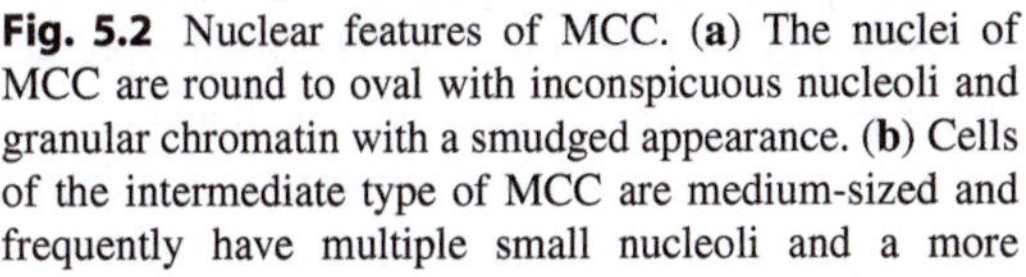

Fig. 5.2 Nuclear features of MCC. (**a**) The nuclei of MCC are round to oval with inconspicuous nucleoli and granular chromatin with a smudged appearance. (**b**) Cells of the intermediate type of MCC are medium-sized and frequently have multiple small nucleoli and a more coarsely granular "salt and pepper" or vesicular chromatin pattern. Numerous mitotic figures and apoptotic cells with prominent desmosomal attachments (*arrows*) are present. Hematoxylin and eosin (H & E) ×400

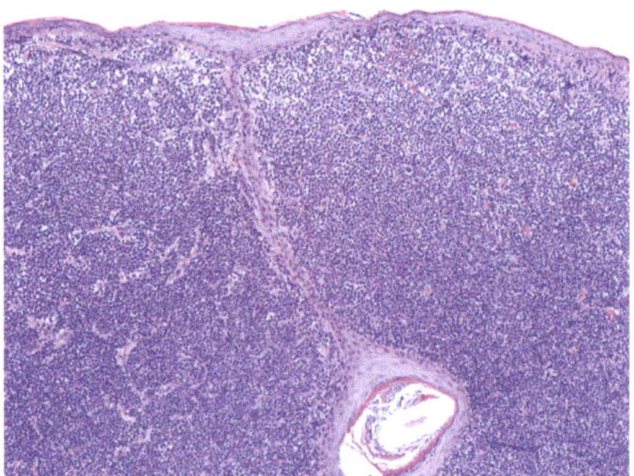

Fig. 5.3 Tumor architecture consisting of sheets of cells filling the dermis. H & E ×100

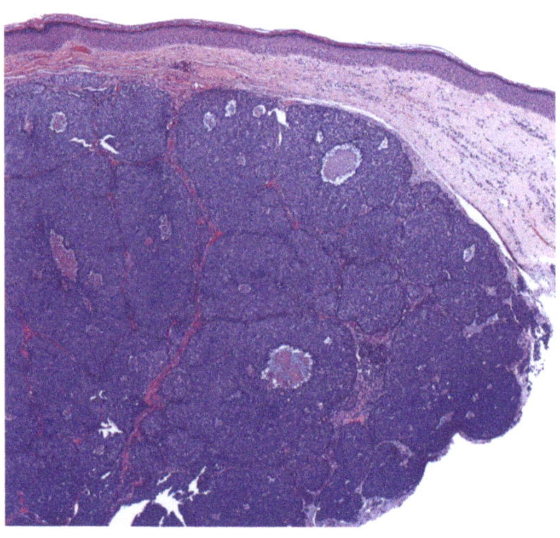

Fig. 5.4 Tumor architecture consisting of nodular aggregations in the dermis. H & E ×40

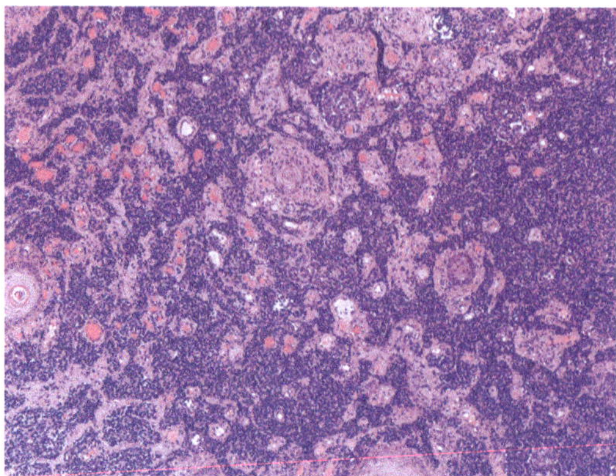

Fig. 5.5 Tumor architecture consisting of interconnecting cords of cells in a trabecular pattern with a highly vascularized stroma and a concurrent squamous proliferation. H & E ×100

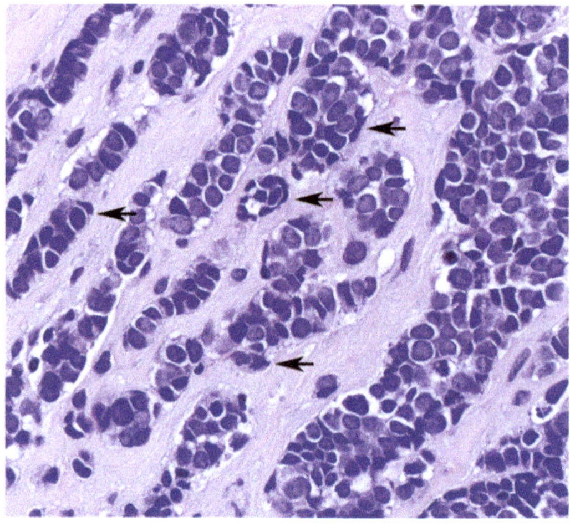

Fig. 5.6 Ball-in-mitt pattern. A central round cell is partially encompassed by one or two adjacent crescentic cells (*arrows*). H & E ×400

with intravascular tumor cells identifiable in 56–93 % of cases [10, 11]. Vascular invasion can typically be observed in conventional sections (Fig. 5.8a), but immunostaining with a vascular marker such as D2-40 is sometimes helpful (Fig. 5.8b).

The stroma surrounding MCC is richly vascular and frequently contains an infiltrate of lymphocytes and plasma cells encompassing or infiltrating the tumor (Fig. 5.9). Dermal collagen bundles range from thin and delicate to thickened and sclerotic. Mucinous stroma is found at least focally in as high as 90 % of cases (Fig. 5.10) [12]. As MCC frequently occurs in sun-exposed sites, marked solar elastosis is often present.

Histopathologic Subtypes

Several pathologic subtypes of MCC have been described in the literature [13]. These subtypes are based primarily on cell size (intermediate or small cell) and tumor architecture (trabecular or diffuse). The majority of tumors fall under the intermediate

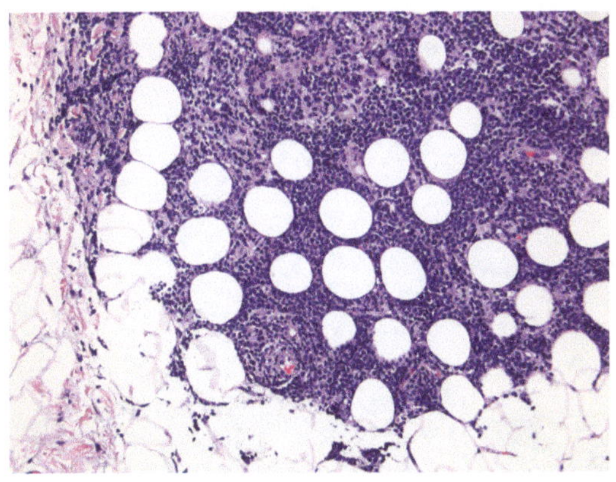

Fig. 5.7 Subcutaneous involvement. Tumor extending into the subcutis with infiltration of neoplastic cells into fat lobules. H & E ×200

cell subtype. Intermediate cell features include cells with moderately large nuclei (10–15 μm) exhibiting an open, granular chromatin pattern that is sometimes referred to as "salt and pepper" chromatin. Many of the cells have multiple micronucleoli (Fig. 5.2). Some degree of nuclear molding, frequently manifesting as the "ball-in-mitt" pattern, is present. The small cell subtype is less common and usually consists of sheets of cells that approximate the size of lymphocytes with hyperchromatic nuclei and inconspicuous nucleoli (Fig. 5.11). A large cell/pleomorphic subtype has also been described (Fig. 5.12) and is rare [14]. Occasionally, tumor cells have a spindled morphology (Fig. 5.13). An infiltrative pattern is present in the majority of MCC and has been associated with decreased survival compared to a nodular growth pattern [15]. Otherwise, there is no prognostic value in separating MCC into subtypes and many cases have overlapping features, e.g., a tumor with both diffuse and trabecular patterns and both small and medium-sized cells. Thus, subtyping MCC is of limited value.

Ultrastructural Features and Immunophenotype

Prior to the development of immunohistochemical stains, electron microscopy played an instrumental role in diagnostic pathology and was key to the characterization of MCC as a type of neuroendocrine carcinoma [4]. The ultrastructural characteristics of MCC with electron microscopy include paranuclear and/or cytoplasmic bundles of tonofilaments (keratin intermediate filaments), cytoplasmic dense-core granules, and desmosomal attachments. The neurosecretory dense-core granules are circular, 80–120 nm, membrane-bound, and located in the peripheral cytoplasm. They vary considerably in number.

The convenience and accessibility of immunohistochemical staining has largely replaced electron microscopy in the diagnosis of MCC. While no immunostain is perfectly sensitive and specific, a select panel of stains can reliably distinguish MCC from its mimics. The immunoreactivity of MCC is summarized in Table 5.1. While many immunostains are available for use in the differential diagnosis of MCC, low molecular weight cytokeratin (e.g., Cam5.2), CK20, and neurofilament yield high diagnostic sensitivity (Fig. 5.14). Negative staining for thyroid transcription factor-1 (TTF-1) helps exclude small carcinoma of the lung and increases specificity. Additional use of immunostains is discussed in the differential diagnosis section.

Lymph Node Involvement

As the regional lymph nodes are the most frequent site of metastasis, sentinel lymph node biopsy (SLNB) has become an important tool in the workup of MCC. Metastatic involvement of lymph nodes ranges from scattered single tumor cells, detectable only by immunohistochemistry, to small or large tumoral aggregations that may efface nodal architecture. Immunohistochemical stains, preferably CK20 or a low molecular weight keratin, should be utilized routinely in SLNB for MCC, as up to 20 % of positive lymph nodes are negative by conventional microscopy alone [16]. Tumor cells may localize to the subcapsular sinus, peripheral parenchyma, or a combination of both (Fig. 5.15). In a prospective analysis of SLNB in MCC, all positive sentinel nodes had involvement of the subcapsular sinus [17]. Eighty percent had involvement of the lymph node parenchyma as well.

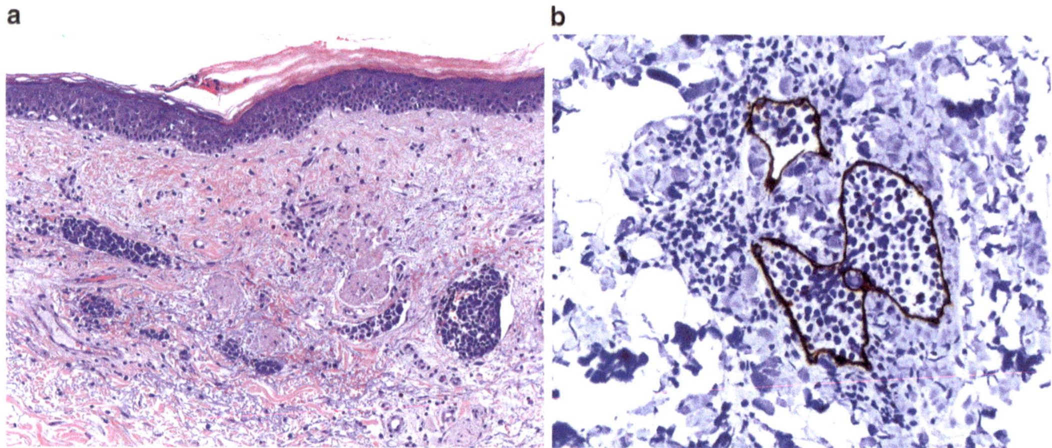

Fig. 5.8 Lymphovascular invasion. (**a**) Tumor cells present in lymphatic vessels near the primary tumor. H & E ×200. (**b**) D2-40 staining outlines lymphatic endothelium surrounding intravascular tumor cells. D2-40 ×200

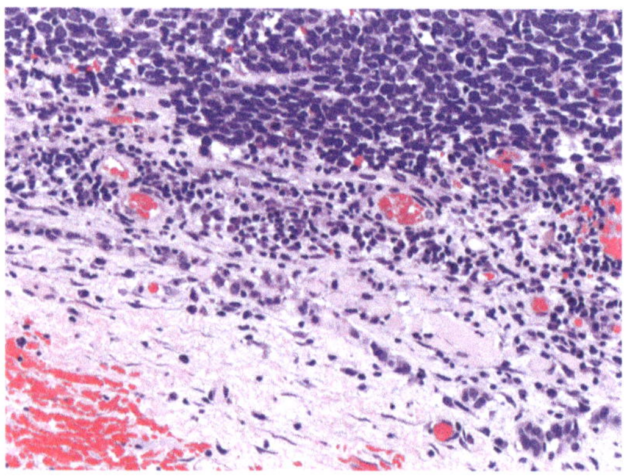

Fig. 5.9 Stroma. Tumor stroma in MCC is vascular with lymphocytes and plasma cells frequently present. Dermal collagen bundles range from thin and delicate to thickened and sclerotic. H & E ×400

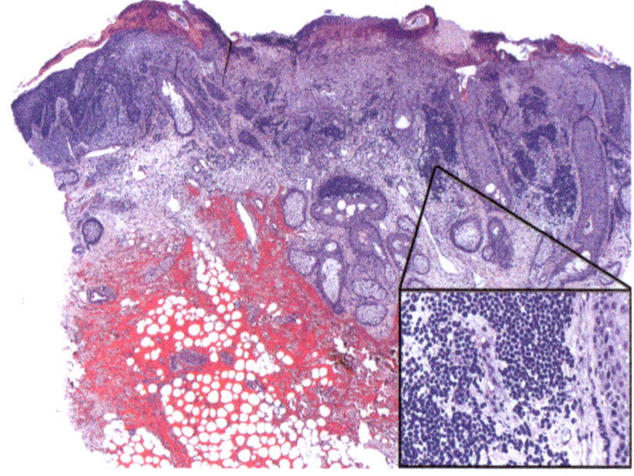

Fig. 5.11 MCC, small cell type. This type of MCC closely resembles an infiltrate of lymphocytes (*inset*). H & E ×40, *inset* ×200

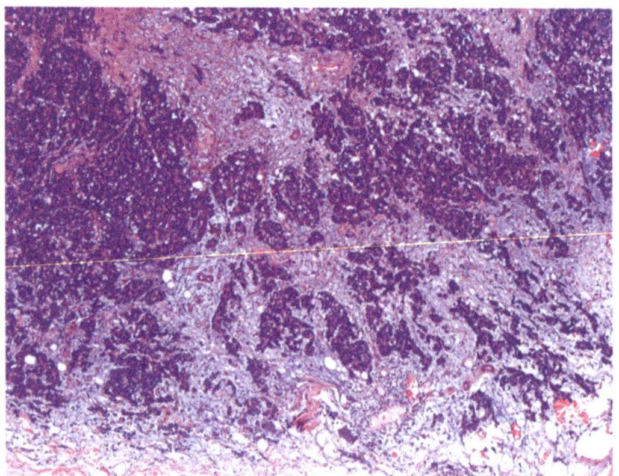

Fig. 5.10 MCC with mucinous stroma. H & E ×100

Recurrent and Metastatic Merkel Cell Carcinoma

The histopathologic features of recurrent MCC are similar to those of primary MCC, with the addition of a scar accompanying the tumor. Within the scar, irregular thin strands of tumor are often interposed among thickened collagen bundles (Fig. 5.16).

In patients with a history of MCC who develop a second lesion of MCC at a distant site, the distinction between metastatic carcinoma and a second primary carcinoma can be very difficult.

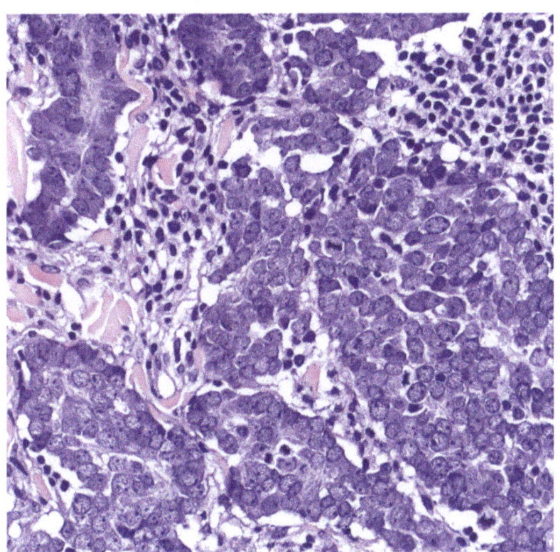

Fig. 5.12 MCC, large cell type. Many of tumor cells are 4–5 times the size of surrounding lymphocytes and some pleomorphic cells are present. H & E ×400

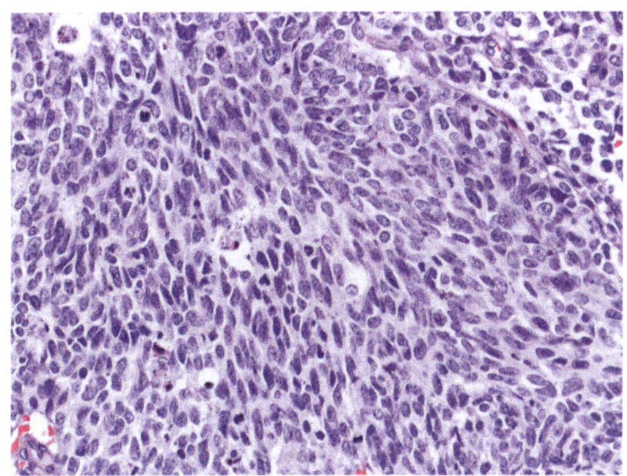

Fig. 5.13 MCC, spindle cell type. Tumor cells have a spindled morphology. The granular chromatin, numerous mitoses, and apoptotic cells are clues to the diagnosis of MCC. H & E ×400

Comparative review of the cytology and immunohistochemical staining pattern of the primary carcinoma can be helpful but is not completely reliable, as tumor phenotype can evolve with progression to metastasis. Molecular techniques such as CGH can be helpful. Sixty to ninety percent of MCCs have chromosomal aberrations detectable by CGH, and more aggressive tumors have been shown to harbor a greater number of aberrations [18, 19]. While characteristic gains or losses at certain chromosomal loci have been found, most tumors have a unique CGH profile. In cases where both the primary and a metastatic lesion were tested, the CGH signatures were nearly identical [19]. This finding has been utilized to distinguish metastatic MCC, which should have a CGH profile resembling that of the primary tumor, from a second primary MCC [20].

Fine Needle Aspiration

Fine needle aspiration (FNA) biopsy can serve as a valuable diagnostic tool in patients with palpable deep soft tissue lesions not easily reached with superficial biopsy techniques. FNA smears of MCC are typically abundantly cellular and reveal discohesive clusters of epithelial cells that may exhibit a pseudorosette pattern. In some cases, there may be a background of necrosis. Artifactual smudging and streaking of nuclei are frequently prominent.

The tumor cells are generally small with scant cytoplasm and high nucleus-to-cytoplasm ratio. Subtle nuclear contour irregularities with finely granular chromatin and multiple small nucleoli are present (Fig. 5.17). Mitotic figures and apoptotic cells are readily identified. Paranuclear "intermediate filament buttons" can be seen on Papanicolaou or Giemsa stains but are best demonstrated via keratin immunostains performed on a cell block.

Additional Features

While MCC is typically a dermal neoplasm, epidermal involvement (Fig. 5.18) occurs in approximately 10 % of cases [21]. MCC limited only to the epidermis is rare and has been referred to as "MCC in situ". A pagetoid pattern with individual cells and small tumor clusters scattered among keratinocytes above the junction is typical of such cases. In addition to epidermotropism, folliculo-tropism may also be seen (Fig. 5.19). One case of primary MCC presenting as a subcutaneous mass has been reported [22]. While MCC presents in the skin in most cases, MCC presenting

Table 5.1 Positive expression of immunomarkers in Merkel cell carcinoma

Cytokeratins		CD		Neuroendocrine markers	
CK20	83 % (546)	CD 10	7 % (15)	Chromogranin	66 % (115)
Cam 5.2	99 % (75)	CD 23	97 % (33)	Synatophysin	76 % (79)
AE1/AE3	78 % (51)	CD 34	0 % (15)	Neuron-specific enolase	80 % (100)
MNF116	100 % (17)	CD 45 (LCA)	0 % (51)	Neurofilament	77 % (412)
Pan keratin	73 % (77)	CD 56	89 % (46)	Bombesin	35 % (20)
CK7	16 % (94)	CD 57	60 % (5)	Vasoactive intestinal peptide	33 % (21)
CK5/6	0 % (13)	CD 99	31 % (45)	PGP9.5	89 % (18)
		CD 117 (KIT)	71 % (137)		
Other					
TTF-1	2 % (116)	BCL-2	80 % (55)		
MCPyV T antigen	73 % (51)	P53	38 % (47)		
p63	58 % (117)	MASH1	0 % (30)		
TdT	68 % (81)	EMA	78 % (36)		
Pax-5	82 % (65)	CEA	0 % (15)		
S-100	4 % (69)	Ber-Ep4	73 % (22)		
HMB45	0 % (6)	Vimentin	8 % (13)		
NKIC3	0 % (6)	Ki-67	47–75 % positivity index		

Percentages were calculated from combining numerous published reports, with the total number of cases tested listed in *parentheses*

within a lymph node in the absence of a cutaneous primary occurs in 15 % of cases [10].

Composite Tumors and Divergent Differentiation

Numerous reports of composite tumors of MCC and SCC have been published. The range spans from MCC with overlying SCC in situ to instances in which invasive SCC and MCC are intimately admixed (Fig. 5.20). As both carcinomas tend to occur in sun-damaged skin, the possibility these represent collision tumors in which the two malignancies arose independently is conceivable. However, the frequency of occurrence (28 % in one series [23]) suggests the relationship goes beyond mere chance. While some may represent coincidence, the hypothesis that these composite carcinomas derive from an epithelial stem cell is appealing. MCC with concurrent SCC does not appear to share the same relationship with Merkel cell polyoma virus infection that non-composite MCC does, possibly reflecting a different oncogenic pathway in these types of tumors.

Multiple reports of MCC occurring in association with basal cell carcinoma (BCC) (Fig. 5.21) [23], benign follicular proliferations including trichoblastoma and follicular cysts [24], and chronic lymphocytic leukemia [25] have been published. Single cases of MCC associated with melanoma [26], atypical fibroxanthoma [27], sebaceous carcinoma [28], and dermatofibrosarcoma protuberans [29] have also been described.

Rarely, MCC exhibits differentiation toward cutaneous adnexa and forms tubular structures and ducts that stain positively with carcinoembryonic antigen (CEA) [30]. This rare finding should not be mistaken for the more common finding of tumor surrounding native eccrine ducts. Multinucleated cells have also been rarely observed in MCC [31]. Rhabdomyoblastic or rhabdomyosarcomatous differentiation has been reported in several case reports (Fig. 5.22) [32], as has leiomyosarcomatous and fibrosarcomatous differentiation [33, 34]. The term Merkel cell

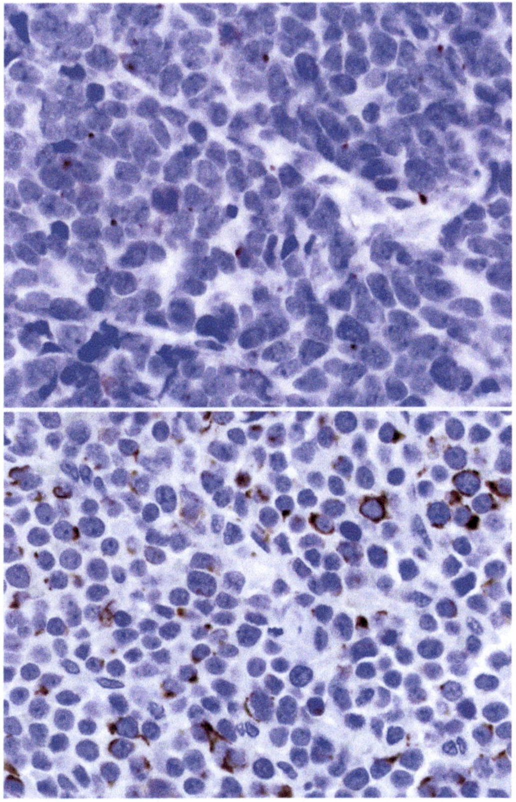

Fig. 5.14 Staining pattern of CK20 and neurofilament. The majority of MCC has a characteristic paranuclear dot pattern of immunostaining for neurofilament (*top*) and CK20 (*bottom*). The cytoplasm of some tumor cells stains diffusely with CK20 as well (*bottom*). *Top*- neurofilatment ×400, *bottom*- CK20 ×400

carcinosarcoma has been used for cases with a spindled sarcomatous component. One report detailing a CK20-positive cutaneous neuroendocrine carcinoma with features of ganglioneuroblastoma could represent MCC with neuroblastoma-like differentiation [35].

Exceptional Stromal Changes

While the stroma of MCC is typically collagenous, hypervascular, and focally mucinous, a minority of MCCs have a prominent fibromyxoid stroma that can mimic the stroma of BCC. Focal desmoplastic change with spindled tumor cells has also been reported [36]. Amyloid deposition in the superficial dermis was reported in one case of intraepidermal MCC [37]. Deposition of basophilic nuclear debris in vessel walls (Azzopardi phenomenon) is occasionally mentioned in reference to MCC but was only identified in 4 % (3/83) of cases in one large series (Fig. 5.23) [38].

Differential Diagnosis

MCC is often referred to as a small blue cell tumor, the differential diagnosis of which includes metastatic neuroendocrine carcinoma, lymphoma, leukemia, neuroblastoma, and Ewing

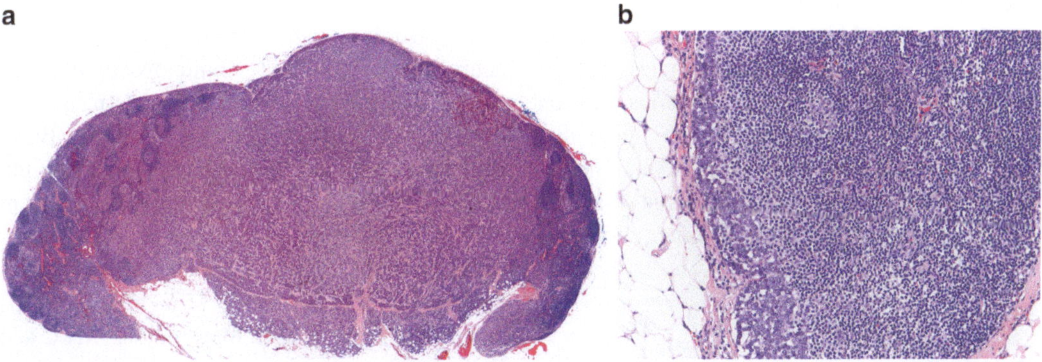

Fig. 5.15 Lymph node involvement. (**a**) Metastastic MCC expands and effaces the center of this lymph node, extending from the subcapsular sinus into the hilum. H & E ×20. (**b**) Metastatic MCC presenting in the subcapsular sinus. H & E ×200

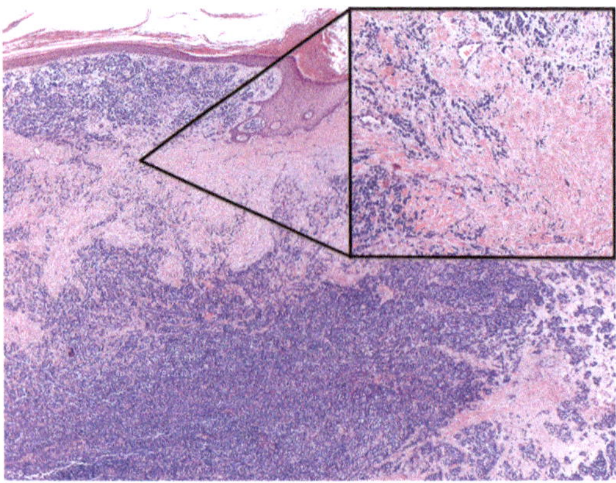

Fig. 5.16 Recurrent MCC. Irregular thin strands of tumor 1–2 cells thick are interposed between thickened collagen bundles of a scar. H & E ×40, *inset*- H & E ×200

sarcoma. In addition, small aggregates of MCC can mimic the melanocytic nests of melanoma or exhibit the peripheral clefting artifact typically associated with BCC. Rarely, the stroma can be extremely hypervascular and hemorrhagic, thus mimicking angiosarcoma (Fig. 5.24). As there is considerable histopathologic overlap in this differential diagnosis, immunohistochemical stains are necessary in the vast majority of cases to confirm the correct diagnosis.

MCC and Other Primary Cutaneous Malignancies

The architectural and cytologic features of MCC usually permit differentiation of MCC from other primary cutaneous malignancies such as melanoma, BCC, SCC, and cutaneous adnexal carcinoma. The round nuclei with finely dispersed chromatin, inconspicuous or small nucleoli, and scant cytoplasm characteristic of MCCs are not usually present in these other cutaneous malignancies.

Melanoma

Clues that favor melanoma over MCC include definitive nest formation (including intraepidermal nests), nuclear pseudoinclusion formation, and finely pigmented cytoplasm. In cases of epidermotropic MCC that do have nest formation, recognizing the nuclear features of MCC can be diagnostically helpful (Fig. 5.18). Immunohistochemical markers such as Melan-A or HMB-45 can be used to recognize melanocytic lineage when the diagnosis is questionable.

Basal Cell Carcinoma

The basophilic appearance and occasional cleft formation seen at the edge of some aggregations of MCC can mimic BCC. In a study of 30 MCCs, approximately 90 % were noted to have associated mucinous stroma and stromal retraction artifact resembling the stroma of BCC [12]. Focal peripheral palisading was noted in 27 %. In addition to these overlapping features between these two carcinomas, BCC can occur concurrently with MCC and lead to misdiagnosis if the entire tumor is not scrutinized (Fig. 5.21). While overlapping features do exist, certain features permit distinction of these two carcinomas in the vast majority of cases utilizing conventional sections alone. Widespread peripheral palisading in BCC is perhaps the most helpful feature. The mitotic index is also typically much lower in BCC. Involvement along the basal epidermis is also a distinguishing feature favoring a diagnosis of BCC, as it is seen only in 10 % or less of MCCs.

In cases with overlapping features, neurofilament or CK20 immunopositivity, particularly in the paranuclear dot pattern, is most useful to distinguish MCC from BCC. Neurofilament has higher overall sensitivity, but CK20 is more commonly utilized. If neurofilament and CK20 are unavailable, use of a low molecular weight keratin, such as Cam5.2, can be considered. Ber-Ep4 is positive in 75 % of MCCs [39] and should never be used to distinguish MCC and BCC. BCCs can express neuroendocrine markers such as neuron-specific enolase and chromagranin in 4 % of cases [40]. In the authors' experience, BCC does not stain with neurofilament.

a

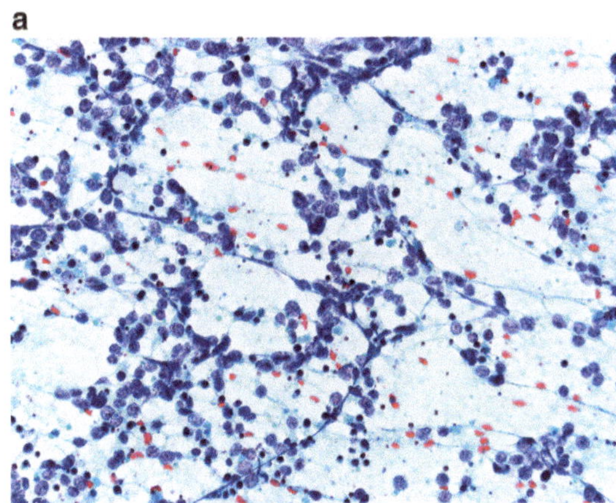

b

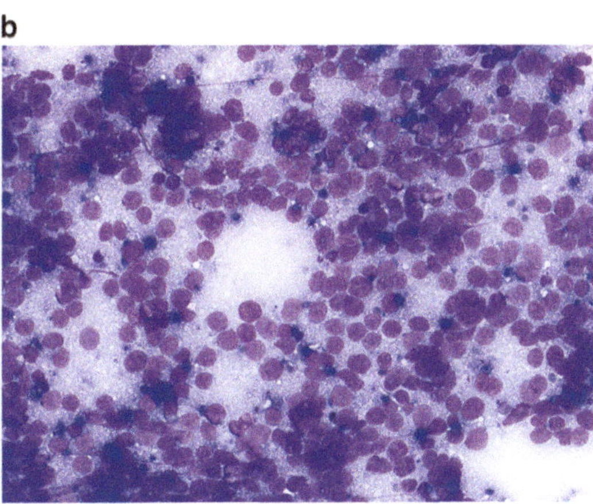

Fig. 5.17 Fine needle aspiration (FNA) biopsy. The smear is hypercellular with discohesive clusters of epithelial cells and smudging/streaking of nuclei. Tumor cells have a high nucleus-to-cytoplasm ratio, finely granular chromatin, and multiple small nucleoli. (**a**) Pap ×400, (**b**) May-Grunwald-Giemsa ×400

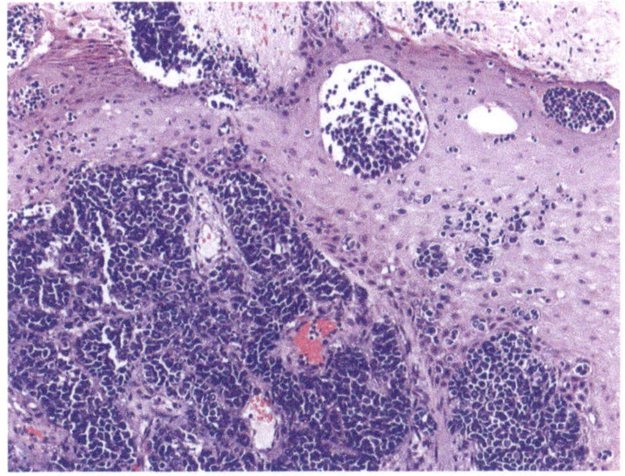

Fig. 5.18 Epidermotropic MCC. Single cells and small collections of MCC in the epidermis can mimic melanocytic nests or Pautrier collections of mycosis fungoides. H & E ×200

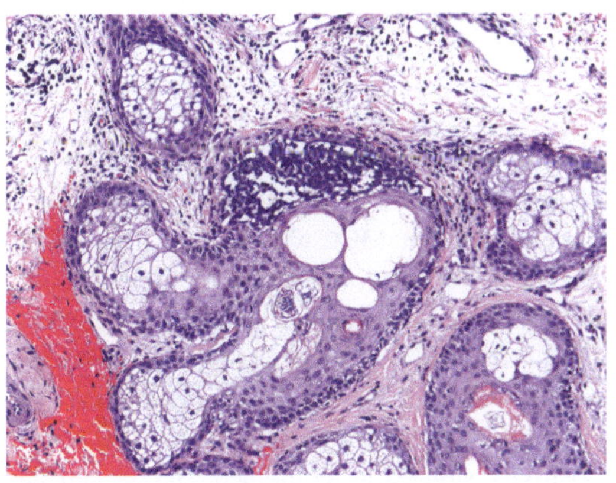

Fig. 5.19 Folliculotropic MCC. H & E ×200

Squamous Cell Carcinoma

Up to 28 % of examples of MCC have associated concurrent SCC [23]. Thus, the potential for a misdiagnosis by overlooking one of the tumor types exists. The component of SCC is usually obvious (Fig. 5.20). If a poorly differentiated tumor is present in the underlying dermis, careful assessment for the possibility of a composite MCC/SCC is advised before assuming the dermal component represents poorly differentiated SCC. As with other primary cutaneous malignancies, the nuclear and cytoplasmic features are usually quite helpful in this differential diagnosis. While both carcinomas feature cells with desmosomes, apoptotic cells, and frequent mitotic figures, SCC tends to be more pleomorphic with scattered dyskeratotic cells containing intense pink cytoplasm. However, in some examples of poorly differentiated SCC, these features are not prominent and immunostains are necessary. The staining approach discussed previously can be employed in this context.

Adnexal Carcinomas and Metastatic Adenocarcinoma

Poorly differentiated metastatic adenocarcinoma can histopathologically mimic MCC (Fig. 5.25).

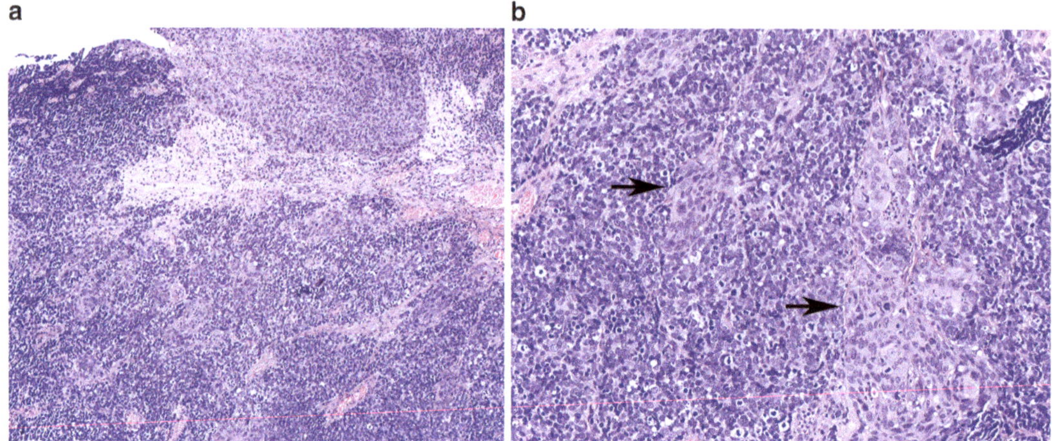

Fig. 5.20 MCC/SCC composite malignancy. (**a**) SCC is present at the top of the image and in small foci juxtaposed throughout the MCC in the dermis. H & E ×100. (**b**) High power view of the MCC (round cells with granular chromatin and scant cytoplasm) intimately associated with the SCC (distinct aggregates of more pleomorphic cells with pink keratinized cytoplasm; *arrows*). There are hints of transition zones between the cell types. H & E ×200

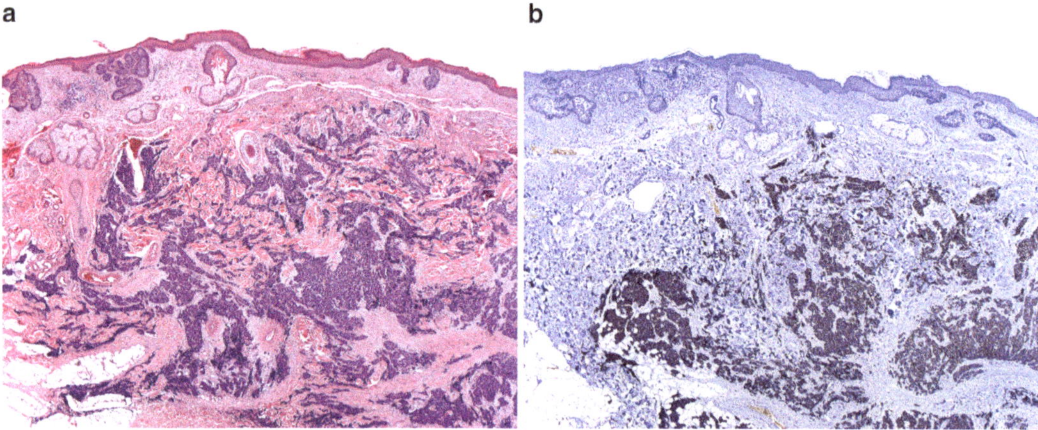

Fig. 5.21 MCC and BCC. (**a**) Superficial BCC is present with prominent peripheral palisading. A basaloid proliferation that lacks significant palisading is present in the subjacent dermis. H & E ×40. (**b**) A CK20 stain strongly labels the MCC, while the BCC is negative. CK20 ×40

The presence of true duct formation is rare in MCC and can be a clue to the diagnosis of a primary cutaneous or metastatic adenocarcinoma. Tumors showing small blue cell morphology with nuclear features of MCC and duct formation require immunostaining for a definitive diagnosis. CK20 or neurofilament dot immunopositivity can be used to distinguish MCC from adenocarcinoma. Some metastatic adenocarcinomas do express CK20 (e.g., colorectal, bladder, and ovarian carcinoma), but do not show the paranuclear dot pattern of MCC and also lack expression of neurofilament. MCC with ductal differentiation has been reported, including a lymphoepithelioma-like appearance with a multinodular pattern of dense lymphocytic inflammation surrounding undifferentiated, closely spaced epithelial cells with CEA, neurofilament, and dot-like keratin positivity suggesting combined Merkel cell and adnexal ductal differentiation [41].

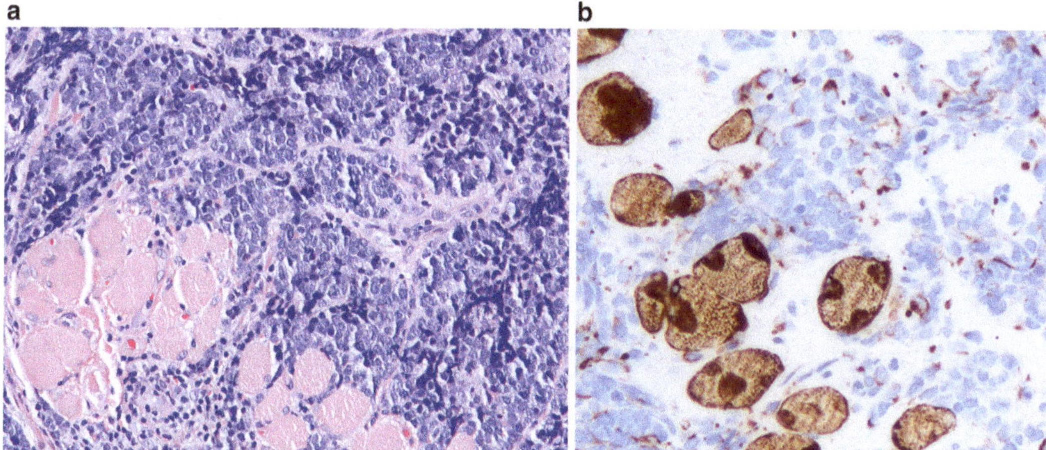

Fig. 5.22 Rhabdomyoblastic differentiation in MCC. (**a**) Basaloid cells with granular chromatin typical of MCC are present in conjunction with large, multi-nucleated cells with bright pink cytoplasm typical of rhabdomyoblasts. H & E ×400. (**b**) Desmin immunostaining is positive in the rhabdomyoblastic population as well as the conventional MCC cells, confirming muscular differentiation. Desmin ×400. (Photos courtesy of Dr. Andrew Folpe)

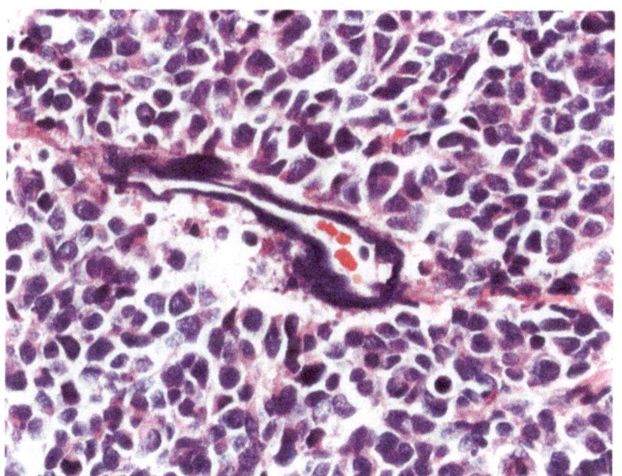

Fig. 5.23 Azzopardi phenomenon. Deposition of basophilic nuclear debris in vessel walls is present in approximately 33 % of small cell lung cancers and 4 % of MCCs. H & E ×400

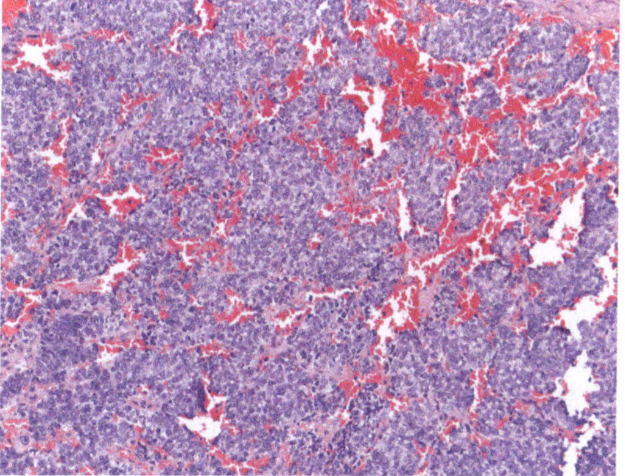

Fig. 5.24 MCC mimicking angiosarcoma. The stroma of this MCC is hypervascular and hemorrhagic resulting in an appearance similar to epithelioid angiosarcoma. Expression of CK20 and lack of vascular markers confirm the diagnosis of MCC. H & E ×200

Metastatic Neuroendocrine Carcinoma, Including Small Cell Lung Carcinoma

MCC belongs to the large family of neuroendocrine tumors that includes small cell carcinomas and carcinoid tumors. Most neuroendocrine tumors have similar histomorphology, making differentiation of MCC from a cutaneous metastasis of an internal neuroendocrine carcinoma quite challenging (Fig. 5.26). Clinical information, especially a past medical history of neuroendocrine carcinoma, can be helpful, as can knowing the anatomic location of the skin lesion. MCC typically occurs in sun-damaged skin on the head and neck or extremities of older adults. Clinical information combined with a small

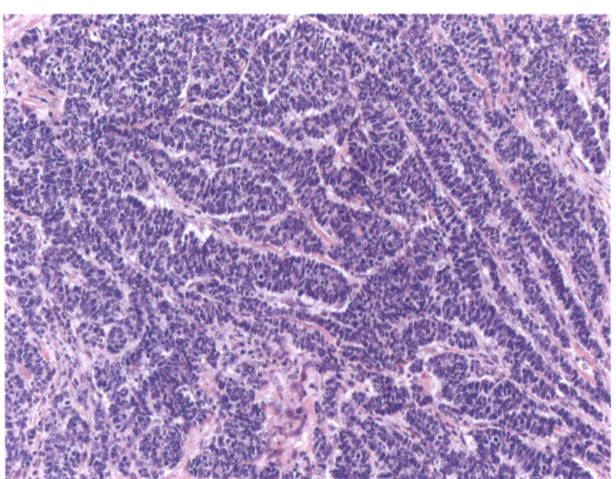

Fig. 5.25 Metastatic adenocarcinoma mimicking MCC. This poorly differentiated colorectal carcinoma lacks definitive duct formation and appears similar to trabecular pattern MCC. Paranuclear dot immunopositivity with CK20 or neurofilament help differentiate MCC from such metastases. H & E ×200

number of immunostains is usually sufficient to correctly differentiate MCC from metastatic neuroendocrine carcinoma. Numerous studies have compared potential markers to differentiate MCC from small cell lung carcinoma, a neuroendocrine carcinoma with a grave prognosis. The combination of CK7 and CK20 with TTF1 is a popular triad of immunostains used to distinguish MCC from metastatic small cell carcinoma of the lung and other internal neuroendocrine carcinomas. These stains are sufficient for a proper diagnosis in the majority of cases.

CK20 shows immunopositivity in roughly 85 % of MCCs. The paranuclear dot pattern strongly supports a diagnosis of MCC. One notable exception is salivary gland small cell carcinoma, which can exhibit a similar CK20 staining pattern. Two cases of small cell carcinoma of the ovary have been reported with this pattern as well [42]. Approximately 15–20 % of MCCs exhibit diffuse CK20 positivity. This is less specific than the paranuclear dot pattern and is seen in metastatic carcinomas from the other sites (e.g., colon, bladder, and ovary). The high sensitivity of CK20 for MCC, combined with a 3 % positivity rate in small cell lung carcinoma, makes this marker extremely useful in differentiating these two tumors. Cytokeratin 7 and TTF1 have the opposite staining pattern of CK20. They are typically negative in MCC and positive in small cell lung carcinoma and are frequently used in conjunction with CK20 (Table 5.2). Neuroendocrine markers such as synaptophysin, chromogranin, and neuron-specific enolase, as well as CD56, stain a high percentage of MCC and small cell lung carcinoma and should not be used to discriminate these two neoplasms.

Perhaps due to a wide range of positivity rates in different studies (20–100 %), neurofilament is often omitted in staining recommendations. The low positivity rates reported by some may result from overlooking the sometimes subtle dot positivity of neurofilament in MCC. In 351 cases of MCC from the authors' institution, neurofilament was positive in 90 % , while CK20 expression was observed in 82 % [43]. A paranuclear dot pattern was observed in 95 % of the positive neurofilament cases and 83 % of the positive CK20 cases. Neurofilament is routinely negative in lung and other small cell neuroendocrine carcinomas, making it particularly useful in this differential diagnosis [44]. Rare reports of CK20-negative, CK7-positive MCC exist, and neurofilament represents a good choice to evaluate tumors with this immunophenotype in which the diagnosis of MCC is suspected [45].

A few studies have explored the differential expression of various neuroendocrine proteins among neuroendocrine tumors to see if they can assist in discriminating specific tumor types. Synaptophysin, chromogranin, neuron-specific enolase, and VIP are variably positive in multiple types of neuroendocrine carcinoma and cannot be reliably used to distinguish MCC from other neuroendocrine carcinomas. One study showed positivity in bombesin, leucine enkephalin, or methionine enkephalin in 6/7 metastatic neuroendocrine carcinomas and 0/21 MCC [46]. However, these immunoreagents are not routinely available for clinical use. Studies exploring differential expression of neuroendocrine markers in cutaneous and internal neuroendocrine carcinomas are few and have had inconsistent results.

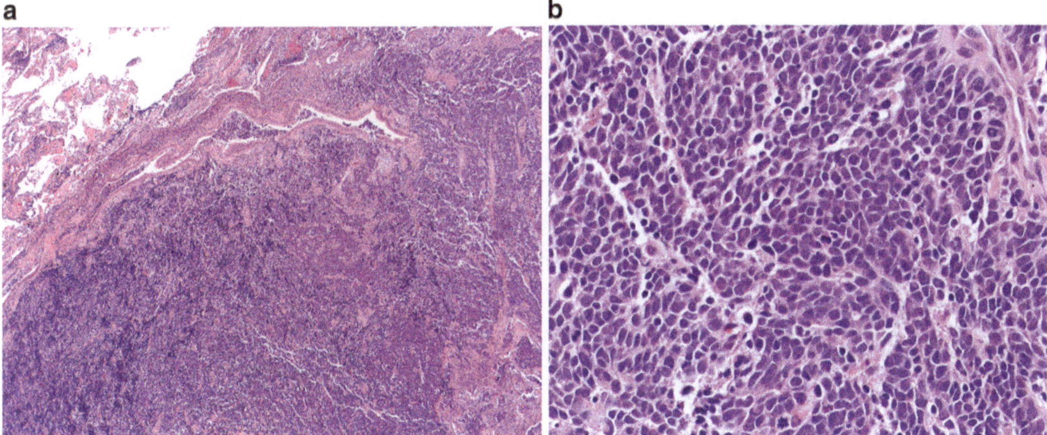

Fig. 5.26 Small cell lung carcinoma. As they are indistinguishable from MCC with routine histopathology, metastases from some internal neuroendocrine tumors, such as this small cell lung carcinoma, require immunostaining for definitive diagnosis. (**a**) H & E ×40, (**b**) H & E ×400

Table 5.2 Differentiating Merkel cell carcinoma and small cell lung carcinoma by immunohistochemistry

	CK20+	CAM 5.2+	CK7+	NF+	TTF-1+
Merkel cell carcinoma	85 % (269)	99 % (75)	16 % (94)	72 % (277)	2 % (116)
Small cell carcinoma, lung	3 % (105)	100 % (10)	67 % (43)	0 % (45)	87 % (79)

The percentage results were obtained from combining numerous published reports, with total number of cases tested listed in *parentheses*
NF neurofilament

Hematologic Infiltrates

Lymphoma and leukemia cutis can have significant clinical and histopathological overlap with MCC. Both are characterized by small, basophilic, round cells in the dermis. In addition, intraepidermal MCC can form discrete collections in the epidermis mimicking the Pautrier collections of mycosis fungoides. As previously mentioned, MCC usually has an associated lymphocyte-predominant inflammatory infiltrate. In rare cases, the inflammatory infiltrate can be quite dense with a follicular growth pattern, thus mimicking a lymphoid neoplasm or cutaneous lymphoid hyperplasia [47].

Some notable histopathologic features can assist in the differential diagnosis of MCC and hematologic malignancies. Leukemia cutis frequently has a peri-adnexal pattern and "single file" arrangement of cells among collagen bundles, neither of which is typical of MCC (Fig. 5.27). Granular cytoplasm seen in some myeloid leukemias and the nuclear features of blasts (open, vesicular chromatin with one or two prominent nucleoli) can also be a clue to the diagnosis of leukemia. A dense lymphocytic infiltrate can be challenging to differentiate from MCC without the assistance of additional stains.

Leukocyte common antigen (CD45) is the most helpful marker in differentiating MCC from hematologic malignancies. It is consistently negative in MCC and stains the vast majority of lymphomas and leukemias, irrespective of lineage. Lymphoblastic lymphoma, which may lack CD45, is a notable exception. Special attention should be given when diagnosing B lymphoblastic lymphoma, which can be CD20 negative, Pax-5 positive, and terminal deoxynucleotidyl

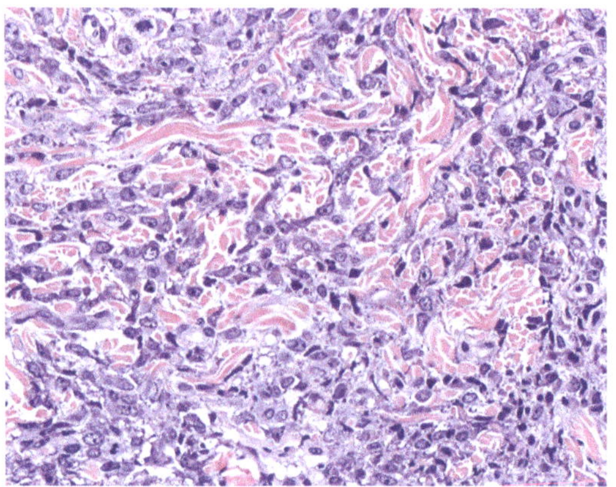

Fig. 5.27 Leukemia cutis (myeloid sarcoma). Prominent arrangement of cells in single file between collagen bundles, granular cytoplasm, and blastic nuclear features present in leukemia cutis help distinguish it from MCC. H & E ×400

transferase (TdT) positive. Pax-5, a nuclear transcription factor, is often present in CD20-negative B cell neoplasms but is also positive in 82 % of MCCs. TdT is used as a blast marker in lymphoma but is positive in 68 % of MCCs. CD56-positive NK cell lymphomas represent another potential pitfall, as CD56 expression is also present in 89 % of MCCs. Keratin stains (e.g., Cam5.2) are negative in lymphomas and should be used in addition to CD45 for differentiating MCC from lymphoma.

Primitive Neuroectodermal Tumor and Ewing Sarcoma

Primitive neuroectodermal tumor (PNET) and Ewing sarcoma belong to a family of tumors with similar cytogenetic abnormalities involving translocation of the EWS gene with Fli-1, ETV1, or ERG. Both have similar histopathologic appearances and can mimic MCC. In comparison to Ewing sarcoma, PNET tends to have more neural features, including rosette formation and positivity for neural markers such as neurofilament, synaptophysin, chromogranin, and S100. CD99 and Fli-1 are positive in most examples of Ewing sarcoma and PNET but are also positive in some MCCs (Table 5.3). Keratin intermediate filaments are detectable in 19 % of PNET/Ewing sarcomas,

Table 5.3 Key diagnostic features

Proliferation of small-/medium-sized basaloid cells with round to oval nuclei
Granular chromatin pattern with inconspicuous or small nucleoli and scant cytoplasm
Nodular or trabecular growth pattern with infiltrative features at the periphery
Dermal-based tumor; epidermotropism in 10 % of cases
High mitotic index with individual apoptotic/necrotic cells
Vascular stroma with variable amounts of collagen and mucin
Frequent lymphovascular invasion
CK20 and neurofilament paranuclear dot immunopositivity

making keratin stains of limited use in this differential diagnosis [48]. Patient age can be a helpful distinguishing factor as tumors of the PNET/Ewing sarcoma family occur primarily in people under age 30, while MCC typically affects older adults. If CD99 positivity is present in tumors in this differential diagnosis, definitive differentiation may require molecular analysis with fluorescence in situ hybridization or polymerase chain reaction for characteristic chromosomal translocations.

Diagnostic Tools Under Development

Comparative Genomic Hybridization

Molecular techniques are becoming increasingly utilized in dermatopathology. Array-based comparative genomic hybridization (aCGH) permits screening of the entire genome for chromosomal copy number gain or loss and can be performed on formalin-fixed paraffin embedded tissue samples. Sixty to ninety percent of examples of MCC have chromosomal aberrations detectable by CGH, with more aggressive tumors harboring a greater number of aberrations [18, 19]. Gain involving chromosome 1 (frequently 1q11 or 1p34) is reported in up to 63 % of cases [49]. Other regions with commonly observed gain include 6p (42 %), 8q (38 %), 5p (32 %), and 3q (33 %). Chromosome 3p is the most frequently reported loss in studies and can be seen in up to

46 % of cases [49]. Loss in 13q (33 %), 5q (21 %), and 10q (33 %) are also commonly found. As recurring patterns of gain and loss are present, detection of these aberrations by CGH could potentially be used as an ancillary test to assist in diagnosis. In addition, while certain gains or losses are found more frequently than others, each individual tumor tends to have a unique CGH profile which can be used to distinguish metastatic MCC from a second primary MCC [20].

Gene Expression Profiling

Analyzing RNA from tumors to explore gene expression levels can provide insight into the oncogenesis of various cancers and assist with tumor classification. One study using cDNA microarrays to analyze the RNA from ten MCC cell lines and four small cell lung carcinoma cell lines identified 17 classifier genes that were capable of discriminating MCC from small cell lung carcinoma [50]. Other differentially expressed genes were able to discriminate different subtypes of MCC. While the more economical immunohistochemical studies are the preferred method for distinguishing MCC from other neoplasms, gene expression profiling could be used in exceptionally difficult cases. Further research in this area may lead to gene classifier systems with prognostic value as well.

Evidence-Based Findings of Prognostic Significance

Histopathologic Prognostic Markers

Numerous studies have explored potential histopathologic findings of prognostic value in MCC. Tumor size and thickness, along with lymphovascular invasion, have been shown to have prognostic value in multiple studies [15]. In a study of 156 patients with MCC, patients with a tumor thickness <5 mm had a 94 % 5-year survival [15]. Those with tumors ranging from 5 to 10 mm, 10 to 20 mm, and >20 mm had 5-year survival rates of 77 %, 61 %, and 44 %, respectively. A similar pattern was present when tumor size, defined as the greatest tumor dimension, was measured. In cases with lymphovascular invasion defined as tumor in vessels outside the main tumor mass, the 5-year survival was 54 % for positive cases and 90 % for negative cases. Tumor growth pattern is another feature found in some studies to hold prognostic value, with infiltrative tumors having a poorer prognosis than ones with a nodular pattern [15]. One study reported an inverse relationship with survival and mitotic rate (univariate analysis) [21], but other studies have not found a similar relationship.

Tumor-Infiltrating Lymphocytes and CD8

Studies assessing the presence of tumor-infiltrating lymphocytes by conventional microscopy are inconsistent, ranging from improved survival [15] to no survival relationship [51] to decreased survival [52]. Due to the conflicting studies, the evidence supporting a prognostic value of tumor-infiltrating lymphocytes identified by routine microscopy is questionable. However, when cytotoxic lymphocytes are specifically identified via CD8 staining, the presence of numerous CD8+ lymphocytes within tumor aggregations does appear to have prognostic value. In a study assessing 146 examples of MCC for intratumoral CD8+ lymphocytes, cases with scores ≥2 (equivalent to approximately 45 or more CD8+ intratumoral lymphocytes/high power field) had a 100 % survival compared to around 60 % survival for cases with a score <2 [51]. The results of this study have not yet been duplicated.

p63

Immunostaining for p63, a member of the p53 family of transcription factors, has the highest reported predictive value of all immunomarkers in MCC. A study of 47 cases with p63 showed a 53 % positivity rate [53]. The 5-year survival rate for positive cases was 7 % compared to 95 %

for negative cases (hazard ratio 22.2). The prognostic value of p63 has been confirmed in a subsequent study as well [54].

Vascular Markers (D2-40, CD34, and CD31)

Lymphovascular invasion is common in MCC, with intravascular tumor cells present in 56–93 % of cases in two large studies [10, 11]. While vascular invasion can frequently be seen in conventional sections, immunohistochemical markers that highlight vascular spaces can increase detection of vascular invasion. A few early studies [21] did not find a significant relationship between lymphovascular invasion and survival, but these studies did not use vascular immunostains to detect invasion. Multiple subsequent studies using vascular immunostains have demonstrated this to be a prognostic marker of significance [10, 11, 15].

The wide variation in the rate at which lymphovascular invasion is reported may stem from the use of different definitions of vascular invasion. In a study of 500 cases of MCC using routine staining supplemented with D2-40 immunostaining, lymphovascular invasion was defined as tumor cells within vessels outside the main tumor mass and was present in 56 % of cases [10]. In a study of 126 cases using conventional microscopy, D2-40, and CD31, vascular invasion was defined as tumor cells within any vessel and was present in 93 % of cases [11]. CD31 detected only four cases that D2-40 did not (so-called blood vascular invasion) and was therefore not responsible for the higher positivity rate. As would be expected, the stricter definition of vascular invasion limited to tumor cells in vessels outside the tumor mass holds stronger prognostic value.

In practice, each case of MCC should be evaluated for lymphovascular invasion in conventional sections. If not detected, additional staining with a vascular marker such as D2-40 or CD34 is warranted. The addition of CD31 appears to yield very minimal benefit. In addition to identifying lymphovascular invasion, vascular markers can also quantify vascular density in a tumor. One study of 36 cases of MCC with CD34 immunostaining found that increased vascular density identified with the immunostain was associated with a worse prognosis [55].

Ki-67/MIB-1

Studies assessing the prognostic value of Ki-67 have produced inconsistent results. A Ki-67 proliferation rate/labeling index greater than 65 % was associated with decreased survival in a univariate analysis in one study but lost statistical significance in the multivariate analysis (hazard ratio 2.9, $p=0.83$) [53]. Similarly, another study reported a significant negative prognostic relationship for Ki-67 rate >50 % and disease-free interval in univariate analysis, but statistical significance was lost in the multivariate analysis [56]. Another study reported a 35 % threshold for Ki-67 positivity and prognostic significance in the development of metastatic disease [57]. In contrast to these studies, numerous studies exist reporting no statistically significant prognostic relationship with Ki-67 labeling index [57].

Merkel Cell Polyomavirus

There are conflicting data regarding the prognostic significance of Merkel cell polyomavirus (MCPyV) status. One study in Finland detected MCPyV DNA by PCR in 80 % of 114 carcinomas. Those with detectable MCPyV had a 5-year survival of 45 % vs. 13 % for MCPyV-negative cases [58]. In a subsequent study, these authors found good correlation with immunopositivity for MCPyV large T antigen and the presence of tumoral MCPyV DNA, both of which corresponded to a favorable prognosis [59]. A study of 174 carcinomas from Germany and Australia did not find a statistically significant prognostic relationship between MCPyV status and survival [60]. While there may be some positive prognostic value in the detection of MCPyV in MCC, conflicting studies necessitate further validation through additional studies before a definitive conclusion can be drawn.

Adhesion Molecules (Cadherins)

Normal Merkel cells adhere to adjacent keratinocytes via desmosome-like attachments involving E- and P-cadherin, desmoglein 2, and desmocollin 2 [61]. In contrast to regular Merkel cells, 90 % of MCCs express N-cadherin and decreased levels of E- and P-cadherin. In a study of 26 cases of MCC with 9 local recurrences and 15 lymph node metastases, 77 % of the primary tumors and 78 % of the recurrences expressed P-cadherin. In contrast, only 33 % of the lymph node metastases expressed P-cadherin ($p=0.006$) [61]. An additional study showed that the presence of P-cadherin in the primary tumor conferred a statistically significant prolonged recurrence-free survival over tumors not expressing P-cadherin [62].

Retinoblastoma and p53

The MCPyV large T antigen interacts with the tumor suppressor retinoblastoma (Rb), which has been found to be elevated in cases with evidence of MCPyV infection [59, 63]. Increased Rb was found to be associated with improved survival in a univariate analysis. When controlling for MCPyV status in a multivariate analysis, Rb was not an independent prognostic factor [59]. A study reporting no significant relationship with MCPyV infection and Rb overexpression has also been published [64].

Expression of p53 reportedly exhibits an expression pattern opposite of Rb and is frequently overexpressed in tumors without evidence of MCPyV. Mutational analysis has confirmed that the majority of the tumors overexpressing p53 do harbor *TP53* mutations [59]. As would be expected, the Finland research group found that p53 overexpression was associated with a decreased disease-specific and overall survival [65]. Patients whose tumors lacked p53 expression and had detectable MCPyV DNA had the best prognosis in their study. The association of increased p53 expression and decreased survival has been reported in other studies as well [66]. Studies reporting no significant prognostic value for p53 have also been published [67].

Miscellaneous Markers

A nuclear immunostaining pattern of survivin, a negative regulator of apoptosis, has been associated with aggressive disease in one small study [68]. Elevated numbers of mast cells detected by a tryptase stain was associated with a less favorable prognosis in a study of 36 cases of MCC [69]. Overexpression of peptidyl-prolyl isomerase (PIN1) [70], CD9 [71], and Patched and Indian hedgehog [72] has been associated with a favorable prognosis in small single studies. Decreased expression of K homology domain-containing protein overexpressed in cancer (KOC) has also been associated with a favorable prognosis in one small study [73].

Conclusions

MCC and other neuroendocrine tumors have histopathologic features that are often characterized as small blue cell tumors. While there are distinguishing features that can help separate these tumors from other entities in that differential diagnosis, the similar appearance of the different types of neuroendocrine tumors, as well as overlapping features with hematologic malignancies and other poorly differentiated carcinomas, typically necessitates the use of confirmatory immunostains for diagnosis. Common pitfalls in the histopathologic differential diagnosis are listed in Table 5.4. With respect to prognosis, there is relatively good evidence that tumor size and thickness, as well as lymphovascular invasion, are reliable prognostic parameters. Some immunostains (p63, CD8+ lymphocytes) have shown promise as prognostic indicators, but the level of evidence for these studies falls in the III–IV range due to the small sample sizes and retrospective nature of these studies. Molecular techniques such as aCGH and expression profiling are powerful tools that permit investigation of pathology at the genetic level and have provided additional diagnostic and prognostic insights in MCC.

Table 5.4 Common diagnostic errors

Overlooking MCC in composite tumors of MCC with SCC or BCC
Misdiagnosis of MCC as BCC due to the presence of a basaloid tumor with crush artifact or a fibromyxoid stroma
Failure to exclude histopathologic mimics, especially metastatic neuroendocrine carcinoma, with proper immunostains
Misinterpreting intraepidermal MCC as a melanocytic proliferation, an epidermotropic lymphocytic infiltrate, or pagetoid SCC in situ
Misinterpreting MCC as lymphoma due to a juxtaposed lymphoid infiltrate
Misinterpreting MCC as large cell lymphoma due to expression of some hematologic markers
Failure to diagnose MCC due to inadequate immunohistochemical workup (i.e., not obtaining additional stains beyond CK20)

References

1. Szeder V, Grim M, Halata Z, Sieber-Blum M. Neural crest origin of mammalian Merkel cells. Dev Biol. 2003;253(2):258–63.
2. Van Keymeulen A, Mascre G, Youseff KK, et al. Epidermal progenitors give rise to Merkel cells during embryonic development and adult homeostasis. J Cell Biol. 2009;187(1):91–100.
3. Toker C. Trabecular carcinoma of the skin. Arch Dermatol. 1972;105(1):107–10.
4. Tang CK, Toker C. Trabecular carcinoma of the skin: an ultrastructural study. Cancer. 1978;42(5):2311–21.
5. De Wolff-Peeters C, Marien K, Mebis J, Desmet V. A cutaneous APUDoma or Merkel cell tumor? A morphologically recognizable tumor with a biological and histological malignant aspect in contrast with its clinical behavior. Cancer. 1980;46(8):1810–6.
6. Hoefler H, Kerl H, Rauch HJ, Denk H. New immunocytochemical observations with diagnostic significance in cutaneous neuroendocrine carcinoma. Am J Dermatopathol. 1984;6(6):525–30.
7. Rocamora A, Badia N, Vives R, Carrillo R, Ulloa J, Ledo A. Epidermotropic primary neuroendocrine (Merkel cell) carcinoma of the skin with Pautrier-like microabscesses. Report of three cases and review of the literature. J Am Acad Dermatol. 1987;16(6):1163–8.
8. Leong AS, Phillips GE, Pieterse AS, Milios J. Criteria for the diagnosis of primary endocrine carcinoma of the skin (Merkel cell carcinoma). A histological, immunohistochemical and ultrastructural study of 13 cases. Pathology. 1986;18(4):393–9.
9. Kuwamoto S, Higaki H, Kanai K, et al. Association of Merkel cell polyomavirus infection with morphologic differences in Merkel cell carcinoma. Hum Pathol. 2011;42(5):632–40.
10. Fields RC, Busam KJ, Chou JF, et al. Five hundred patients with Merkel cell carcinoma evaluated at a single institution. Ann Surg. 2011;254(3):465–73; discussion 473–465.
11. Kukko HM, Koljonen VS, Tukiainen EJ, Haglund CH, Bohling TO. Vascular invasion is an early event in pathogenesis of Merkel cell carcinoma. Mod Pathol. 2010;23(8):1151–6.
12. Ball NJ, Tanhuanco-Kho G. Merkel cell carcinoma frequently shows histologic features of basal cell carcinoma: a study of 30 cases. J Cutan Pathol. 2007;34(8):612–9.
13. Plaza JA, Suster S. The Toker tumor: spectrum of morphologic features in primary neuroendocrine carcinomas of the skin (Merkel cell carcinoma). Ann Diagn Pathol. 2006;10(6):376–85.
14. Leong AS, Dixon BR. Bidirectional differentiation in a large cell pleomorphic primary endocrine carcinoma of the skin (a variant of malignant Merkel cell tumour). Pathology. 1986;18(2):256–61.
15. Andea AA, Coit DG, Amin B, Busam KJ. Merkel cell carcinoma: histologic features and prognosis. Cancer. 2008;113(9):2549–58.
16. Fields RC, Busam KJ, Chou JF, et al. Recurrence and survival in patients undergoing sentinel lymph node biopsy for merkel cell carcinoma: analysis of 153 patients from a single institution. Ann Surg Oncol. 2011;18(9):2529–37.
17. Koljonen V, Bohling T, Virolainen S. Tumor burden of sentinel lymph node metastasis in Merkel cell carcinoma. J Cutan Pathol. 2011;38(6):508–13.
18. Larramendy ML, Koljonen V, Bohling T, Tukiainen E, Knuutila S. Recurrent DNA copy number changes revealed by comparative genomic hybridization in primary Merkel cell carcinomas. Mod Pathol. 2004;17(5):561–7.
19. Paulson KG, Lemos BD, Feng B, et al. Array-CGH reveals recurrent genomic changes in Merkel cell carcinoma including amplification of L-Myc. J Invest Dermatol. 2009;129(6):1547–55.
20. Ahronowitz IZ, Daud AI, Leong SP, et al. An isolated Merkel cell carcinoma metastasis at a distant cutaneous site presenting as a second 'primary' tumor. J Cutan Pathol. 2011;38(10):801–7.
21. Skelton HG, Smith KJ, Hitchcock CL, McCarthy WF, Lupton GP, Graham JH. Merkel cell carcinoma: analysis of clinical, histologic, and immunohistologic features of 132 cases with relation to survival. J Am Acad Dermatol. 1997;37(5 Pt 1):734–9.
22. Sarma DP, Heagley DE, Chalupa J, Cox M, Shehan JM. An unusual clinical presentation of merkel cell carcinoma: a case report. Case Report Med. 2010; 2010:905414.
23. Walsh NM. Primary neuroendocrine (Merkel cell) carcinoma of the skin: morphologic diversity and implications thereof. Hum Pathol. 2001;32(7): 680–9.

24. Battistella M, Durand L, Jouary T, Peltre B, Cribier B. Primary cutaneous neuroendocrine carcinoma within a cystic trichoblastoma: a nonfortuitous association? Am J Dermatopathol. 2011;33(4):383–7.
25. Barroeta JE, Farkas T. Merkel cell carcinoma and chronic lymphocytic leukemia (collision tumor) of the arm: a diagnosis by fine-needle aspiration biopsy. Diagn Cytopathol. 2007;35(5):293–5.
26. Forman SB, Vidmar DA, Ferringer TC. Collision tumor composed of Merkel cell carcinoma and lentigo maligna melanoma. J Cutan Pathol. 2008;35(2):203–6.
27. Youker SR, Billingsley EM. Combined Merkel cell carcinoma and atypical fibroxanthoma. J Cutan Med Surg. 2005;9(1):6–9.
28. Tanahashi J, Kashima K, Daa T, Yada N, Fujiwara S, Yokoyama S. Merkel cell carcinoma co-existent with sebaceous carcinoma of the eyelid. J Cutan Pathol. 2009;36(9):983–6.
29. Tilkorn DJ, Lehnhardt M, Hauser J, et al. Merkel cell carcinoma metastasis and dermatofibrosarcoma protuberans presenting as a collision tumour: a case report and review of the literature. J Med Case Reports. 2009;3:7493.
30. Gould E, Albores-Saavedra J, Dubner B, Smith W, Payne CM. Eccrine and squamous differentiation in Merkel cell carcinoma. An immunohistochemical study. Am J Surg Pathol. 1988;12(10):768–72.
31. Hallman JR, Shaw JA, Geisinger KR, Loggie BW, White WL. Cytomorphologic features of Merkel cell carcinoma in fine needle aspiration biopsies. A study of two atypical cases. Acta Cytol. 2000;44(2):185–93.
32. Adhikari LA, McCalmont TH, Folpe AL. Merkel cell carcinoma with heterologous rhabdomyoblastic differentiation: the role of immunohistochemistry for Merkel cell polyomavirus large T-antigen in confirmation. J Cutan Pathol. 2012;39(1):47–51.
33. Cooper L, Debono R, Alsanjari N, Al-Nafussi A. Merkel cell tumour with leiomyosarcomatous differentiation. Histopathology. 2000;36(6):540–3.
34. Tan KB, Murali R, Karim RZ, et al. Merkel cell carcinoma with fibrosarcomatous differentiation. Pathology. 2008;40(3):314–6.
35. Vanchinathan V, Marinelli EC, Kartha RV, Uzieblo A, Ranchod M, Sundram UN. A malignant cutaneous neuroendocrine tumor with features of Merkel cell carcinoma and differentiating neuroblastoma. Am J Dermatopathol. 2009;31(2):193–6.
36. Kossard S, Wittal R, Killingsworth M. Merkel cell carcinoma with a desmoplastic portion. Am J Dermatopathol. 1995;17(5):517–22.
37. Hashimoto K, Lee MW, D'Annunzio DR, Balle MR, Narisawa Y. Pagetoid Merkel cell carcinoma: epidermal origin of the tumor. J Cutan Pathol. 1998;25(10):572–9.
38. Vazmitel M, Michal M, Kazakov DV. Merkel cell carcinoma and Azzopardi phenomenon. Am J Dermatopathol. 2007;29(3):314–5.
39. Acebo E, Vidaurrazaga N, Varas C, Burgos-Bretones JJ, Diaz-Perez JL. Merkel cell carcinoma: a clinicopathological study of 11 cases. J Eur Acad Dermatol Venereol. 2005;19(5):546–51.
40. George E, Swanson PE, Wick MR. Neuroendocrine differentiation in basal cell carcinoma. An immunohistochemical study. Am J Dermatopathol. 1989;11(2):131–5.
41. Rosso R, Paulli M, Carnevali L. Neuroendocrine carcinoma of the skin with lymphoepithelioma-like features. Am J Dermatopathol. 1998;20(5):483–6.
42. Rund CR, Fischer EG. Perinuclear dot-like cytokeratin 20 staining in small cell neuroendocrine carcinoma of the ovary (pulmonary-type). Appl Immunohistochem Mol Morphol. 2006;14(2):244–8.
43. Wong A, McCalmont T. Neurofilament is superior to CK20 for the identification of Merkel cell carcinoma: A review of 351 cases. J Cutan Pathol. 2012;39(1):97.
44. Shah IA, Netto D, Schlageter MO, Muth C, Fox I, Manne RK. Neurofilament immunoreactivity in Merkel-cell tumors: a differentiating feature from small-cell carcinoma. Mod Pathol. 1993;6(1):3–9.
45. Calder KB, Coplowitz S, Schlauder S, Morgan MB. A case series and immunophenotypic analysis of CK20-/CK7+ primary neuroendocrine carcinoma of the skin. J Cutan Pathol. 2007;34(12):918–23.
46. Wick MR, Millns JL, Sibley RK, Pittelkow MR, Winkelmann RK. Secondary neuroendocrine carcinomas of the skin. An immunohistochemical comparison with primary neuroendocrine carcinoma of the skin ("Merkel cell" carcinoma). J Am Acad Dermatol. 1985;13(1):134–42.
47. Bastian BC, Kreipe HH, Brocker EB. Primary neuroendocrine carcinoma of the skin with an unusual follicular lymphocytic infiltrate of the dermis. Am J Dermatopathol. 1996;18(6):625–8.
48. Machado I, Navarro S, Lopez-Guerrero JA, Alberghini M, Picci P, Llombart-Bosch A. Epithelial marker expression does not rule out a diagnosis of Ewing's sarcoma family of tumours. Virchows Arch. 2011;459(4):409–14.
49. Van Gele M, Leonard JH, Van Roy N, et al. Combined karyotyping, CGH and M-FISH analysis allows detailed characterization of unidentified chromosomal rearrangements in Merkel cell carcinoma. Int J Cancer. 2002;101(2):137–45.
50. Van Gele M, Boyle GM, Cook AL, et al. Gene-expression profiling reveals distinct expression patterns for classic versus variant Merkel cell phenotypes and new classifier genes to distinguish Merkel cell from small-cell lung carcinoma. Oncogene. 2004;23(15):2732–42.
51. Paulson KG, Iyer JG, Tegeder AR, et al. Transcriptome-wide studies of merkel cell carcinoma and validation of intratumoral CD8+ lymphocyte invasion as an independent predictor of survival. J Clin Oncol. 2011;29(12):1539–46.
52. Mott RT, Smoller BR, Morgan MB. Merkel cell carcinoma: a clinicopathologic study with prognostic implications. J Cutan Pathol. 2004;31(3):217–23.
53. Asioli S, Righi A, Volante M, Eusebi V, Bussolati G. p63 expression as a new prognostic marker in Merkel cell carcinoma. Cancer. 2007;110(3):640–7.
54. Hall B, Pincus L, Yu S, Oh D, Wilson A, McCalmont T. Immunohistochemical prognostication of Merkel

cell carcinoma: p63 expression but not polyomavirus status correlates with outcome. J Cutan Pathol. 2012; 39(10):911–7.
55. Ng L, Beer TW, Murray K. Vascular density has prognostic value in Merkel cell carcinoma. Am J Dermatopathol. 2008;30(5):442–5.
56. Llombart B, Monteagudo C, Lopez-Guerrero JA, et al. Clinicopathological and immunohistochemical analysis of 20 cases of Merkel cell carcinoma in search of prognostic markers. Histopathology. 2005; 46(6):622–34.
57. Koljonen V, Tukiainen E, Haglund C, Bohling T. Proliferative activity detected by Ki67 correlates with poor outcome in Merkel cell carcinoma. Histopathology. 2006;49(5):551–3.
58. Sihto H, Kukko H, Koljonen V, Sankila R, Bohling T, Joensuu H. Clinical factors associated with Merkel cell polyomavirus infection in Merkel cell carcinoma. J Natl Cancer Inst. 2009;101(13):938–45.
59. Sihto H, Kukko H, Koljonen V, Sankila R, Bohling T, Joensuu H. Merkel cell polyomavirus infection, large T antigen, retinoblastoma protein and outcome in Merkel cell carcinoma. Clin Cancer Res. 2011;17(14): 4806–13.
60. Schrama D, Peitsch WK, Zapatka M, et al. Merkel cell polyomavirus status is not associated with clinical course of Merkel cell carcinoma. J Invest Dermatol. 2011;131(8):1631–8.
61. Werling AM, Doerflinger Y, Brandner JM, et al. Homo- and heterotypic cell-cell contacts in Merkel cells and Merkel cell carcinomas: heterogeneity and indications for cadherin switching. Histopathology. 2011;58(2):286–303.
62. Vlahova L, Doerflinger Y, Houben R, et al. P-cadherin expression in Merkel cell carcinomas is associated with prolonged recurrence-free survival. Br J Dermatol. 2012;166(5):1043–52.
63. Bhatia K, Goedert JJ, Modali R, Preiss L, Ayers LW. Merkel cell carcinoma subgroups by Merkel cell polyomavirus DNA relative abundance and oncogene expression. Int J Cancer. 2010;126(9):2240–6.
64. Houben R, Schrama D, Alb M, et al. Comparable expression and phosphorylation of the retinoblastoma protein in Merkel cell polyoma virus-positive and negative Merkel cell carcinoma. Int J Cancer. 2010; 126(3):796–8.
65. Waltari M, Sihto H, Kukko H, et al. Association of Merkel cell polyomavirus infection with tumor p53, KIT, stem cell factor, PDGFR-alpha and survival in Merkel cell carcinoma. Int J Cancer. 2011;129(3): 619–28.
66. Carson HJ, Reddy V, Taxy JB. Proliferation markers and prognosis in Merkel cell carcinoma. J Cutan Pathol. 1998;25(1):16–9.
67. Feinmesser M, Halpern M, Fenig E, et al. Expression of the apoptosis-related oncogenes bcl-2, bax, and p53 in Merkel cell carcinoma: can they predict treatment response and clinical outcome? Hum Pathol. 1999;30(11):1367–72.
68. Kim J, McNiff JM. Nuclear expression of survivin portends a poor prognosis in Merkel cell carcinoma. Mod Pathol. 2008;21(6):764–9.
69. Beer TW, Ng LB, Murray K. Mast cells have prognostic value in Merkel cell carcinoma. Am J Dermatopathol. 2008;30(1):27–30.
70. Lill C, Schneider S, Pammer J, et al. Significant correlation of peptidyl-prolyl isomerase overexpression in merkel cell carcinoma with overall survival of patients. Head Neck. 2010;33(9):1294–300.
71. Woegerbauer M, Thurnher D, Houben R, et al. Expression of the tetraspanins CD9, CD37, CD63, and CD151 in Merkel cell carcinoma: strong evidence for a posttranscriptional fine-tuning of CD9 gene expression. Mod Pathol. 2010;23(5):751–62.
72. Brunner M, Thurnher D, Pammer J, et al. Expression of hedgehog signaling molecules in Merkel cell carcinoma. Head Neck. 2010;32(3):333–40.
73. Pryor JG, Simon RA, Bourne PA, Spaulding BO, Scott GA, Xu H. Merkel cell carcinoma expresses K homology domain-containing protein overexpressed in cancer similar to other high-grade neuroendocrine carcinomas. Hum Pathol. 2009;40(2):238–43.

Part III

Therapy

Local Excision (Primary, Recurrent Disease)

6

Melanie Warycha and Murad Alam

Introduction and History

Merkel cell carcinoma was first described by Toker in 1972 as "trabecular carcinoma" and later characterized as an aggressive tumor of neuroendocrine origin, arising as an asymptomatic erythematous to violaceous papule or nodule on sun-exposed skin [1]. Since this initial report, at least 2,000 cases of Merkel cell carcinoma have been reported in the literature, with an estimated 1,400 new cases diagnosed each year in the United States [2, 3]. While advances in the molecular biology and pathogenesis of Merkel cell carcinoma have been recently elucidated, the rarity of this tumor has prevented establishment of validated prognostic indicators and treatment guidelines [4]. In fact, management decisions up to this point remain controversial and have been based primarily on retrospective case reports and case series, with no prospective randomized trials to date. While wide surgical excision with margins of at least 2–3 cm was initially recommended for primary treatment of this tumor, many reports have since shown histopathologic clearance with even narrower margins. Mohs surgery has also emerged as an effective treatment modality for primary Merkel cell carcinoma. In this chapter, we comprehensively review the surgical management of Merkel cell carcinoma and offer an evidence-based treatment algorithm by which to manage this aggressive tumor.

M. Warycha
Mount Kisco Medical Group, Department of Dermatology, 110 South Bedford Road, Mount Kisco, NY 10549, USA
e-mail: melanie.warycha@gmail.com

M. Alam (✉)
Department of Dermatology, Northwestern University, 676 North St. Clair Street, Suite 1600, Chicago, IL 60611, USA
e-mail: m-alam@northwestern.edu

Patient Selection

Prior to proceeding with surgery, it is important to have the histopathology reviewed by a dermatopathologist with adequate experience in identifying Merkel cell carcinoma. As certain histopathologic criteria, like lymphovascular invasion and mitotic rate, have been associated with survival, it is important to have this information documented [5, 6]. Once the diagnosis has been confirmed, patients with primary Merkel cell carcinoma should be promptly referred for surgical evaluation, including either standard wide excision or Mohs surgery, the data for which will be presented later in this chapter. In devising a treatment strategy, the size of the tumor should be assessed as this will help guide whether a surgical approach is feasible or not, keeping in mind that most lesions will need at least a 1 cm margin to achieve histopathologic clearance. A detailed medical and surgical history should also be obtained. Given that these tumors often occur in the elderly, comorbidities need to be considered, with patients referred for presurgical clearance

M. Alam et al. (eds.), *Merkel Cell Carcinoma*, DOI 10.1007/978-1-4614-6608-6_6,

when warranted. A comprehensive skin examination is useful, with focused attention on the presence or absence of satellite lesions, in-transit metastases, and mucosal or eye involvement. A lymph node examination may reveal nodal metastases, which are common, and may alter treatment. Anticoagulant medications that are not medically necessary, including such supplements as garlic, fish oil, and vitamin E, in addition to alcohol, may be discontinued at least 1 week prior to the procedure. In planning the surgery and eventual repair, especially when the tumor is on the head and neck, efforts are typically made to preserve anatomic function and limit disfigurement. The extent of the procedure and anticipated cosmetic outcome is discussed thoroughly with the patient prior to surgery so that reasonable expectations can be set and questions answered. Some physicians may prefer to delay repair until final histopathologic clearance has been confirmed by additional tests or special stains. Given the multitude of treatment options available for Merkel cell carcinoma, including surgery, radiation therapy, and chemotherapy, it is advisable to consider a multidisciplinary approach in the management of this tumor. It may be prudent to seek early consultation from various specialties, including as appropriate dermatology, surgical oncology, plastic surgery, oncology, radiation oncology, otolaryngology, or ophthalmology, in order to formulate a plan of care. This is particularly relevant in patients who present with locally unresectable lesions, for which data regarding the appropriate treatment strategy is lacking, or those who are too ill to undergo extensive procedures. When available, participation in a multidisciplinary tumor board may facilitate collaboration and expedite treatment.

Although the role of sentinel lymph node biopsy in the management of Merkel cell carcinoma is discussed in detail in a separate chapter, the 2012 NCCN Guidelines now recommend this procedure in primary Merkel cell carcinomas of the trunk and extremities (as a qualifier, the NCCN Guidelines are neither prescriptive or comprehensive nor forward-looking, but rather are a reporting of the most prevalent current therapeutic approaches at the relatively small number of participating cancer centers) [7]. Given the unpredictable lymphatic drainage patterns of the head and neck, with resultant high rates of false negativity, sentinel lymph node biopsy is not yet universally recommended for patients with primary Merkel cell carcinoma occurring in these locations, although this option is reasonable to consider and discuss with the patient. In fact, some institutions recommend sentinel lymph node biopsy for all patients with Merkel cell carcinoma, irrespective of its primary site. If the decision to undergo sentinel lymph node biopsy has been made, this procedure should be scheduled either before or concurrently with surgical excision or Mohs surgery in order to ensure reliable results.

Treatment of Primary Carcinoma

According to the 2012 NCCN Guidelines, local wide excision with 1–2 cm margins to fascia of muscle or pericranium is advised for the treatment of primary Merkel cell carcinoma, with the goal of negative surgical margins [7]. If necessary, re-excisions are recommended until margins are clear, but functional and anatomic distortions are ideally minimized. Given the high risk of local and lymph node recurrences, some surgeons may opt to take an additional 5–10 mm margin beyond histologic clearance [8]. In addition to local wide excision, Mohs surgery can also be considered for primary Merkel cell carcinoma, and in fact, may be preferred in cases where surgical margins are close to the periphery or remain positive [7]. Mohs surgery can be particularly advantageous for tumors with clinically indistinct margins or those located on the head and neck, particularly in the periocular or perioral region, where tissue sparing is of utmost concern. If Mohs surgery is selected, the diagnosis of Merkel cell carcinoma is routinely established based on formalin-fixed sections prior to the Mohs procedure [9]. Lastly, a modified Mohs surgery procedure where the final margin is sent for permanent sections, and repair is delayed until clear margins are confirmed, is also an acceptable treatment strategy.

Evidence-Based Findings

To date, randomized controlled trials evaluating surgical margins or comparing wide local excision to Mohs surgery in the treatment of primary Merkel cell carcinoma do not exist. Much of the current data on management of Merkel cell carcinoma is derived from retrospective reviews, case reports, and case series. In attempting to critically analyze the existing literature, several challenges arise. First, the rarity of this tumor has restricted accumulation of sample sizes large enough to perform meaningful statistical analyses, with most studies being underpowered. Second, the lack of standardized treatment regimens, outcome measures, and staging systems makes direct comparisons between publications difficult. Furthermore, only a handful of studies specifically comment on the risk for recurrence and disease-specific survival in patients who were treated with surgery alone. This may be due to the fact that a significant number of patients have advanced disease that warrants aggressive management, including a combination of surgery, lymphadenectomy, adjuvant radiation, and/or chemotherapy, thus making it difficult to separately assess the impact of surgery. Lastly, case series with larger sample sizes are often from tertiary referral centers, where selection bias may be a concern. Despite these inherent shortcomings, important information has been derived from these retrospective analyses and has proven invaluable in guiding treatment decisions. Below, several key observations and findings regarding the surgical management of primary Merkel cell carcinoma are discussed.

Common Approaches

Mohs Micrographic Surgery

A handful of studies have studied the use of Mohs surgery as a surgical treatment option for patients with primary Merkel cell carcinoma. Mohs surgery is a staged procedure in which frozen sections are examined to render a complete histologic assessment of the surgical margin, including lateral and deep margins. The principle of Mohs surgery relies on the fact that nonmelanoma skin cancers grow as contiguous tumors. Based on the available data, the recurrence rates for Merkel cell carcinoma after Mohs surgery compare favorably with those after wide local excision, as will be discussed below. This secondarily also suggests that early Merkel cell carcinoma grows in a contiguous pattern. That being said, more data is needed to validate this observation [8].

In a retrospective analysis of 13 patients with Merkel cell carcinoma (mean tumor diameter of 2.98 cm) treated with Mohs surgery at the Mayo clinic from 1975 to 1995, negative margins were achieved in 12 of 13 patients. Ten cases were histologically clear after one stage, one case after two stages, and one case after three stages. One patient with negative surgical margins who developed locally persistent disease was cleared after a second Mohs surgery procedure and remained disease-free at 84 months. Four of 12 patients with negative surgical margins underwent postoperative radiation and were disease-free at a mean follow-up time of 2 years. Four of the eight patients who did not undergo radiation treatment developed regional metastases at a mean follow-up time of 36 months. Overall, the recurrence rate in this cohort was 42 % (one local recurrence and four regional nodal metastases), which was similar to recurrence rates for patients undergoing wide local excision in this study [8].

A larger collaborative retrospective study by Boyer et al. included 45 patients with primary Merkel cell carcinoma, of which 25 were treated with Mohs surgery alone, 8 with Mohs surgery and radiation to the primary site, 12 with Mohs surgery and radiation to the primary site and regional lymph node basin, and 3 with Mohs surgery and either adjuvant chemotherapy or elective regional lymph node dissection. Of note, this study only included cases where tumor free margins were achieved following Mohs surgery. Overall, 48 % of tumors required less than a 1 cm margin, 25 % needed more than a 2 cm margin, and 12 % more than a 3 cm margin. In the group of patients treated with Mohs surgery alone, a local recurrence rate of 16 % was observed, including one recurrence contiguous with the primary excision scar and three in-transit metastases. In addition, four lymph node metastases (16 %) and two distant metastases (8 %) were observed as first sites of treatment failure. In patients treated with Mohs surgery and radiation, there were no cases of recurrence in the scar or in-transit metastases, although three lymph node metastases and one distant metastasis at sites of initial treatment failure were documented. The mean time to development of in-transit, lymph node, and distant metastases was 9, 11.4, and 15.7 months, respectively. Overall, there was no statistically significant difference across the treatment groups in the proportion of patients who developed local recurrences, in-transit metastases, lymph node metastases, or distant metastases. Similarly, there was no statistically significant difference in overall survival, overall disease-specific survival, relapse-free survival, or disease-free survival. This, of course, is in the context of treatment arms with small sample sizes [10]. The cumulative recurrence rate after Mohs surgery in this study compares favorably with those reported after wide local excision (4–14 %) [3, 10].

Eight cases of Merkel cell carcinoma treated with a modified Mohs technique utilizing permanent sections at the Scripps Health Hospitals from 1985 to 1996 were reviewed by Gollard et al. The average number of stages required for histologic clearance was 1.4, with an average margin of 1.5 cm (1.2 cm on the face and 1.9 cm on extremities). Three of the eight cases were treated with Mohs surgery alone, two on the head and neck and one on the extremity, with an average tumor size of 0.9 cm. None of these patients experienced recurrence. The remaining five patients received adjuvant radiation treatment (average tumor size 1.2 cm, three located on the head and neck, two on the extremity), and one of these went on to develop a lymph node recurrence and one a skin recurrence at 8 and 10 months, respectively. Mean follow-up time for this study was 37 months. No local recurrences were noted [11].

A retrospective study of nine patients with cutaneous Merkel cell carcinoma and one with mucosal involvement treated with Mohs surgery with or without adjuvant treatment at the University of Wisconsin-Madison from 1982 to 1999 was conducted by Snow et al. Negative histologic margins were not attained in one patient with mucosal involvement (of the nasal septum). Of the nine cutaneous cases, two developed local recurrences located on the scalp and temple, although these were large tumors, with Mohs surgery postoperative defect sizes of 6 cm and 3.5 cm, respectively. An additional two patients developed lymph node metastases. Overall, four of ten patients died of disease at a mean follow-up time of 2.7 years [12].

Although these initial studies describing small cohorts of Merkel cell carcinoma patients treated with Mohs surgery are promising, more data are needed to further elucidate the role of Mohs surgery in the surgical management of primary Merkel cell carcinoma and to see if Mohs offers a recurrence or survival advantage over wide local excision.

Wide Local Excision

Historically, many authors had recommended wide local excision with margins between 2.5 and 3 cm as the standard treatment for primary Merkel cell carcinoma. This algorithm was derived largely from an early retrospective analysis of 38 Merkel cell carcinoma patients treated at the Memorial Sloan–Kettering Cancer Center. In this study, increased local recurrence rates were observed in patients in whom surgical margins of 3 cm or less were taken. Despite the fact that this was only a trend and not a statistically significant finding ($p=0.16$), this convention of taking 2.5–3 cm margins remained pervasive as the treatment of choice for many years [13]. Given more recent data based on larger cohorts and more critical analyses, however, these surgical margins have been challenged. In fact, the association between margin status and outcome has been questioned. In 2005, an updated review based on the Memorial Sloan–Kettering Cancer Center registry was performed. In this study, data on surgical margin status was available on 196 patients with Merkel cell carcinoma. Negative margins were achieved in 185 (94 %) of 196 patients, and the average margin width was only 1.1 cm. Furthermore, local recurrence developed in 15 (8 %) of the 185 patients who underwent a margin-negative excision and in 2 (18 %) of the 11 patients who underwent a margin-positive excision ($p=0.31$). The study authors concluded that obtaining a surgical margin of more than 1 cm was not associated with a decreased local recurrence rate (<1 cm, 9 % local recurrence rate vs. ≥1 cm, 10 % local recurrence rate, $p=0.83$) [14]. Shifting forward to the most recent and comprehensive publication based on this registry, the outcomes of 412 patients with Merkel cell carcinoma diagnosed between 1969 and 2010 (with prospective enrollment from 2001), with a median tumor size of 1.3 cm, were analyzed. Of 324 patients with an intact primary tumor at presentation, 299 (92 %) had a margin-negative excision (including one amputation and one treated with Mohs surgery). Among those with a margin-negative excision, the median primary tumor excision margin width was 1 cm. In concordance with earlier analyses, surgical margin status was not associated with overall survival on multivariate analysis, with a median follow-up time of 3 years [5, 15]. Although publications based on large cohorts offer several advantages over smaller studies, including improved internal validity, these are limited by being single-institution findings and need to be validated on a more general population. To this end, a smaller study from Australia supports the recent MSKCC conclusions. In a retrospective review of Australian patients diagnosed with Merkel cell carcinoma between 1992 and 2004, 60 of 73 (82 %) patients had negative margins after wide local excision. In this analysis, neither the minimum margin of excision or involvement of the surgical margin after re-excision were significantly associated with survival on univariate or multivariate analyses at a median follow-up time of 23 months. Interestingly, disease in the surgical margin after the first excision was an independent predictor of survival, although this was of borderline significance ($p=0.049$) [16]. Conflicting results have been presented by Tai et al. who conducted a multicenter retrospective review of 145 cases of Merkel cell carcinoma treated between 1988 and 2007. In this study, a negative resection margin was found to be a statistically significant predictor of cause-specific survival and overall survival on multivariate analysis, with a median follow-up of 21.5 months. However, the median margin needed for histologic clearance was not provided [17]. Similarly, in a retrospective analysis of 95 consecutive patients with Merkel cell carcinoma who presented to the National Cancer Institute of Milan between 1980 and 2006, negative margins after wide local excision were associated with decreased recurrence and improved survival on multivariate analysis at a median follow-up time of 65 months. Wide local excision at this single institution was defined as margins of at least 2 cm whenever possible, although the investigators noted that achieving clear margins often necessitated re-excision [18]. Thus, although randomized controlled trials are lacking, recommendations for 1–2 cm margins to fascia of muscle or pericranium for the treatment of primary Merkel cell carcinoma as proposed by the NCCN appear a justified and reasonable surgical approach based on the available data to date [7].

Several retrospective reviews have also provided important information regarding the incidence of recurrence in Merkel cell carcinoma patients treated with surgery alone. In a retrospective review of 38 patients presenting to the Queensland Radium Institute between 1981 and 1991 for primary treatment of Merkel cell carcinoma, 34 of the 38 patients were treated with surgery alone with at least a 5 mm margin, with 15 of these 34 patients undergoing re-excision due to margin uncertainty and 2 of the 34 patients receiving lymph node dissections. The primary tumor could not be assessed in the remaining four patients, and thus they were treated with a combination of lymph node dissections and/or excision of skin metastases. In this study, all 38 patients developed relapse of disease at a median follow-up time of 20 months, with the pattern of first recurrence as follows: 2 with local recurrences, 27 with nodal recurrences, 6 with a combination of local and nodal recurrences, and 3 with a combination of nodal and distant recurrences, with a overall median time to recurrence of 5.5 months. Unfortunately, since the final margin status of patients after surgical excision was not reported, it is unclear if local disease control was attained even after re-excisions [19]. In a separate study of 36 patients with Merkel cell carcinoma who presented to the Department of Defense Medical System and St. Louis University Health Sciences Center from 1983 to 1996, there was a statistically significant higher rate of locoregional and distant recurrences in patients who underwent simple excision ($n = 18$) vs. wide excision ($n = 15$), with wide excision defined as having a margin greater than or equal to 2.5 cm. A multivariate analysis accounting for confounding factors, however, was not performed. The average time to locoregional and distant recurrence was determined to be 7.8 and 8.5 months, respectively, with a mean follow-up time of 31 months [20]. In a retrospective case series by O'Connor et al., 41 patients with clinically localized Merkel cell carcinoma were treated at the Mayo clinic from 1975 to 1995 and underwent wide local excision of 2.5–3 cm margins with no adjuvant treatment. In this sample, recurrent disease adjacent to the scar was documented in 13 of 41 (32 %) patients and regional metastases in 20 of 41 (49 %) patients, with a mean follow-up time of 60 months. Data on margin status was not provided [8]. Although conclusions are difficult to reach based on these data, the reviewed retrospective studies do confirm the high propensity for Merkel cell carcinoma to recur, often within a few months after diagnosis. Thus, adjuvant treatment beyond surgical interventions may be warranted as is discussed in a separate chapter.

Treatment of Recurrent Disease

While guidelines regarding the treatment of primary Merkel cell carcinoma remain controversial, even less data is available as to the optimal management of recurrent disease. Because of Merkel cell carcinoma's aggressive clinical course, it is not uncommon for patients with recurrent disease to partake of all available treatment options, including a combination of surgery, radiation, and chemotherapy [2]. As such, the NCCN Guidelines recommend individualized treatment for those patients presenting with local and regional recurrences. When available, clinical trials may be appropriate for those with disseminated disease. The treatment strategies utilized in 46 patients with recurrent Merkel cell carcinoma were presented in a small retrospective review by Eng et al. Of 25 patients who sought treatment of their disease, seven received local re-excision only, three received locoregional radiation only, one received chemotherapy only, and the remaining patients received a combination of surgery, radiation, and/or chemotherapy. In patients for which surgery was the sole treatment modality, a 57 % overall survival was noted at a median follow-up time after recurrence of 15 months. The authors proposed individualized multimodality therapy for patients presenting with recurrent Merkel cell carcinoma, including comprehensive salvage surgery for locally or nodally recurrent disease, if possible [21]. In another retrospective case series of 36 patients with Merkel cell carcinoma treated between 1984 and 1994 at the Netherlands Cancer Institute and the Heinrich-Heine-University Dusseldorf, 20 (61 %) patients developed locoregional recurrence. Of these, nine patients underwent salvage therapy with surgical resection and adjuvant radiation, with three alive with no evidence of disease, three alive with disease, and three dead from unrelated conditions at last follow-up. Five patients with unresectable recurrences were treated with radiation alone, and of these, three died of metastatic disease, one remains alive without disease at 6.6 years follow-up, and one is lost to follow-up [22]. Given the dearth of studies on recurrent Merkel cell carcinoma, with only small samples in these two retrospective series, it is nearly impossible to formulate an ideal treatment strategy for patients with recurrent disease. As emphasized before, an individualized plan of care is generally devised using a multidisciplinary approach, incorporating a combination of surgery, radiation, and chemotherapy, as deemed appropriate, and in close consultation with the patient.

Conclusions

- Randomized trials are not yet available to help guide surgical management of primary or recurrent Merkel cell carcinoma. The rationale behind treatment decisions is thus predominantly based on retrospective case series.
- Primary Merkel cell carcinoma should be treated early and aggressively with either wide surgical excision or Mohs surgery with the endpoint of clear surgical margins.
- While the most appropriate surgical margins remain to be determined, the NCCN currently recommends local wide excision with 1–2 cm margins to fascia of muscle or pericranium or Mohs surgery for the treatment of primary Merkel cell carcinoma.
- To date, there are no controlled trials comparing recurrence and/or survival rates in primary Merkel cell carcinoma patients treated with wide surgical excision vs. Mohs surgery.
- Based on retrospective reviews, Mohs surgery yields comparable recurrence and survival data as that published for wide surgical excision. However, more data is needed to further define the role of Mohs surgery in the surgical management of primary Merkel cell carcinoma.
- Although no definitive management strategy for recurrent Merkel cell carcinoma exists, aggressive treatment is advocated, including a combination of surgery, radiation, and/or chemotherapy.

References

1. Zhan FQ, Packianathan VS, Zeitouni NC. Merkel cell carcinoma: a review of current advances. J Natl Compr Canc Netw. 2009;7:333–9.
2. Ruan JH, Reeves M. A Merkel cell carcinoma treatment algorithm. Arch Surg. 2009;144(6):582–5.
3. Bichakjian CK, Lowe L, Lao CD, et al. Merkel cell carcinoma: critical review with guidelines for multidisciplinary management. Cancer. 2007;110:1–12.
4. Kuwamoto S. Recent advances in the biology of Merkel cell carcinoma. Hum Pathol. 2011;42(8):1063–77.
5. Fields RC, Busam KJ, Chou JF, et al. Five hundred patients with Merkel cell carcinoma evaluated at a single institution. Ann Surg. 2011;254(3):465–75.
6. Skelton HG, Smith KJ, Hitchcock CL, et al. Merkel cell carcinoma: analysis of clinical, histologic, and immunohistologic features of 132 cases with relation to survival. J Am Acad Dermatol. 1997;37:734–9.
7. National Comprehensive Cancer Network. NCCN Guidelines for treatment of Merkel cell carcinoma. 2012. http://www.nccn.org/professionals/physician_gls/f_guidelines.asp. Accessed 10 Oct 2012.
8. O'Connor WJ, Roenigk RK, Brodland DG. Merkel cell carcinoma: comparison of Mohs micrographic surgery and wide excision in eight-six patients. Dermatol Surg. 1997;23:929–33.
9. Roenigk RK, Goltz RW. Residents' corner: Merkel cell carcinoma—a problem with microscopically controlled surgery. J Dermatol Surg Oncol. 1986;12(4):332–6.
10. Boyer JD, Zitelli JA, Brodland DG, D'Angelo G. Local control of primary Merkel cell carcinoma: review of 45 cases treated with Mohs micrographic surgery with and without adjuvant radiation. J Am Acad Dermatol. 2002;47:885–92.
11. Gollard R, Weber R, Kosty MP, et al. Merkel cell carcinoma: review of 22 cases with surgical, pathologic, and therapeutic considerations. Cancer. 2000;88:1842–51.
12. Snow SN, Larson PO, Hardy S, et al. Merkel cell carcinoma of the skin and mucosa: report of 12 cutaneous cases with 2 cases arising from the nasal mucosa. Dermatol Surg. 2001;27:165–70.
13. Yiengpruksawan A, Coit DG, Thaler HT, et al. Merkel cell carcinoma prognosis and management. Arch Surg. 1991;126:1514–9.
14. Allen PJ, Bowne WB, Jaques DP, et al. Merkel cell carcinoma: prognosis and treatment of patients from a single institution. J Clin Oncol. 2005;23:2300–9.
15. Fields RC, Busam KJ, Chou JF, et al. Recurrence after complete resection and selective use of adjuvant therapy for stage I through III Merkel cell carcinoma. Cancer. 2012;118(13):3311–20.
16. Jabbour J, Cumming R, Scolyer RA, et al. Merkel cell carcinoma: assessing the effect of wide local excision, lymph node dissection, and radiotherapy on recurrence and survival in early-stage disease—results from a review of 82 consecutive cases diagnosed between 1992 and 2004. Ann Surg Oncol. 2007;14(6):1943–52.
17. Tai P, Yu E, Assouline A, et al. Management of Merkel cell carcinoma with emphasis on small primary tumors—a case series and review of the current literature. J Drugs Dermatol. 2010;9(2):105–10.
18. Bajetta E, Celio L, Platania M, et al. Single-institution series of early-stage Merkel cell carcinoma: long-term outcomes in 95 patients managed with surgery along. Ann Surg Oncol. 2009;16:2985–93.

19. Meeuwissen JA, Bourne RG, Kearsley JH. The importance of postoperative radiation therapy in the treatment of Merkel cell carcinoma. Int J Radiat Oncol Biol Phys. 1995;31(2):325–31.
20. Kokoska ER, Kokoska MS, Collins BT, et al. Early aggressive treatment for Merkel cell carcinoma improves outcome. Am J Surg. 1997;174:688–93.
21. Eng TY, Naguib M, Fuller CD, et al. Treatment of recurrent Merkel cell carcinoma: an analysis of 46 cases. Am J Clin Oncol. 2004;27:576–83.
22. Muller A, Keus R, Neumann N, et al. Management of Merkel cell carcinoma: case series of 36 patients. Oncol Rep. 2003;10(3):577–85.

Lymph Node Procedures of the Head and Neck

7

Chase M. Heaton and Steven J. Wang

Introduction and History

The head and neck is the most common location to diagnose Merkel cell carcinoma (MCC) with a reported incidence of 30–50 % of all cases found there due to the fact that the disease has a predilection to occur on sun-exposed skin [1, 2]. However, up to 5 % of disease can be located on mucous membranes as well [3]. As when seen in other locations throughout the body, MCC tends to present in the seventh or eighth decade of life, most frequently in the elderly and those who are immunosuppressed. With its aggressive behavior and potential for primary site recurrence, locoregional spread, and distant metastasis, diagnosis and treatment should be paramount when MCC occurs in this lymphatic-rich location.

Epidemiology

Within the head and neck, epidemiological traits of MCC parallel those of the disease in other locations throughout the body with an increasing incidence. Roughly 1,500 cases of MCC in all sites are diagnosed yearly with up to 50 % of lesions located on the head neck. It has a predilection for men with a reported predominance of 1.1–2.5:1; and by race, nearly all cases are in Caucasians [4–6]. Rarely does the disease manifest at ages younger than 65 with most lesions identified in patients greater than 75 [3]. As previously mentioned, MCC has a predilection for sun-exposed skin. Agelli demonstrated a higher incidence of MCC in climates with more sun exposure by noting differences in MCC incidence within cities of varying ultraviolet B (UVB) indices [4]. From these findings, the most common patient presentation is an elderly Caucasian male with a history of sun exposure. Immunosuppression also increases the risk of developing MCC. Studies have shown a nearly eightfold increase in risk HIV patients and tenfold increase risk in organ transplant patients [7, 8]. There is also a predilection for earlier development of MCC in this patient population, with one study showing nearly 30 % of cases diagnosed before the age of 50 [8].

Risk Factors

MCC of the head and neck shares the same risk factors as with the disease seen in other parts of the body. Both UVB exposure and immunosuppression, whether acquired as in HIV or iatrogenic in the immunosuppressed transplant patient, appear to be independent risk factors for the

C.M. Heaton
Department of Otolaryngology - Head and Neck Surgery, University of California, San Francisco, 2233 Post Street, 3rd Floor, San Francisco, CA 94115, USA
e-mail: cheaton@ohns.ucsf.edu

S.J. Wang (✉)
Department of Otolaryngology - Head and Neck Surgery, University of California, San Francisco, 2380 Sutter Street, Box 1703, San Francisco, CA 94115, USA
e-mail: swang@ohns.ucsf.edu

M. Alam et al. (eds.), *Merkel Cell Carcinoma*, DOI 10.1007/978-1-4614-6608-6_7,

development of MCC. There is also a growing suspicion of a suspected viral etiology for the disease. A recently discovered polyomavirus, appropriately penned Merkel cell polyomavirus (MCP), has been suspected to contribute to the majority of cases of MCC [9]. In this study, eight of ten MCC specimens were found to have the virus while only 8 and 16 % of control tissues bore the virus. Their infected rate of 80 % has been replicated in multiple studies with similar rates between 50 and 80 % [10–12]. Within the eight specimens positive for MCP, six demonstrated integration of the virus in the tumor DNA.

Presentation

In the head and neck, MCC typically presents as a rapidly growing, skin nodule. It is often painless and rarely involves the epidermis, which may give it the appearance of being shiny displaying a range of color from flesh-colored to violaceous. Occasionally, ulceration may be present in more advanced tumors. Patients often seek medical attention because the lesion is growing rapidly or the overlying skin has begun to breakdown. Common locations include the cheeks, nose, eyelids, periocular, and perioral regions [13, 14]. Occasionally MCC may metastasize from a skin primary to the oropharyngeal mucosa [15]. The differential for lesions with these characteristics is quite broad, and for this reason, as well as the fact that MCC overall remains quite rare, the clinical diagnosis remains challenging. Most commonly confused diagnoses are amelanotic melanoma and basal cell carcinoma. In order to aid the physician in diagnosis, the mnemonic "AEIOU" developed by Heath et al. has gained much popularity in use during the clinical workup: Asymptomatic (no tenderness on palpation), rapidly Expanding (doubling in <3 months), Immunosuppression, Older than 50, and Ultraviolet exposed skin [1]. MCC lesions vary in size from a few millimeters up to 5 cm. Within the head and neck, lesions of MCC are most often diagnosed before they reach 2 cm in size. Taken together, these clinical characteristics are not all specific to MCC, and for this reason, no established criteria exist for purely clinical diagnosis. Suspicion and prompt biopsy remain the mainstays for definitive diagnosis.

Workup

Due to the propensity of MCC to progressively spread from primary site to regional lymph nodes to then distant sites, an expedited workup via a multidisciplinary team approach is necessary to ensure the best treatment when a suspicion of MCC exists [16]. Prompt biopsy of the lesion with H&E staining is used to obtain pathologic diagnosis. Imaging with MRI or CT is often recommended for initial staging of the disease. Octreotide scanning and PET imaging have also been used with reported success. Various treatment options then exist including surgery, radiation, and chemotherapy. However, as noted in the current National Comprehensive Cancer Network (NCCN) treatment guidelines, surgery is the primary treatment modality for MCC of the head and neck [17]. Appropriate surgery includes a wide local excision with negative margins, with or without a sentinel lymph node biopsy (SLNB) or elective lymph node dissection in patients with clinically negative lymph node basins. When clinically apparent lymph nodes are present and confirmed on biopsy, a therapeutic lymphadenectomy and/or radiation/chemotherapy is preferred. Post surgical treatment modalities include adjuvant radiation and chemotherapy for control of local and regional disease.

Anatomy

Following pathologic diagnosis of MCC, surgical treatment options must be explored. The presence of clinically positive lymph nodes in draining nodal basins will determine the extent of the lymphadenectomy performed. Guidelines for type of lymph node dissection mirror those seen in other cancers of the head and neck. It is therefore important to know the lymphatic drainage patterns of head and neck subsites. In patients with clinically negative lymph nodes,

SLNB is most often performed. Again, understanding of lymphatic drainage is important to help to localize the sentinel lymph node once in the operating room. The head and neck region is divided in to six lymph node levels with the addition of the peri-parotid and external jugular lymph node basins. Level I encompasses the submental and submandibular area, a prime drainage site for oral cavity cancers (specifically the floor of month, anterior tongue, and mandibular ridge) and the lower lip. Levels II–IV are oriented in a vertical fashion along the sternocleidomastoid muscle. Most scalp and face lesions drain into these nodal basins, with level II being the first level involved. MCC involving the cheek over the parotid gland would be expected to first drain to the intra-parotid lymph nodes and level II. Level V encompasses the posterolateral neck, also known as the posterior triangle. Posterior scalp and neck primaries have the highest predilection for metastases to this nodal region. Level VI may harbor thyroid or laryngeal cancer metastases and therefore does not pertain to discussion of MCC. The peri-parotid lymph nodes are found anterior to the external ear and may be surrounding or within the underlying parotid tissue. The external jugular lymph node chain follows the path of the superficial external jugular vein and is very important in the drainage of cutaneous based MCC lesions. As most MCCs are on the face, scalp, and mucous membranes, certain nodal basins carry a higher predilection of lymph node metastases. Lymph node basins I, II, III, IV, and V, as well as the peri-parotid and external jugular lymph nodes are most often involved in lymphadenectomy procedures, including SLNB. Rarely is lymph node level VI explored in lymphadenectomy procedures for MCC.

Patient Selection

As with any surgical procedure, patient selection is critical. Risk factors that portend a poor surgical outcome in lymphadenectomy procedures include smoking history, alcohol use, prior head or neck radiation, and poor nutritional status. However, in the case of MCC, the presence of these risk factors would not delay or prevent the use of surgical treatment given its necessity in multimodality management. The risks of head and neck lymphadenectomy procedures must then be thoroughly explained to the patient. The rich lymphatics of the head and neck are in close relation to many vital and important structures, including cranial nerves, vessels, and salivary glands. An understanding of these risks is paramount prior to an operation. Appropriate preoperative clearance is also required as MCC patients are elderly and often have comorbid conditions.

Preoperative Considerations

A thorough preoperative physical exam should be performed. The skin of the scalp, face, ears, and neck should be examined for MCC satellite lesions, coexisting primary lesions, or associated basal and squamous cell carcinomas. Having a propensity for deep invasion, a complete cranial nerve exam should be performed to assess the relationship of the primary tumor to underlying structures. Specific attention to the facial nerve should be critical. Depending on location, referral to an ophthalmologist for a complete eye exam may be necessary. Mucosal surfaces should be examined for synchronous lesions. Finally, a thorough examination of lymph node basins should be performed to assess N status.

Postoperative Considerations

Postoperative considerations should also be explored in patient selection prior to surgery. To prevent postoperative complications, patients should be ambulatory by postoperative day 1 to decrease the risk of pneumonia and deep vein thromboses. Depending on the extent of the lymphadenectomy procedure performed, closed suction drains are often placed at the end of the case—SLNB procedures are often limited enough to not require drain placement. Physical therapy is often required after surgery of the head and neck due to retraction on neck muscles and their associated nerves. While most therapy sessions take place in the hospital and often do not need long-term follow-up, some patients may need home physical therapy services.

Depending on the site of the MCC primary, wide local excisions often require innovative and wide-ranging reconstructive techniques. The patient should expect to be involved in daily wound care with close clinical follow-up during the immediate postoperative period. Patients must be explained the significance the surgery will have on their physical appearance. If concern exists regarding the how the patient will handle potential disfigurement, referral to an appropriate therapist may be needed.

Staging Procedures

After a new diagnosis of MCC of the head and neck is made, pathologic staging of the disease is the next priority. Accurate staging of head and neck MCC is often difficult and presents a unique dilemma; 75 % of patients present as clinically N0, but it is presumed that 16–50 % of patients will eventually develop regional disease which was likely present at initial presentation [5, 18–20]. Various studies have quoted between 11 and 43 % of patients who are clinically N0 have occult micrometastatic disease [19, 21, 22]. Therefore, some type of assessment of the regional nodal basins should be performed at the time of diagnosis. Various options exist including imaging using PET/CT, MRI, or ultrasound; SLNB; or elective neck dissection.

Elective Lymphadenectomy

With the increasing acceptance of SLNB followed by adjuvant radiation and/or chemotherapy, the role of elective lymphadenectomy for the N0 neck remains controversial and has diminished in practice [23]. Due to the aggressive nature of MCC and the propensity for early locoregional spread, prior literature recommended prophylactic lymphadenectomy for all N0 patients, especially if unfavorable prognostic factors—large tumor size, lymphatic invasion, and increased mitotic activity—coexist [20, 24–26]. In a cohort of 33 patients, Kokoska et al. found that patients who underwent elective lymphadenectomy had locoregional and distant recurrence rates of 0 % and 9 %, respectively, as compared to 91 and 68 % in those who did not undergo prophylactic lymph node excisions [24]. Allen et al. noted that elective lymphadenectomy was the only factor associated with an improved relapse-free survival rate [19]. Specific to the head and neck, Goepfert et al. in 1984 recommended an elective radical neck dissection be performed due to their studied high rate of nodal recurrence. In the case of midline lesions, bilateral neck dissections are recommended [20]. Others recommend elective lymph node dissection only in specific cases. Silva et al. recommended this treatment modality if the primary tumor was >2 cm in size or showed microscopic evidence of an aggressive nature [27]. Now, with advances in radiolocalization of sentinel nodes, targeted nodal biopsies are becoming first line treatment for N0 necks with increasing frequency and are recommended by the NCCN guidelines [17].

Sentinel Lymph Node Biopsy

The current NCCN practice guidelines for MCC nodal staging in the newly diagnosed N0 patient recommend SLNB. Many studies have confirmed its ability to detect the presence or absence of nodal disease with success rates nearing or at 100 % [21, 22, 28–32]. A recent meta-analysis confirmed the accuracy of SLNB, reporting only one patient out of 35 who had a false-negative result on SLNB who soon after experienced disease recurrence. Because of this they concluded that SLNB is a reliable technique to determine lymph node status in patients who are clinically N0 [30]. Another recent meta-analysis demonstrated that one third of patients whose disease would have been understaged clinically or radiographically were detected to have spread of MCC and therefore received appropriate treatment to that nodal basin that otherwise may have been withheld [31]. Because of their findings, they concluded that SLNB should be routinely performed in all patients with MCC as it is an important factor in prognosis and directed therapy. However, these numbers are based on MCC of all sites and specifically note the difficulty in sentinel node isolation in head and neck surgery. Due to the complex and variable lymphatic drainage patterns of the head and neck, NCCN guidelines make clear that SLNB is less reliable and is therefore not mandatory [17]. A study from 2007 noted this variability by comparing serial lymphoscintigraphy scans of patients scheduled for SLNB for MCC and melanoma of the head or neck. Eight out of 25 patients showed discordance in lymphoscintigraphy studies in identification of lymph drainage pathways. They concluded that patterns of lymphatic drainage in the head and neck not only vary between patients but often may vary with time in a single patient [32]. Opponents of SLNB for MCC also note differences in lymphatic drainage pathways between MCC and melanoma. It is believed that MCC may have a propensity to drain via subcutaneous lymphatics as well as intradermal lymphatics. Subsequently, possible micrometastatic disease may be missed.

SLNB for Head and Neck MCC

Despite these considerations, and due to the success, accuracy, and standardization of SLNB for melanoma of the head and neck, many surgeons have employed this staging modality with variable success in patients with MCC. This use is rooted in the belief that SLNB may provide accurate staging information without the morbidity associated with an elective lymphadenectomy and is likely more accurate in detection of micrometastases than imaging studies [33]. Review of the literature suggests a wide range of experiences with SLNB for MCC of the head and neck. The Dana Farber Cancer Institute experience reported only a 45 % success rate in isolating the sentinel lymph node [30].

Conversely, a smaller retrospective study involving ten patients with head and neck MCC identified the sentinel node in 100 % of cases and reported a positive node in 20 % which mirrors the rate of occult nodal metastases as reported in prior studies [18]. With this success rate and low rate of complications, they concluded that SLNB should be considered a reliable and safe technique for regional staging of MCC of the head and neck. A University of Miami experience also isolated the sentinel lymph node in ten patients with clinically N0 MCC of the head and neck. Of those with negative sentinel lymph nodes by pathology, only one patient developed recurrent disease. Positivity of lymph nodes in the other patients directed future adjuvant treatment. They concluded that SLNB provides accurate identification of lymph node drainage patterns and aids in planning future treatment if positive [34]. Further identification of the accuracy of SLNB was seen in a small case series of eight patients with N0 MCC of the head and/or neck. They concluded due to the high success rate and low false negatives, SLNB for MCC is a viable staging option [22]. In addition to the studied success rates and accuracy of SLNB for MCC of the head and neck, proponents of the procedure also note that the nearly 50 % of N0 patients who do not have regional disease will be spared the morbidity of an elective lymphadenectomy.

Preoperative Discussion

Once it is decided that SLNB will be performed, a detailed conversation is critical with the patient regarding the logistics and risks of the procedure. At our institution, patients are scheduled for a lymphoscintigraphy scan in the nuclear medicine department no more than 24 h prior to their operation. ^{99m}Technetium radiolabeled sulfur colloid is injected intradermally in four quadrants circumferentially around the prior biopsy site or tumor. This radiocolloid is taken up in lymphatic channels and concentrated in lymph nodes. Fifteen to 30 min after injection, lymphoscintigraphy using a gamma camera system is performed allowing for static and dynamic imaging of lymphatic drainage and localization of sentinel nodes. Serial single photon emission computed tomography (SPECT-CT) images are obtained as the sulfur colloid may take up to an hour and half to collect in the sentinel nodes. Due to the complex three-dimensional anatomy of the lymph node basins of the head and neck, as well as the frequent close proximity of the primary site and the draining nodal basins, it is the authors' opinion that SPECT-CT imaging for localization of head and neck sentinel lymph nodes should be utilized in all cases. Other than minor pain associated with the slightly acidic nature of the radionucleotide injection, very few risks are associated with the procedure. Radiation exposure is minimal due to the small amount of radiocolloid injected. Allergic reactions may occur but are extremely rare and often minor. An allergy assessment should be performed prior to the examination.

Operative Technique

Once in the operating room, standard preparation for a neck dissection is performed. This includes proper positioning enabling an unobstructed view of the neck and surface landmarks. A shoulder roll placed under the patient is often used to help in proper positioning. Anesthetic considerations include withholding use of paralytic to allow the surgeon to assess proximity of dissection to critical nerves. Depending on the site of expected dissection, appropriate nerve monitoring should be used, including facial nerve monitoring when operating near the parotid gland. Care should be taken in posterolateral dissections to avoid injuring the spinal accessory nerve.

Prior to sterile prepping and draping of the patient, some surgeons prefer to inject methylene blue at the site of the primary lesion. Similar to the intradermal injections done in nuclear medicine for lymphoscintigraphy, the dye will follow the associated lymphatic networks draining the lesion. Once incisions have been made, it may be possible to more easily visualize lymphatic channels with the blue dye marker.

A gamma probe is then used to localize the sentinel nodes. Equipment selection is based on hospital and surgeon preference. Probes are available in multiple sizes and tip diameters depending on the ergonomical design needed for examining the specific nodal basins. Wireless probes using Bluetooth technology clear the operative field of obstructing wires. All probes are sterile and available for use in the operating field. Touchscreen control units with audio feedback are also available and widely used.

The skin incision is then planned for the SLNB following localization of the sentinel node with the gamma probe. Bearing in mind that a positive sentinel node biopsy may require further surgery, skin incisions should be appropriately placed with consideration of the need for a completion procedure (example, parotidectomy or completion neck dissection). Incisions should be planned in natural skin creases for the best cosmetic results. A planned skin incision for the primary lesion should also be formulated obtaining at least 1–2 cm margins around the tumor. The skin is then injected with local anesthetic and the surgical field is prepped and draped in a sterile fashion.

Once the skin incision has been completed through the platysma muscle layer, the gamma probe is used to localize the radiocolloid tracer in the sentinel node. There are no defined numerical criteria with which to base successful location of the sentinel node. Often, surgeons search for nodes with the highest absolute value displayed on the gamma probe unit relative to the background radiation levels. Additional node excision continues until the background radiation levels are less than 10 % of the count of the highest node.

Pitfalls

Proponents of SLNB suggest that patients with no disease of the sentinel node on biopsy are spared the morbidity of a completion lymphadenectomy procedure. However, adjuvant radiation treatment is often recommended as false-negative sentinel node biopsies, assumed due to regional recurrence, have been reported. Warner et al. reported recurrence in five of six patients who had negative SLNB not followed by adjuvant radiation [29]. Schmalbach et al. noted regional recurrence in one of eight patients with a false-negative SLNB with a mean follow-up interval of 34 months [18]. Other studies that report low or no evidence of false-negative biopsies do not report their length of follow-up or are have short follow-up intervals [21, 28, 30]. The propensity for multi-node involvement of locoregional spread of MCC is a suspected reason for the high rate of occult nodal involvement in the head and neck [20, 33, 35]. In addition, due to the variable lymphatic drainage of the head and neck, occult disease may be missed during SLNB. Finally, as previously mentioned, MCC has a tendency to drain via dermal and subcutaneous lymphatics. It is therefore possible that lymphoscintigraphy may not isolate the sentinel lymph node associated with the correct drainage pathway of the primary lesion. Despite these findings, most centers still continue to perform SLNB and consider it an important staging tool in evaluation of MCC.

Therapeutic Procedures

Surgical excision is the primary treatment modality for cutaneous MCC of the head and neck. Adjuvant radiation therapy and chemotherapy have also been used with little difference in retrospective data regarding locoregional control and metastatic inhibition. The rarity of the disease makes prospective studies of these treatment modalities difficult to study. In this section, we will discuss the role of primary surgical therapy for the treatment of MCC of the head and neck.

Primary Lesions

For the primary cutaneous tumor, NCCN guidelines recommend excision with 1–2 cm margins down to investing fascia or muscle [17]. Prior studies have recommended more generous margins of at least 2–3 cm [20, 23, 24]. In a small study of 18 patients by Gillenwater et al., there was no difference in locoregional control or survival based on margins obtained [13]. A study by Allen et al. demonstrated that negative margins were obtained in 94 % of their patients at an average margin width of 1.1 cm. The recurrence rate for their margin-negative patients was 8 % as compared to 18 % for margin-positive patients. Their conclusion was that the goal of wide local excision should be to obtain negative margins without concern for what margin width is obtained [36]. Further studies have confirmed that larger margin widths do not correlate with locoregional recurrence rates [36, 37]. In cases with close and/or positive margins or larger primary tumors, postoperative radiation therapy is often recommended and used.

Reconstruction Principles of Primary Lesions

The recommended 1–2 cm margins for lesions of the head and neck make for a formidable reconstructive challenge. The goal of excision is to, most importantly, obtain negative margins and, secondarily, to preserve the function and aesthetic of the face. When planning surgical excision of the primary lesion, potential reconstruction techniques should be considered. To facilitate a successful and aesthetically pleasing reconstruction, specific attention should be focused on the aesthetic units of the face and associated relaxed skin tension lines. Various local flaps exist for reconstruction and defect coverage depending on the location of the primary lesion. Preoperative discussion with the patient regarding reconstruction plan is important as meticulous wound care and clinic follow-up may be necessary. NCCN guidelines recommend immediate reconstruction in most cases, though staged reconstruction techniques may be required if time is needed to ensure negative margins prior to performing an extensive reconstruction [17, 34]. Split thickness skin grafts should be used to aid in recurrence monitoring if primary closure is not feasible [17].

The N+ Patient

NCCN guidelines direct treatment in patients with clinically apparent nodal disease of the head and neck [17]. Following palpation of a suspicious lymph node, fine-needle aspiration (FNA) biopsy should be performed. A biopsy positive for MCC warrants further diagnostic work up with appropriate imaging for evaluation of further locoregional disease as well as metastases. Negative biopsy results should be followed by an excisional biopsy of the suspicious node to avoid the consequences of a potentially false-negative FNA. In N+ patients without evidence of distant metastatic disease, a multidisciplinary discussion should be held to determine further treatment strategies. Current treatment modalities include a comprehensive nodal dissection and/or radiation therapy.

If the treatment modality chosen for the N+ patient is surgery, a comprehensive nodal dissection would be recommended. Traditionally, a modified radical neck dissection would be performed. This surgery entails dissection of all lymph node basins (I–V) with sparing of the internal jugular vein, sternocleidomastoid muscle, and/or the spinal accessory nerve. The location of the primary tumor would determine what other nodal basins should be dissected. Lesions of the pre-auricular skin or scalp would likely also require a parotidectomy to remove periparotid lymph nodes that may be involved with tumor.

Radiation in Head and Neck MCC

When performing a wide local excision of a head and neck MCC primary lesion in the absence of a SLNB, NCCN guidelines recommend adjuvant radiation therapy to the primary site, nodal beds, and in-transit lymphatic pathways. If an SLNB is performed, consideration of adjuvant radiation therapy to the nodal basin or completion lymphadenectomy procedures may be recommended despite the nodal status discovered on SLNB [17]. The debate on the best treatment modality for control of locoregional lymphatic spread of MCC is long-standing. Many authors have considered surgery alone superior [19, 26, 36]. Other studies have concluded the opposite stating that radiation therapy alone is sufficient [13, 38–41]. Proponents of combined treatment (surgery and radiotherapy) have concluded that combining the two treatment modalities leads to the best patient results [24, 25, 42, 43]. In a large study conducted on 110 patients with MCC of the head and neck, the addition of adjuvant radiotherapy with wide local excision of the primary lesion greatly increased the disease-free survival median length from 8 to 34 months [44]. This study substantiated the effects of adjuvant radiation treatment on disease-free survival seen in earlier studies (6 months vs. 23 months) [42]. Despite prior work, a debate regarding the role of radiation therapy still exists. Larger prospective studies will likely be needed to further delineate the roll of radiotherapy in MCC of the head and neck.

References

1. Heath M, Jaimes N, Lemos B, Mostaghimi A, Wang LC, Penas PF, et al. Clinical characteristics of Merkel cell carcinoma at diagnosis in 195 patients: the AEIOU features. J Am Acad Dermatol. 2008;58: 375–81.
2. Akhtar S, Oza KK, Wright J. Merkel cell carcinoma: report of 10 cases and review of the literature. J Am Acad Dermatol. 2000;43:755–67.
3. Agelli M, Clegg LX. Epidemiology of primary Merkel cell carcinoma in the United States. J Am Acad Dermatol. 2003;49:832–41.
4. Hodgson NC. Merkel cell carcinoma: changing incidence trends. J Surg Oncol. 2005;89:1–4.
5. Reichgelt BA, Visser O. Epidemiology and survival of Merkel cell carcinoma in the Netherlands. A population-based study of 808 cases in 1997–2007. Eur J Cancer. 2010;47(4):579–85.
6. Miller RW, Rabkin CS. Merkel cell carcinoma and melanoma: etiological similarities and differences. Cancer Epidemiol Biomarkers Prev. 1999;8:153–8.
7. Lanoy E, Costagliola D, Engels EA. Skin cancers associated with HIV infection and solid-organ transplantation among elderly adults. Int J Cancer. 2010;26(7):1724–31.
8. Penn I, First MR. Merkel's cell carcinoma in organ recipients: report of 41 cases. Transplantation. 1999; 68(11):1717–21.
9. Feng H, Shuda M, Chang Y, Moore PS. Clonal integration of a polyomavirus in human Merkel cell carcinoma. Science. 2008;319:1096–100.
10. Duncavage EJ, Le BM, Wang D, Pfeifer JD. Merkel cell polyomavirus: a specific marker for Merkel cell carcinoma in histologically similar tumors. Am J Surg Pathol. 2009;33:1771–7.
11. Duncavage EJ, Zehnbauer BA, Pfeifer JD. Prevalence of Merkel cell polyomavirus in Merkel cell carcinoma. Mod Pathol. 2009;22:516–21.

12. Carter JJ, Paulson KG, Wipf GC, Miranda D, Madeleine MM, et al. Association of Merkel cell polyomavirus-specific antibodies with Merkel cell carcinoma. J Natl Cancer Inst. 2009;101:1510–22.
13. Gillenwater AM, Hessel AC, Morrison WH, et al. Merkel cell carcinoma of the head and neck: effect of surgical excision and radiations on recurrence and survival. Arch Otolaryngol Head Neck Surg. 2001; 127:149–54.
14. Brisset AE, Olsen KD, Kasperbauer JL, et al. Merkel cell carcinoma of the head and neck: a retrospective case series. Head Neck. 2002;24:982–8.
15. Reichel OA, Mayr D, Issing WJ. Oropharyngeal metastasis of a Merkel cell carcinoma of the skin. Eur Arch Otorhinolaryngol. 2003;260:258–60.
16. Sarnaik AA, Lien MH, Nghiem P, Bichakjian CK. Clinical recognition, diagnosis, and staging of Merkel cell carcinoma, and the role of the multidisciplinary team. Curr Probl Cancer. 2010;34:38–46.
17. National Comprehensive Cancer Network (NCCN). Merkel cell carcinoma treatment guidelines (updated annually). www.nccn.org.
18. Schmalbach CE, Lowe L, et al. Reliability of sentinel lymph node biopsy for regional staging of head and neck Merkel cell carcinoma. Arch Otolaryngol Head Neck Surg. 2005;131:610–4.
19. Allen PJ, Zhang ZF, Coit DG. Surgical management of Merkel cell carcinoma. Ann Surg. 1999;229:97–105.
20. Goepfert H, Remmler D, et al. Merkel cell carcinoma (endocrine carcinoma of the skin) of the head and neck. Arch Otolaryngol. 1984;110:707–12.
21. Ames SE, Krag DN, Brady MS. Radiolocalization of the sentinel lymph node in Merkel cell carcinoma: a clinical analysis of seven cases. J Surg Oncol. 1998; 67:251–4.
22. Alex JC. The application of sentinel node radiolocalization to solid tumors of the head and neck: a 10-year experience. Laryngoscope. 2004;114:1–19.
23. Hitchcock CL, Bland KI, Laney RG, et al. Neuroendocrine (Merkel cell) carcinoma of the skin: its natural history, diagnosis, and treatment. Ann Surg. 1988;207:201–7.
24. Kokoska ER, Kokoska MS, Collins BT, et al. Early aggressive treatment of Merkel cell carcinoma improves outcome. Am J Surg. 1997;174:688–93.
25. Shaw JH, Rumball E. Merkel cell tumour: clinical behaviour and treatment. Br J Surg. 1991;78:138–42.
26. Yiengpruksawan A, Coit DG, Thaler HT, et al. Merkel cell carcinoma: prognosis and management. Arch Surg. 1991;126:1514–9.
27. Silva EG, Mackay B, Goepfert H, et al. Endocrine carcinoma of the skin (Merkel cell carcinoma). Pathol Annu. 1984;19:1–30.
28. Hill ADK, Brady MS, Coit DG. Intraoperative lymphatic mapping and sentinel lymph node biopsy for Merkel cell carcinoma. Br J Surg. 1999;86:518–21.
29. Warner RE, Quinn MJ, et al. Management of Merkel cell carcinoma: the roles of lymphoscintigraphy, sentinel lymph node biopsy and adjuvant radiotherapy. Ann Surg Oncol. 2008;15:2509–18.
30. Mehrany K, Otley CC, et al. A meta-analysis of the prognostic significance of sentinel lymph node status in Merkel cell carcinoma. Dermatol Surg. 2002;28:113–7.
31. Gupta SG, Wang LC, et al. Sentinel lymph node biopsy for evaluation and treatment of patients with Merkel cell carcinoma. Arch Dermatol. 2006;142: 685–90.
32. Willis AI, Ridge JA. Discordant lymphatic drainage patterns revealed by serial lymphoscintigraphy in cutaneous head and neck malignancies. Head Neck. 2007;29:979–85.
33. Gonzalez RJ, Padhya TA, Cherpelis BS, Prince MD, Aya-Ay ML, Sondak VK, et al. The surgical management of primary metastatic Merkel cell carcinoma. Curr Probl Cancer. 2010;34:77–96.
34. Shnayder Y, Weed DT, Arnold DJ, et al. Management of the neck in Merkel cell carcinoma of the head and neck: University of Miami experience. Head Neck. 2008;30:1559–65.
35. Lawenda BD, Thiringer JK, Foss RD, et al. Merkel cell carcinoma arising in the head and neck. Am J Clin Oncol. 2001;24:35–42.
36. Allen PJ, Bowne WB, Jacques DP, et al. Merkel cell carcinoma: prognosis and treatment of patients from a single institution. J Clin Oncol. 2005;23:2300–9.
37. Bichakjian CK, Lowe L, Loa CD, et al. Merkel cell carcinoma: critical review with guidelines for multidisciplinary management. Cancer. 2007;110:1–12.
38. Morrison WH, Peters LJ, Silva EG, et al. The essential role of radiation therapy in securing locoregional control of Merkel cell carcinoma. Int J Radiat Oncol Biol Phys. 1990;19:583–91.
39. Meeuwisen JA, Bourne RG, Kearsley JH. The importance of postoperative radiation therapy in the treatment of Merkel cell carcinoma. Int J Radiat Oncol Biol Phys. 1995;31:325–31.
40. Suntharalingam M, Rudoltz MS, Mendenhall WM. Radiotherapy for Merkel cell carcinoma of the skin of the head and neck. Head Neck. 1995;17:96–101.
41. Mendenhall WM, Mendenhall CM, Mendenhall NP. Merkel cell carcinoma. Laryngoscope. 2004;114: 906–10.
42. Veness MJ, Morgan GJ, Gebski V. Adjuvant locoregional radiotherapy as best practice in patients with Merkel cell carcinoma of the head and neck. Head Neck. 2005;27:208–16.
43. Lewis KG, Weinstock MA, Weaver AL, et al. Adjuvant local irradiation for Merkel cell carcinoma. Arch Dermatol. 2006;142:693–700.
44. Clark JR, Veness MJ, Gilbert R, et al. Merkel cell carcinoma of the head and neck: is adjuvant radiotherapy necessary? Head Neck. 2007;29:249–57.

Lymph Node Procedures of the Trunk and Extremities

8

Julian Kim

Introduction and History

For most solid tumors, lymph node status is an important prognostic factor which suggests that the cancer is no longer localized and has the potential for systemic micrometastatic spread. In patients with Merkel cell carcinoma, regional lymphatic metastasis portends a poor prognosis. Lymph node positive patients are either Stage IIIA (micrometastases in regional lymph node) or Stage IIIB (macrometastases in regional lymph node) and the corresponding survival is significantly worse than patients who have node negative disease. Analysis of 1,034 patients within the Surveillance, Epidemiology and End Results Program (SEER) demonstrated a 5-year relative survival rate of 59 % in patients with nodal metastases as compared to 75 % in patients with node negative Merkel cell carcinoma [1]. A single institution series published from Memorial Sloan Kettering in 2005 in 251 patients demonstrated a 5-year disease-specific survival of 52 % for patients with Stage III disease as compared to 81 % and 67 % for patients with Stage I and II node negative disease, respectively [2]. Of note is that of patients who were eventually determined to have nodal metastases confirmed by histopathology, those who presented with clinically node negative disease had a better disease-specific survival than patients who presented with palpable, clinically suspicious regional lymph nodes. These data directly support the concept that knowledge of nodal status carries important prognostic information. Additionally, there is indirect evidence that identification of nodal disease when it is micrometastatic portends a better prognosis than diagnosis of macrometastatic or clinically evident nodal disease.

J. Kim (✉)
Department of Surgery, University Hospitals Case Medical Center, LKSD 5047, 11100 Euclid Avenue, Cleveland, OH 44106, USA
e-mail: julian.kim@UHhospitals.org

Historical Progression of Lymph Node Procedures for Patients with Merkel Cell Carcinoma

The rare nature of Merkel cell carcinoma has precluded prospective randomized trials to determine the benefit related to lymph node procedures. Thus, most of the evidence supporting the use of lymph node procedures relates to either single institutional studies or translation of evidence from experience with patients with melanoma. In patients who present with palpable metastatic disease to the regional lymph nodes without evidence of distant metastatic spread, regional lymphadenectomy or complete lymph node dissection of the axilla or groin serves two functions. First, clearance of regional nodal metastatic disease improves local control. Progression of regional nodal metastases in the axilla can lead to fixation of the tumor mass to the underlying chest wall which can lead to severe pain. In more advanced cases, progression of nodal disease in

M. Alam et al. (eds.), *Merkel Cell Carcinoma*, DOI 10.1007/978-1-4614-6608-6_8,

the axilla can result in disabling lymphedema of the upper extremity. In the most extreme cases, occlusion of the axillary vein and invasion into the brachial plexus can lead to a nonfunctional limb which is insensate and at risk for life-threatening infectious complications. Typically lymphadenectomy prior to development of disabling axillary nodal metastases can significantly reduce the risk of losing local control of disease resulting in these disabling symptoms. Similar principles apply to those patients who present with inguinal nodal metastases, where the risk of lymphedema is equally as high.

In addition to improving local control of disease, complete lymphadenectomy has the theoretical potential to improve or prolong survival. Unfortunately, since there is a paucity of cases of Merkel cell carcinoma, the study of the impact of lymphadenectomy on survival is not possible in the setting of a prospective, randomized study. However, as mentioned previously there is single institution data from Memorial Sloan Kettering Cancer Center which suggests that resection of lymph nodes in settings where the metastatic disease is microscopic and clinically non-palpable appeared to result in an improved survival over patients who underwent lymphadenectomy for palpable, macroscopic disease [2].

Development of techniques to identify patients with microscopic, subclinical metastatic disease to the regional lymph nodes for both prognostic and therapeutic purposes lead to the development of lymphatic mapping and sentinel lymph node biopsy (SLNB). This technique was first described in patients with penile cancer, where lymphatic mapping was performed by injecting a traceable liquid (blue dye or radioactive sulfur colloid) near the primary tumor site. The injected material then traveled through the same lymphatic channels that would mimic lymphatic spread of the penile carcinoma cells and be trapped within the first regional lymph node—the *sentinel lymph node* [3]. Proof-of-concept that lymphatic mapping and SLNB could reliably identify the first set of lymph nodes within a regional draining basin that could contain metastatic disease followed in prospective studies in patients with breast cancer and melanoma [4–8]. Positive results from these larger studies lead investigators to explore the role of SLNB as a method of identifying subclinical micrometastatic disease in patients with Merkel cell carcinoma.

Table 8.1 Published series of sentinel lymph node biopsy (SLNB) in patients with Merkel cell carcinoma

References	Number of patients	Sentinel node metastases
Allen et al. [2]	71	16
Ames et al. [9]	7	3
Hill et al. [10]	18	2
Maza et al. [11]	23	11
Rodrigues et al. [13]	6	3
Mehrany et al. [15]	60	20

Several single institutional series as well as a meta-analysis of the use of SLNB in patients with Merkel cell carcinoma have demonstrated that subclinical regional nodal metastatic disease can be identified (Table 8.1) [9–14]. The meta-analysis of a total of 60 patients demonstrated that in 20 patients (33 %), subclinical regional nodal metastases were identified. Importantly, those patients who had nodal metastases that were clinically not suspected preoperatively had a 19-fold increased odds of recurrence or metastasis as compared to patients who had a negative sentinel lymph node [15]. Although it can be debated whether completion of lymph node dissection in patients with a positive sentinel lymph node results in improved Merkel cell-specific survival, the prognostic information gained from sentinel node biopsy has now defined its use in the standard treatment pathway in patients with Merkel cell carcinoma.

Patient Selection for Lymphatic Mapping and Sentinel Lymph Node Biopsy

Controversy exists as to whether all patients with Merkel cell carcinoma should undergo SLNB. As a general rule, when evaluating a patient for any type of procedure, an assessment of the risk of the procedure, the potential benefits of the procedure and the alternatives to the procedure are weighed in aggregate. The sentinel node biopsy in addition to the wide local excision of the Merkel cell carcinoma adds cost, risk related to prolonged operative time, deeper dissection and need for additional anesthesia and risks related to infectious complications. The risk of lymphedema is variable depending upon whether the location of the sentinel node is in the axilla or the inguinal region, but can be estimated to be around 2–3 % [16, 17]. Clearly the risks of prolonged anesthesia will be variable depending on the patient's age and more importantly comorbidities, which can be significant in the older patient population which acquires Merkel cell carcinoma. As with any diagnostic test, if it is determined that the results of the test will not alter management of the patient such as in patients with advanced age and poor overall health, the utility of the test simply to predict outcome may be limited. However, for patients who are able to tolerate the anesthesia required for SLNB, the benefits of accurate prognostic information seem to outweigh the risks of the procedure.

The primary debate about whether all patients with Merkel cell carcinoma should undergo SLNB revolves around patients with primary tumors with a size of less than 1 cm. A previous single institution study demonstrated that in analysis of 95 patients with Merkel cell carcinoma who had SLNB, there was no subgroup of patients based upon tumor thickness and growth pattern that could be predicted to have a positive sentinel lymph node rate of less than 15 % [18]. However, more recently a review of 346 patients identified with Merkel cell carcinoma entered into the Department of Veterans Affairs database between 1995 and 2006 demonstrated that in 213 patients who underwent wide local excision and evaluation of the draining lymph node basin (either by physical examination or SLNB), only two patients with primary tumor size less than 1 cm were found to have regional lymph node metastases, and both of these patients had clinically palpable nodes [19]. This concept is being debated and it should be noted that in terms of patient selection, the lower rate of sentinel lymph node metastases in patients with tumor size less than 1 cm should be considered when evaluating the potential benefit of SLNB in this patient subset [20].

Staging Procedures: Technical Aspects of Lymphatic Mapping and Sentinel Lymph Node Biopsy

Lymphatic mapping and SLNB is a procedure which requires planning and the appropriate resources to achieve an optimal result. Nuclear medicine physicians are necessary in the event that radionuclide is used as the mapping agent for proper preparation and handling of the radioactive materials as well as interpretation of the imaging studies (lymphoscintigraphy) to determine location of the sentinel nodes. The surgeon must have experience in lymphatic mapping using either radionuclide with a hand-held gamma probe or visual mapping using vital blue dye. Finally, the pathologist must have a consistent method of sectioning and staining sentinel nodes for determination of metastatic disease. Most hospitals have these resources available due to development of lymphatic mapping programs for patients with breast cancer and melanoma, where SLNB is considered standard of care for patients with early stage disease. If these resources do not exist at a hospital, a decision must be made whether to proceed with the procedure using vital blue dye only or refer the patient to a medical center that has processes and resources in place to achieve expected outcomes.

Injection Technique and Lymphatic Mapping

Lymphatic mapping for cutaneous malignancies is typically performed by intradermal injection in close proximity to the primary lesion. Vital blue dye (Lymphazurin®) is FDA approved for lymphatic mapping and can be injected in the operating room immediately prior to lymphatic mapping. Since vital blue dye has a low molecular weight, it travels through the lymphatic channels rapidly and can deposit within the sentinel node within seconds to minutes. Intradermal injection with a small gauge needle generates high pressure within the lymphatic channels which helps the migration of dye to the sentinel

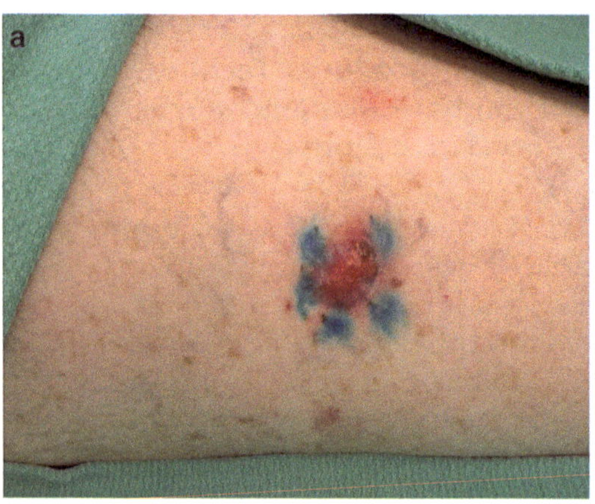

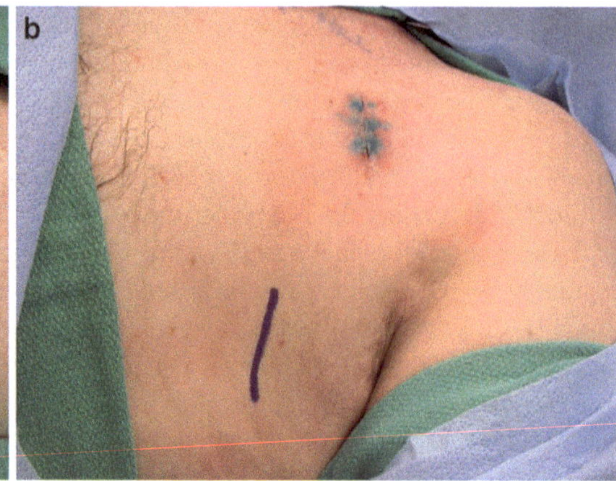

Fig. 8.1 Intradermal injection of vital blue dye. Note how the volume and location of the injection is limited to skin which will be incorporated into the wide excision. (**a**) Injection around existing lesion in the lower extremity. (**b**) Injection around a previous diagnostic narrow excision scar

node. Gentle massage of the injection site following injection will also assist in migration of blue dye into the sentinel node. The volume of injection is somewhat limited to the intradermal nature of the injection, and it must be stressed that intradermal injection of the dye must be limited to areas of skin which will be incorporated within the wide local excision of the Merkel cell carcinoma (Fig. 8.1). Failure to excise injected skin will result in tattoo of the residual skin which may be discolored for a prolonged period of time. In instances where the primary Merkel cell carcinoma has been narrowly excised, the injections can be performed adjacent to the excision scar.

Lymphatic mapping using vital blue dye can be performed in a variety of ways. Initial attempts at lymphatic mapping utilized serial transverse incisions spaced several centimeters apart starting close to the injection site and identification of the blue lymphatic channel which would terminate in the regional nodal basin within the sentinel nodes. In instances where lymphatic drainage is predictable, such as proximal anterior thigh or upper chest, a single incision can be performed in the inguinal or axillary region respectively to identify the sentinel lymphatic and blue stained sentinel nodes. However, a limitation of using vital blue dye alone for mapping of primary lesions of the distal extremity or mid-trunk are the variations in lymphatic drainage such that the location of the sentinel lymph node is not easily predictable. In these instances the use of radiolabeled injected materials and lymphoscintigraphy are warranted.

Injection of radiolabeled lymphatic mapping agents allows for imaging to be performed in order to confirm anticipated sites of sentinel lymph nodes as well as to identify sites that could not have been readily identified with use of vital blue dye alone [21, 22]. Examples of various draining patterns identified by lymphoscintigraphy are illustrated in Fig. 8.2. As examples, it is not uncommon for lesions of the distal extremity to drain not only to the regional axillary or inguinal locations but in addition the brachial or popliteal locations. These sites would likely not be identified if lymphatic mapping was performed using blue dye alone.

Although injection of radiolabeled lymphatic mapping agents is performed in a similar peritumoral distribution as vital blue dye, the radiolabeled agents usually take longer to migrate to the sentinel lymph node. In addition, the time associated with the lymphoscintigraphy can cause a prolonged waiting time (up to 2 h) for the patient. The most commonly used mapping agent is technetium 99 labeled sulfur colloid (^{99m}Tc) [9]. Since the colloid particles vary in size, it is not uncommon to perform filtration to reduce the particle size which effectively decreases the migration time from the injection site to the sentinel node. Typically injection of ^{99m}Tc and lymphoscintigraphy are

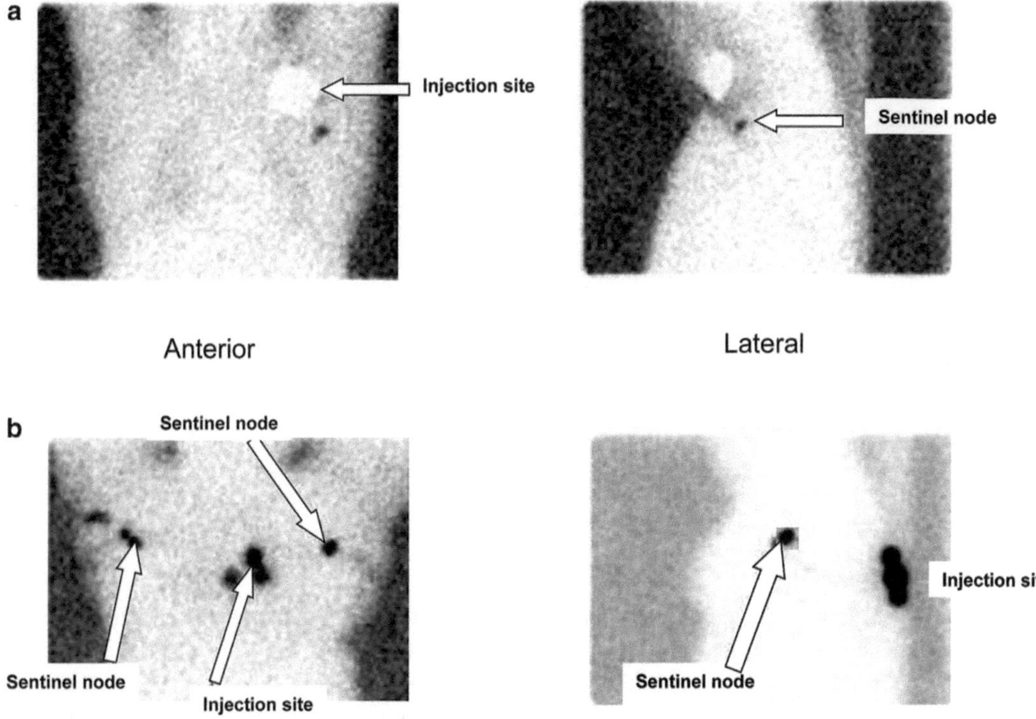

Fig. 8.2 Lymphoscintigraphy images associated with lymphatic drainage patterns following injection of radiolabeled mapping agent at the primary tumor site. (**a**) Injection site is in the upper chest and migrates to a sentinel node in the ipsilateral axilla. (**b**) Injection site is in the mid-back and migrates to sentinel nodes in both right and left axillae

performed on the morning of surgery, and immediately after lymphatic mapping and sentinel node biopsy are performed in the operating room.

Sentinel Lymph Node Biopsy

Sentinel lymph nodes are detected either using a hand-held radiation detecting probe or intraoperative visualization of vital blue dye stained lymph nodes. Standard incisions are performed in the axilla (lower transverse) or inguinal (oblique) regions such that if the sentinel lymph node demonstrates metastatic disease, the incision can be extended for a completion lymph node dissection. Transcutaneous assessment using the handheld gamma probe can confirm the general location of the radioactive sentinel lymph node prior to incision (Fig. 8.3). Individual sentinel lymph nodes are excised, radioactive counts recorded, and then they are placed into buffered formalin solution separately for histopathologic evaluation. Any lymph node with radioactive counts within 10 % of the lymph node with the highest count would be considered a sentinel lymph node and should be removed [23]. Complications related to SLNB include infection, seroma, and paresthesias and are estimated to occur in approximately 5 % of patients [24]. Lymphedema rates will vary depending upon whether the sentinel node biopsy is axillary or inguinal and are estimated anywhere from 2 to 5 % [17, 24].

Histopathologic Assessment of Sentinel Lymph Nodes

The technique of histopathologic assessment of the sentinel lymph nodes will directly impact the proportion of sentinel nodes in which micrometastatic disease is identified. Studies in patients with both breast cancer and melanoma have demonstrated that serial thin sectioning of sentinel

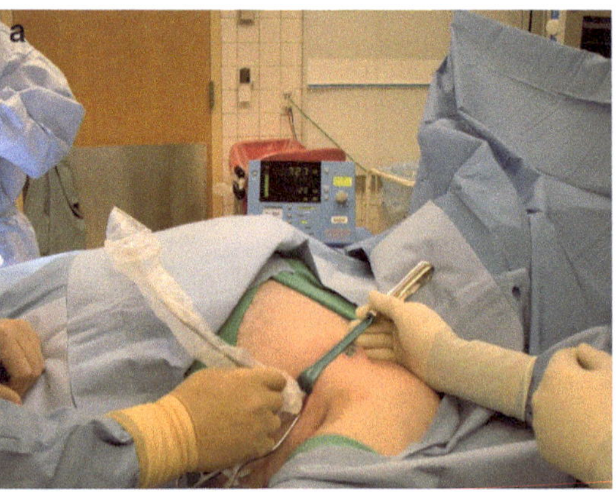

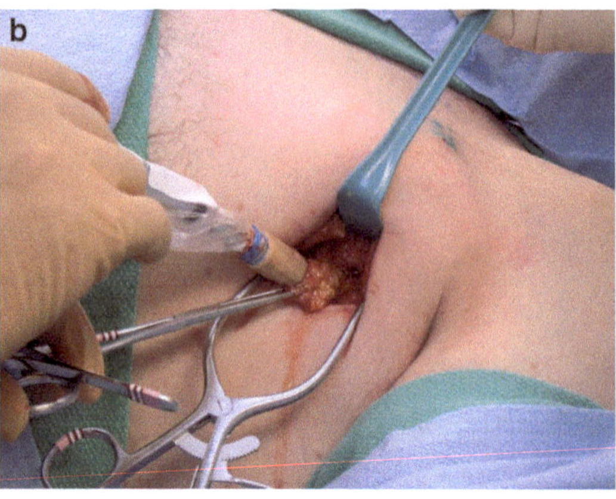

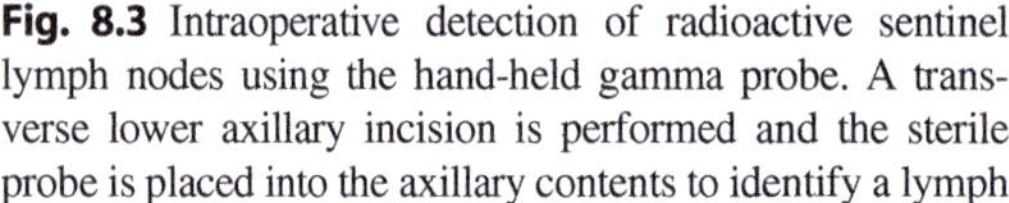

Fig. 8.3 Intraoperative detection of radioactive sentinel lymph nodes using the hand-held gamma probe. A transverse lower axillary incision is performed and the sterile probe is placed into the axillary contents to identify a lymph node with increased radioactive counts. (**a**) Probe with sterile sheath is placed in the axilla while radioactive counts appear on the control box in the background. (**b**) Radioactive sentinel node is identified using the hand-held gamma probe

lymph nodes and the use of immunohistochemical techniques increases the detection of micrometastases, resulting in stage migration. Interestingly, after many years of study, the use of serial sectioning and immunohistochemistry in sentinel lymph nodes in patients with breast cancer is no longer recommended, but these techniques are still recommended in the assessment of sentinel lymph nodes from patients with melanoma. There are few reports of the use of serial sectioning and immunohistochemistry in sentinel lymph nodes from patients with Merkel cell carcinoma [25]. As expected, there appeared to be an increase in the detection of micrometastases using immunohistochemistry as compared to routine hematoxylin and eosin staining.

Less Common Approaches and Their Indications

The easiest staging procedure for determination of whether there is lymph node metastasis from a primary Merkel cell carcinoma is palpation of the regional lymph nodes. Although these techniques have low sensitivity and specificity, in patients who present with palpable regional lymphadenopathy, fine needle aspiration, or core needle biopsy of the palpable node either with or without ultrasound guidance can confirm the diagnosis of metastatic Merkel cell carcinoma to the regional lymph nodes and alleviate the need for SLNB for staging purposes. In patients with no palpable evidence of metastatic nodal disease, high resolution ultrasound has been used to evaluate for the presence of metastatic disease in regional lymph nodes as well as computed tomography (CT), magnetic resonance imaging (MRI), or positron emission tomography (PET) scan. These techniques can identify subclinical lymph node metastases and may provide a noninvasive method of regional lymph node staging which may be useful in patients who are not candidates for surgical lymph node biopsy. However, it is generally recommended that any abnormal appearing lymph node undergoes a tissue biopsy to confirm the presence of metastatic Merkel cell carcinoma prior to making any further treatment decisions.

Therapeutic Procedures: Complete Axillary and Inguinal Lymph Node Dissections

Complete regional lymph node dissections as mentioned previously can be undertaken to serve two purposes. First, in patients who present with bulky nodal metastases with no evidence of distant metastases, complete lymph node dissection can palliate symptoms of pain and discomfort

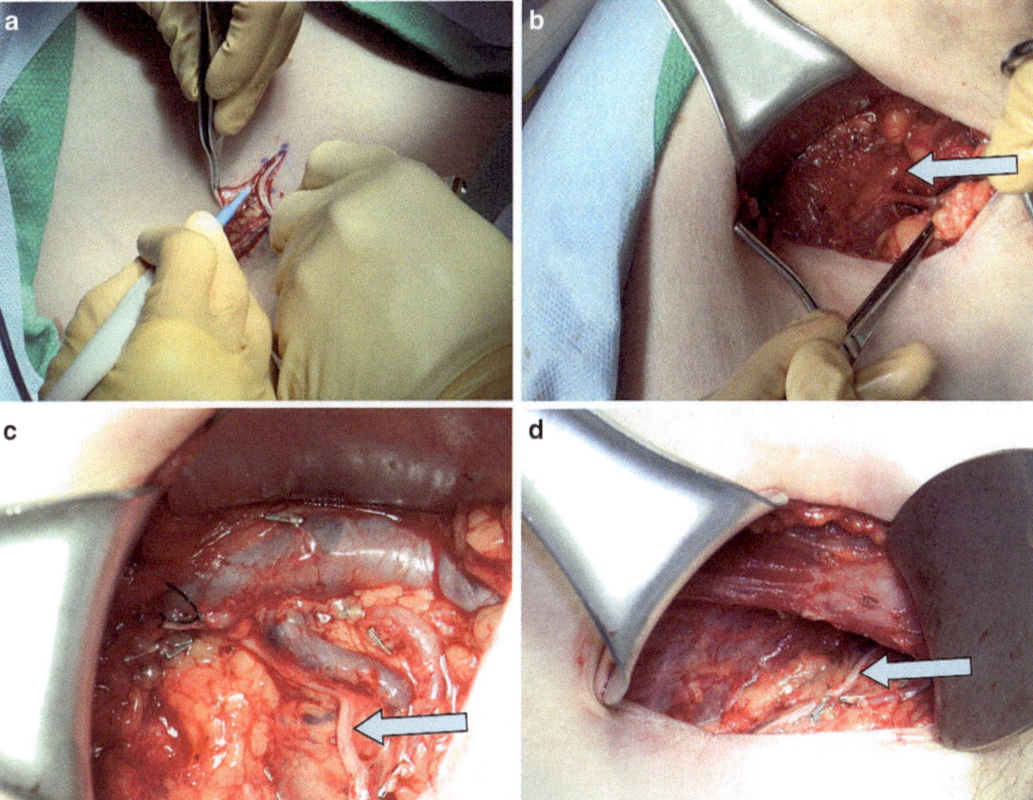

Fig. 8.4 Axillary lymph node dissection technique. (**a**) Lower transverse axillary incision incorporates the previous SLNB incision. (**b**) Lymph node fat pad dissected to expose the axillary vein superiorly (*arrow*). (**c**) Completion of dissection exposes the thoracodorsal nerve (*arrow*). (**d**) Long thoracic nerve is preserved (*arrow*) running parallel to the serratus anterior muscle

related to nodal disease as well as reduce the risk of progression to unresectable disease fixed to the underlying tissues. Second, complete lymph node dissection in patients with micrometastatic disease affords the possibility of improving long-term survival. As mentioned previously, no studies to date have determined that elective lymph node dissection in this situation improves survival for patients with Merkel cell carcinoma, primarily based upon the lack of a prospective, randomized study to address this issue.

Axillary Lymph Node Dissection Technique

Patients who are being offered complete axillary lymph node dissection for therapeutic purposes should be aware preoperatively of the risks associated with the procedure as part of the informed consent process. Large series estimate the risk of lymphedema at 5–15 % for upper extremity, but these rates generally increase with the addition of nodal basin external beam radiation [26]. Most studies that compare lymphedema rates of patients who had SLNB alone vs. those that progressed to have complete lymph node dissection demonstrate a higher proportion of patients with lymphedema.

Operative photos of the technique of axillary dissection are illustrated in Fig. 8.4. A lower transverse incision is performed which incorporates the previous SLNB incision. The axillary fat pad is identified by incising the fascia at the lateral edge of the pectoralis major and minor muscles and retracting them medially. The axillary vein is identified at the superior aspect of the field and long thoracic and thoracodorsal nerves are preserved. The lymph node fat pad is then dissected from the serratus anterior muscle medially, the subscapular muscle posteriorly, the latissimus dorsi muscle laterally, and then placed into a buffered formalin solution for histopathology. A closed suction drain is placed and patients rarely require blood transfusion.

Nerve complications related to axillary dissection include injury to the long thoracic nerve which can result in "winged scapula" and to the thoracodorsal nerve which can result in weakness of shoulder abduction and elevation of the arm. These are rare complications in experienced surgeons hands but can occur as a result of traction or thermal injury. A branch of the intercostobrachial nerve is usually divided resulting in paresthesia of the upper inner arm.

Inguinal Lymph Node Dissection

Preoperative preparation of the patient for short-term and long-term complications related to inguinal lymph node dissection is extremely important to increase compliance and manage expectations. Risks of infectious wound complications and lymphedema are typically reported to be significantly higher following inguinal lymph node dissection as compared to axillary lymph node dissection and is estimated to approximate 50–65 % of patients [27]. Many of these complications are short-term such that ambulation is maintained long-term, but quality of life may be affected long-term in patients with significant lower extremity lymphedema.

The inguinal lymph node dissection technique is illustrated in Fig. 8.5. The incision is vertical in the infrainguinal location and incorporates the previous SLNB incision. Skin flaps are raised at the level of the superficial thigh fascia and the inguinal ligament is exposed at the superior portion of the field. All fatty tissue and superficial lymph nodes are removed from the lower abdominal wall. The femoral sheath is incised to expose the common femoral artery and vein. The lymph nodes are removed from the common and superficial femoral vessels and the greater saphenous vein is preserved if possible. Lymph nodes are removed from the deep thigh muscles posteriorly, the sartorius muscle laterally, and the adductor compartment medially. The femoral nerve is not dissected and better left untouched. After the lymph node fat pad is removed, the sartorius muscle can be mobilized and detached from the anterior superior iliac spine such that it can be rotated medially to cover the exposed femoral vessels. The sartorius muscle flap is then sutured to the inguinal ligament to complete the operation and the skin flaps are approximated over closed suction drains. Although motor nerve injury is extremely uncommon, division of cutaneous nerves during inguinal lymph node dissection is common and typically results in paresthesias of the anterior upper thigh.

Less Common Approaches and Their Indications

There are alternative therapies to complete lymph node dissection in patients with either a positive sentinel lymph node or those with bulky metastatic nodal disease. Observation with no further nodal therapy is one option for patients with a microscopically positive sentinel lymph node. Although there are small series that have demonstrated regional nodal recurrence following SLNB alone in patients with Merkel cell carcinoma, a large prospective randomized study in melanoma is ongoing looking at whether completion lymph node dissection adds benefit to SLNB alone. This idea is based upon data from a large randomized study in patients with melanoma with thickness greater than 1.5 mm underwent SLNB. The average number of sentinel nodes removed was 2.2 and the average number of lymph nodes with metastatic disease was 1.6 [28]. These and other data which suggest that the percentage of patients with metastatic disease in non-sentinel nodes is small provide the rationale to consider observation following sentinel node biopsy.

External beam radiation therapy is a modality which can be extremely effective in controlling Merkel cell carcinoma and will be discussed extensively in Chap. 9. There is evidence from smaller trials that radiation therapy given to nodal basins either following SLNB alone or in patients

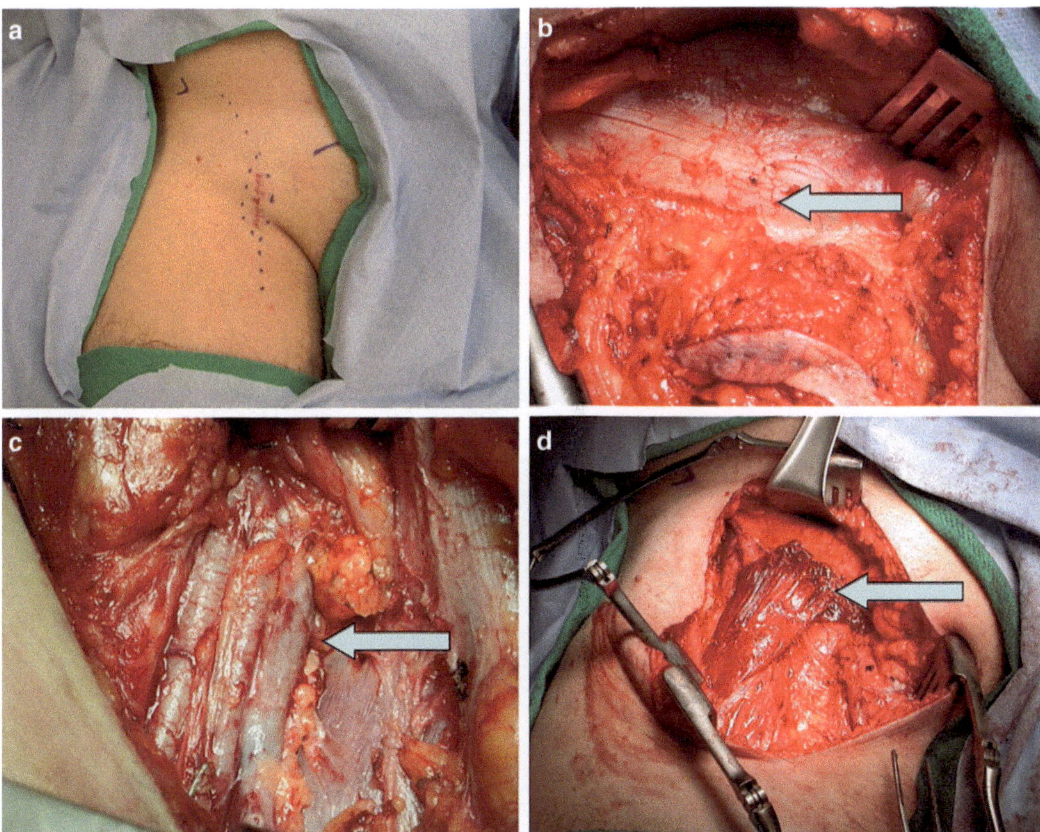

Fig. 8.5 Inguinal lymph node dissection. (**a**) Inguinal incision. (**b**) Lymph node fat pad dissected to expose inguinal ligament (*arrow*). (**c**) Exposed common femoral vessels after lymph node removal (*arrow* points to femoral vein medially). (**d**) Sartorius muscle flap coverage of the femoral vessels (*arrow*)

with bulky metastatic disease as an alternative to surgery result in favorable clinical results [29–31]. Again, lack of prospective randomized data on the use of radiation as an adjuvant or alternative to nodal procedures makes definitive recommendations challenging.

Diagnostic or Treatment Techniques Under Development

Two newer diagnostic techniques which deserve mention is the use of single-photon emission computed tomography (SPECT) imaging to assist with identification of sentinel lymph nodes and the development of a novel carrier substance Tilmanocept®. Nuclear medicine physicians at University Hospitals Seidman Cancer Center in Cleveland, Ohio have developed SPECT imaging in conjunction with lymphoscintigraphy to provide anatomic localization to sentinel nodes preoperatively. In instances where the primary tumor overlies the nodal basin or the injection of radionuclide obscures the nodal basins (such as in the head and neck), it is sometimes difficult to accurately identify a sentinel lymph node by lymphoscintigraphy, which is essentially a planar view from either anterior, posterior, or lateral projection (Fig. 8.6). SPECT imaging combined with lymphoscintigraphy allows for anatomic localization of sentinel nodes and assists the surgeon during preoperative planning.

In addition, a novel carrier agent Tilmanocept® has currently progressed through Phase III studies and is being evaluated by the FDA for approval for lymphatic mapping. Tilmanocept® is a carbohydrate-based carrier which is labeled with 99m-Tc and used as an alternative to sulfur colloid.

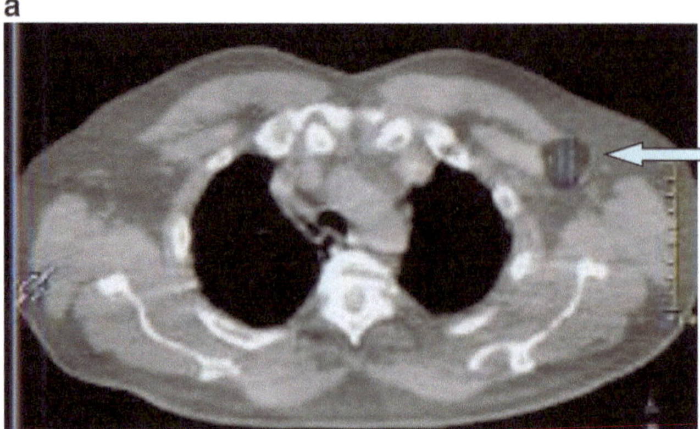

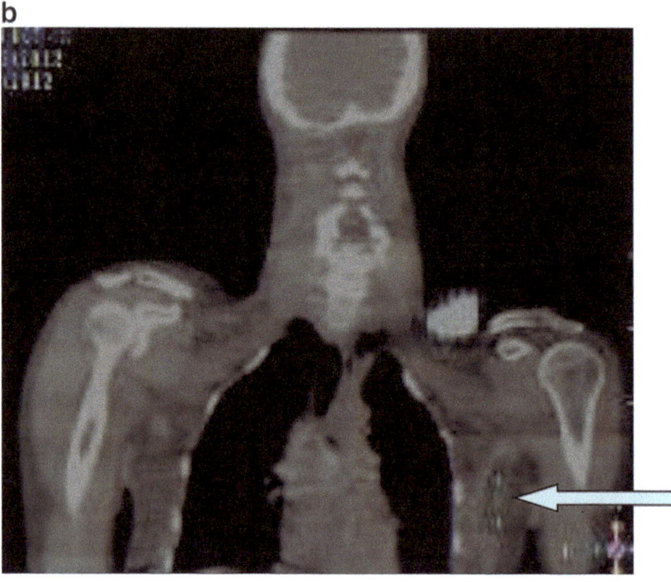

Fig. 8.6 SPECT imaging of sentinel nodes of axilla. (**a**) Sentinel node of axilla (*arrow*). (**b**) Injection site in left supraclavicular region with sentinel lymph node in left axillary region (*arrow*)

The results of the use of Tilmanocept® in a Phase II study demonstrated that it was at least equivalent to vital blue dye in identification of the sentinel node in patients with breast cancer and melanoma [32]. This novel agent has a lower molecular weight than sulfur colloid and thus may have a theoretical advantage of reduced migration time from injection site to the sentinel node.

Evidence-Based Findings

Currently there is no Level I evidence of the utility and/or benefit of lymph node procedures in patients with Merkel cell carcinoma. However, two large prospective randomized trials of SLNB in patients with breast cancer and melanoma may provide valuable insight. In both studies, the presence of metastatic disease in the sentinel lymph node was an independent predictor of survival [28, 33]. Interestingly, although micrometastases identified by immunohistochemistry was prognostic in patients with melanoma, it was not in patients with breast cancer [34]. Thus although it is likely that metastatic disease within the sentinel node is prognostic, it appears that the prognostic significance of micrometastases identified by immunohistochemistry may be disease-specific.

In terms of the impact of SLNB followed by completion lymph node dissection on overall survival, the results again vary by disease type. In patients with breast cancer, there was no evidence that addition of completion lymph node dissection in patients who had a positive SLNB improved survival. In patients with melanoma, sentinel node biopsy did not improve survival as compared to observation in all patients. However, in the subset of patients with a positive lymph node, immediate early complete lymph node dissection after identification of the positive sentinel node resulted in improved survival as compared to patients who underwent delayed lymph node dissection when they did not have an initial SLNB and developed a palpable nodal metastasis. Interestingly, the number of positive sentinel nodes was higher in node positive patients who underwent delayed lymph node dissection as compared to those who underwent immediate dissection. Thus, although there is Level I evidence of outcomes related to SLNB and complete lymph node dissection in patients with breast cancer and melanoma, the findings are somewhat disease-specific, and the translation of these findings in patients with Merkel cell carcinoma should be done with caution.

Conclusions

In summary, the following conclusions can be drawn concerning lymph node procedures for patients with Merkel cell carcinoma based upon direct evidence or evidence extrapolated from similar procedures in patients with melanoma:

- Lymph node metastases carry important prognostic information in patients with Merkel cell carcinoma (Level II)
- SLNB accurately identifies micrometastatic disease in patients who are clinically node negative (Level II)
- Complete lymph node dissections may provide palliation for patients who are node positive and have the potential to improve survival (Level III)
- External beam radiotherapy to the regional lymph nodes either alone or in combination with lymph node procedures may result in favorable clinical outcome (Level III)

References

1. Agelli M, Clegg LX. Epidemiology of primary Merkel cell carcinoma in the United States. J Am Acad Dermatol. 2003;49(5):832–41.
2. Allen PJ, Bowne WB, Jaques DP, Brennan MF, Busam K, Coit DG. Merkel cell carcinoma: prognosis and treatment of patients from a single institution. J Clin Oncol. 2005;23(10):2300–9.
3. Essner R, Conforti A, Kelley MC, et al. Efficacy of lymphatic mapping, sentinel lymphadenectomy, and selective complete lymph node dissection as a therapeutic procedure for early-stage melanoma. Ann Surg Oncol. 1999;6(5):442–9.
4. Fowler Jr JE. Sentinel lymph node biopsy for staging penile cancer. Urology. 1984;23(4):352–3.
5. Giuliano AE. Mapping a pathway for axillary staging: a personal perspective on the current status of sentinel lymph node dissection for breast cancer. Arch Surg. 1999;134(2):195–9.
6. Haigh PI, Giuliano AE. Role of sentinel lymph node dissection in breast cancer. Ann Med. 2000;32(1):51–6.
7. Hsueh EC, Hansen N, Giuliano AE. Intraoperative lymphatic mapping and sentinel lymph node dissection in breast cancer. CA Cancer J Clin. 2000;50(5):279–91.
8. Lee JH, Essner R, Torisu-Itakura H, Wanek L, Wang H, Morton DL. Factors predictive of tumor-positive nonsentinel lymph nodes after tumor-positive sentinel lymph node dissection for melanoma. J Clin Oncol. 2004;22(18):3677–84.
9. Ames SE, Krag DN, Brady MS. Radiolocalization of the sentinel lymph node in Merkel cell carcinoma: a clinical analysis of seven cases. J Surg Oncol. 1998;67(4):251–4.
10. Hill AD, Brady MS, Coit DG. Intraoperative lymphatic mapping and sentinel lymph node biopsy for Merkel cell carcinoma. Br J Surg. 1999;86(4):518–21.
11. Maza S, Trefzer U, Hofmann M, et al. Impact of sentinel lymph node biopsy in patients with Merkel cell carcinoma: results of a prospective study and review of the literature. Eur J Nucl Med Mol Imaging. 2006;33(4):433–40.
12. Pan D, Narayan D, Ariyan S. Merkel cell carcinoma: five case reports using sentinel lymph node biopsy and a review of 110 new cases. Plast Reconstr Surg. 2002;110(5):1259–65.
13. Rodrigues LK, Leong SP, Kashani-Sabet M, Wong JH. Early experience with sentinel lymph node mapping for Merkel cell carcinoma. J Am Acad Dermatol. 2001;45(2):303–8.
14. Wasserberg N, Feinmesser M, Schachter J, Fenig E, Gutman H. Sentinel-node guided lymph-node dissection for Merkel cell carcinoma. Eur J Surg Oncol. 1999;25(4):444–6.
15. Mehrany K, Otley CC, Weenig RH, Phillips PK, Roenigk RK, Nguyen TH. A meta-analysis of the prognostic significance of sentinel lymph node status in Merkel cell carcinoma. Dermatol Surg. 2002;28(2):113–7; discussion 117.

16. Golshan M, Martin WJ, Dowlatshahi K. Sentinel lymph node biopsy lowers the rate of lymphedema when compared with standard axillary lymph node dissection. Am Surg. 2003;69(3):209–11; discussion 212.
17. Wrone DA, Tanabe KK, Cosimi AB, Gadd MA, Souba WW, Sober AJ. Lymphedema after sentinel lymph node biopsy for cutaneous melanoma: a report of 5 cases. Arch Dermatol. 2000;136(4):511–4.
18. Schwartz JL, Griffith KA, Lowe L, et al. Features predicting sentinel lymph node positivity in Merkel cell carcinoma. J Clin Oncol. 2011;29(8):1036–41.
19. Stokes JB, Graw KS, Dengel LT, et al. Patients with Merkel cell carcinoma tumors < or = 1.0 cm in diameter are unlikely to harbor regional lymph node metastasis. J Clin Oncol. 2009;27(23):3772–7.
20. Sarnaik AA, Zager JS, Cox LE, Ochoa TM, Messina JL, Sondak VK. Routine omission of sentinel lymph node biopsy for Merkel cell carcinoma <= 1 cm is not justified. J Clin Oncol. 2010;28(1):e7.
21. Uren RF, Howman-Giles R, Chung DK, Morton RL, Thompson JF. The reproducibility in routine clinical practice of sentinel lymph node identification by preoperative lymphoscintigraphy in patients with cutaneous melanoma. Ann Surg Oncol. 2007;14(2):899–905.
22. Sian KU, Wagner JD, Sood R, Park HM, Havlik R, Coleman JJ. Lymphoscintigraphy with sentinel lymph node biopsy in cutaneous Merkel cell carcinoma. Ann Plast Surg. 1999;42(6):679–82.
23. Liu LC, Parrett BM, Jenkins T, et al. Selective sentinel lymph node dissection for melanoma: importance of harvesting nodes with lower radioactive counts without the need for blue dye. Ann Surg Oncol. 2011;18(10):2919–24.
24. Wrightson WR, Wong SL, Edwards MJ, et al. Complications associated with sentinel lymph node biopsy for melanoma. Ann Surg Oncol. 2003;10(6):676–80.
25. Allen PJ, Busam K, Hill AD, Stojadinovic A, Coit DG. Immunohistochemical analysis of sentinel lymph nodes from patients with Merkel cell carcinoma. Cancer. 2001;92(6):1650–5.
26. McLaughlin SA, Wright MJ, Morris KT, et al. Prevalence of lymphedema in women with breast cancer 5 years after sentinel lymph node biopsy or axillary dissection: objective measurements. J Clin Oncol. 2008;26(32):5213–9.
27. Carlson JW, Kauderer J, Walker JL, et al. A randomized phase III trial of VH fibrin sealant to reduce lymphedema after inguinal lymph node dissection: a Gynecologic Oncology Group study. Gynecol Oncol. 2008;110(1):76–82.
28. Morton DL, Thompson JF, Cochran AJ, et al. Sentinel-node biopsy or nodal observation in melanoma. N Engl J Med. 2006;355(13):1307–17.
29. Bischof M, van Kampen M, Huber P, Wannenmacher M. Merkel cell carcinoma: the role of radiation therapy in general management. Strahlenther Onkol. 1999;175(12):611–5.
30. Fenig E, Brenner B, Katz A, Rakovsky E, Hana MB, Sulkes A. The role of radiation therapy and chemotherapy in the treatment of Merkel cell carcinoma. Cancer. 1997;80(5):881–5.
31. Garneski KM, Nghiem P. Merkel cell carcinoma adjuvant therapy: current data support radiation but not chemotherapy. J Am Acad Dermatol. 2007;57(1):166–9.
32. Leong SP, Kim J, Ross M, et al. A phase 2 study of (99m)Tc-tilmanocept in the detection of sentinel lymph nodes in melanoma and breast cancer. Ann Surg Oncol. 2011;18(4):961–9.
33. Giuliano AE, Hunt KK, Ballman KV, et al. Axillary dissection vs no axillary dissection in women with invasive breast cancer and sentinel node metastasis: a randomized clinical trial. JAMA. 2011;305(6):569–75.
34. Giuliano AE, Hawes D, Ballman KV, et al. Association of occult metastases in sentinel lymph nodes and bone marrow with survival among women with early-stage invasive breast cancer. JAMA. 2011;306(4):385–93.

Radiation Therapy (Primary and Recurrent Disease)

9

William R. Silveira and Sue S. Yom

Summary

Radiation therapy (RT) plays an essential role in the multimodal treatment of all stages of Merkel cell carcinoma (MCC). In this chapter, we review the evidence demonstrating the radiosensitivity of MCC, the basis for current treatment recommendations for primary MCC, and principles for oncologic decision-making for recurrent and metastatic MCC. Case examples are presented to illustrate the role of RT in management. Evidence-based findings regarding definitive and adjuvant (postoperative) RT are discussed. Finally, future directions and new techniques under development are described.

Introduction

The radiosensitivity of MCC was established in the 1980s. Observations regarding the remarkable responsiveness of this tumor type led to RT's current crucial role in the local and regional control of MCC. Prior to this, treatment had primarily involved wide surgical excision when feasible.

W.R. Silveira (✉) • S.S. Yom
Department of Radiation Oncology, University of California, San Francisco, 1600 Divisadero Street, Suite H1031, San Francisco, CA 94115, USA
e-mail: silveiraww@radonc.ucsf.edu; yoms@radonc.ucsf.edu

Cotlar et al. [1] examined eight patients treated initially by surgical resection followed by adjuvant RT and found that the tumor was highly radiosensitive. Despite a successful outcome in just one patient, there was only a single failure within eight irradiated fields. The sensitivity of MCC to radiation was also demonstrated clinically in patients with regional and distant nodal disease. Long-term survival was achieved in one patient with axillary disease treated with post-dissection RT to 45 Gy [2]. Raaf et al. conducted a review of the literature including case reports, with conclusions supporting the utility of RT due to the excellent treatment responses of recurrent and metastatic MCC [2]. In another small, early retrospective study examining four patients with MCC, three of them had a complete response to radiation delivered to the primary tumor at a median follow-up of 1.5 years. There was also early evidence that postoperative nodal irradiation provided excellent regional control [3].

In general terms, the response of MCC to radiation is impressive. However, a moderate variation in clinical response has been observed clinically in patients treated for macroscopic disease. This variability has been quantified in MCC cell lines [4]. Experiments show that MCC cell lines produce a range in the surviving fraction at 2 Gy from 0.21 to 0.45 with an average of 0.30, which is very close to that of small cell lung cancer (SCLC). Samples derived from one tumor showed variability in the surviving fraction, supporting the notion that MCC can develop areas of radioresistance.

M. Alam et al. (eds.), *Merkel Cell Carcinoma*, DOI 10.1007/978-1-4614-6608-6_9,

The observed radiosensitivity of MCC in the laboratory and the clinic opened up an opportunity to obviate the need for massive resection. Furthermore, it was felt that RT should be considered a reasonable alternative for patients who refused surgery or were unresectable due to anatomical considerations or comorbidities.

Treatment of Primary Carcinoma

Radiation therapy techniques for treating MCC involve mainly low energy electrons and photons, sometimes in combination with higher energy photons depending on the depth of disease to be irradiated. Radiation treatment fields are often quite generously planned, using margins up to 2–5 cm of normal tissue in areas of concern.

Radiation therapy for MCC at UCSF includes targeting the primary tumor site, satellite or in-transit areas, and regional lymphatics [5]. Involved nodal areas may be detected surgically or radiographically by computed tomography (CT), positron emission tomography (PET), or magnetic resonance imaging (MRI). Coverage includes the primary surgical bed or residual gross tumor, draining lymphatics, and the regional lymph nodes with 2–3 cm margins. At UCSF, typical radiation doses for macroscopic disease or microscopic disease with positive surgical resection margins range from 56 to 60 Gy, with additional boosts of 4–6 Gy depending on tumor bulk. Areas with uninvolved or close surgical margins are treated to a dose of 50 Gy. The field is typically drawn with a 5 cm margin around the tumor or tumor bed, with smaller boost fields using 3 cm margins. Lymph nodes at risk within a draining nodal basin which do not harbor detectable disease but which are located within 20 cm of the primary site are treated to 46–50 Gy. The total dose is divided into daily sessions giving 1.8–2.0 Gy per fraction. Treatment is 5–6 weeks in duration, depending on the total dose and fractionation.

Radiation dose was initially chosen from experience and historical reasons. Most studies recommend doses between 50 and 60 Gy and show excellent tumor response and control. However, detailed investigations into the ideal dose are lacking due to the rare nature of MCC. Foote et al. [6] investigated the effects of dose on relapse patterns for MCC. These data suggest that there were no in-field failures within the tumor bed or regional lymph nodes for doses above 50 Gy. The authors also use their data to argue that 50 Gy is adequate for adjuvant and prophylactic treatments, but that 55 Gy is more suitable for gross disease. Finally, they suggest a 4 cm radial margin about the primary disease site. Hui et al. [7] used a multivariate analysis to show that dose was predictive of locoregional control, using a cutoff of 45 Gy as a distinction between palliative and radical treatment. Radiation doses for definitive treatment have ranged from 40 to 60 Gy in 20–30 fractions. In a palliative setting, where the hope is to control pain, tumor bleeding, and mass effect, excellent response has been achieved with doses as low as 25 Gy in a small number of patients [8].

For primary MCC located in the head and neck, the ipsilateral lymph nodes are treated prophylactically and bilateral treatment is reserved for those lesions that approach the midline. Intensity-modulated radiation therapy (IMRT), which allows for a more conformal dose distribution, may be utilized for complex plans involving the head and neck. Less sophisticated three-dimensional techniques may be used for other sites as appropriate.

The temporal aspects of RT are very important. Treatment delays can affect outcomes in a measurable way, owing to the aggressive nature of MCC. Progression of disease was found in 41 % of patients waiting a median of 24 days for therapy [9]. The subset of those to be treated with adjuvant RT was found to have even longer delays, with a median of 41 days to the initial consultation. It is imperative to evaluate and begin treatment as soon as possible for those with MCC.

Toxicity is anticipated to be acceptable or moderate in most patients. The most common side effects are fatigue, dermatitis, and localized edema. However, more potent radiation-induced toxicities can include acute mucosal or cutaneous reactions in the head and neck region or severe moist desquamation in the axilla or groin. These toxicities will often resolve in the 1 or 2 months following the conclusion of RT. Only rarely will toxicity create the need for a break in treatment.

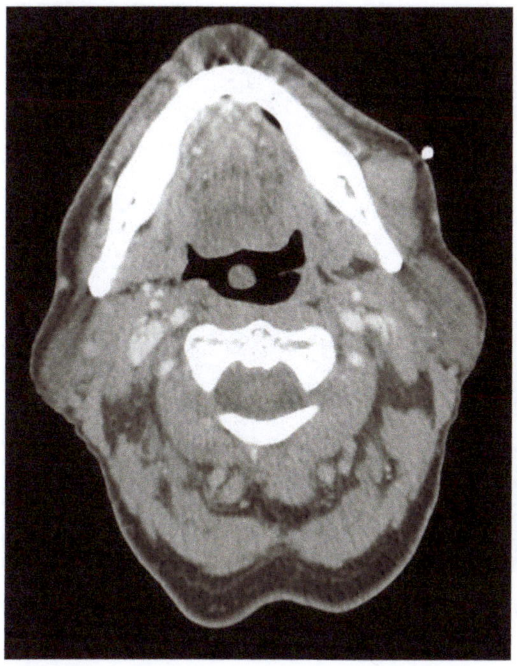

Fig. 9.1 CT with contrast showing a mass adjacent to the left masseter

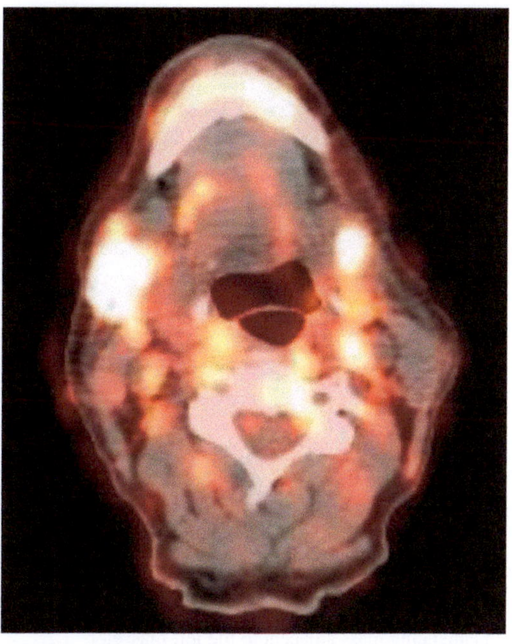

Fig. 9.2 PET/CT neck (axial) showing right and left-sided FDG-avid lymphadenopathy

Example: Head and Neck MCC

A 66-year-old Caucasian man noticed a stable lesion on his central philtrum for several months. He developed swelling on the left face and under the mandible. Screening CT imaging at that time revealed an enhancing soft tissue mass in the face anterior to the left masseter measuring 1.8 cm in diameter (Fig. 9.1) with associated bilateral neck lymph nodes that were considered suspicious. An excisional biopsy of the lesion at the philtrum confirmed MCC. A fine needle aspiration biopsy of the left facial lymph node also showed MCC.

Dual-modality PET/CT with diagnostic-quality contrast-enhanced head and neck CT confirmed FDG avidity in the left lower facial node. There were also bilateral submandibular lymph nodes that were FDG-avid (Fig. 9.2). No distant metastatic disease was identified. Anatomic imaging was ordered for presurgical planning. MRI of the neck with gadolinium enhancement showed the left facial node measuring 3.1 cm, a left submandibular node measuring 1.6 cm and a right submandibular node measuring 3.2 cm (Figs. 9.3 and 9.4).

The patient underwent surgery of the primary lesion that involved wide excision of the 1.2 cm lesion at the philtrum with reconstruction of the lip defect by plastic surgery. He also underwent a modified left radical neck dissection with a partial parotidectomy and a right selective neck dissection. Pathology showed that the primary was 0.9 cm in greatest diameter and the closest peripheral margin was 2.5 cm with the closest deep margin less than 1 mm. There was nodal involvement in two level IB lymph nodes and one right level I lymph node with extracapsular extension. The final stage was pT1N1M1a. He recovered well from his surgery but unfortunately a right sided facial lymph node became enlarged and palpable in the immediate postoperative period.

The patient was treated with IMRT. Tumor delineation was achieved by fusing the MRI and PET imaging with the radiation planning CT. A custom-fitted thermoplastic mesh mask was used to reproduce the patient's daily position accurately. Figure 9.5 shows representative axial, sagittal, and coronal slices of the planning CT with isodose lines. The progressing right sided facial node was treated definitively

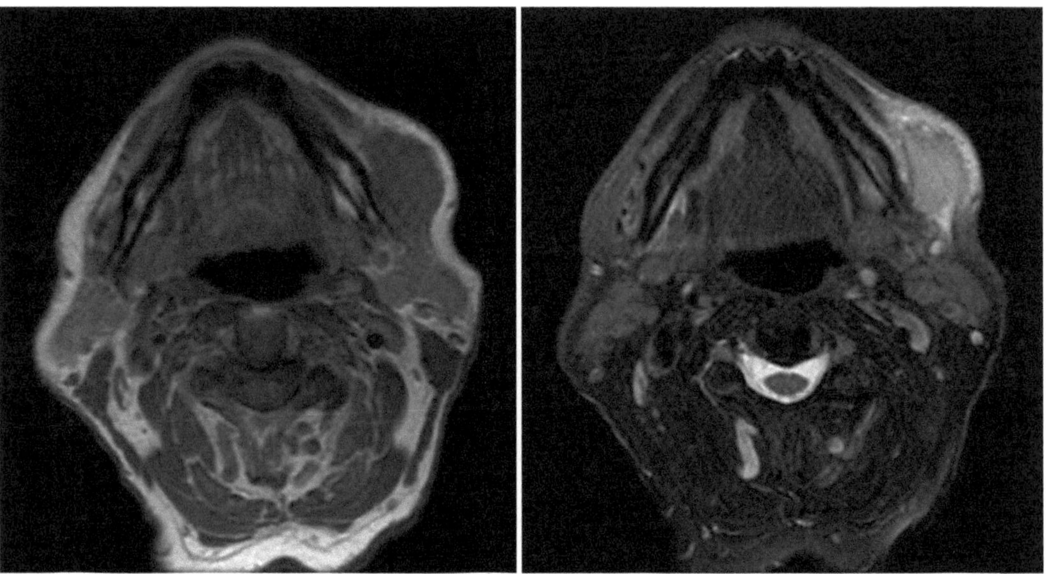

Fig. 9.3 Magnetic resonance imaging (MRI) neck. *Left*: T1 pre-gadolinium. *Right*: T1 post-gadolinium demonstrates an enhancing mass adjacent to the left masseter

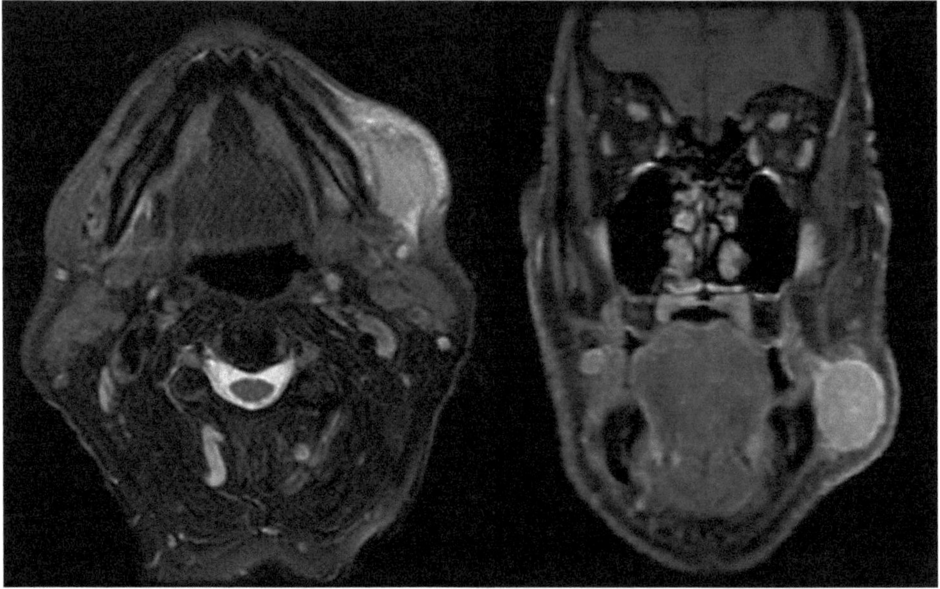

Fig. 9.4 MRI with contrast and fat suppression. The *left* and *right images* show axial and coronal slices through one of the enhancing left nodal metastases, respectively

to a wide-field dose of 60 Gy in 30 fractions, boosted to 66 Gy just around the gross disease. The dissected, involved lymph node regions in the right and left upper neck were treated to 60 Gy due to the extracapsular extension. The remainder of the regional head and neck lymphatics received prophylactic doses of approximately 54 Gy. The treatment was given as an integrated treatment over the course of 30 treatment sessions. The patient tolerated the treatment fairly well with the expected acute mucositis and dry desquamation of the skin.

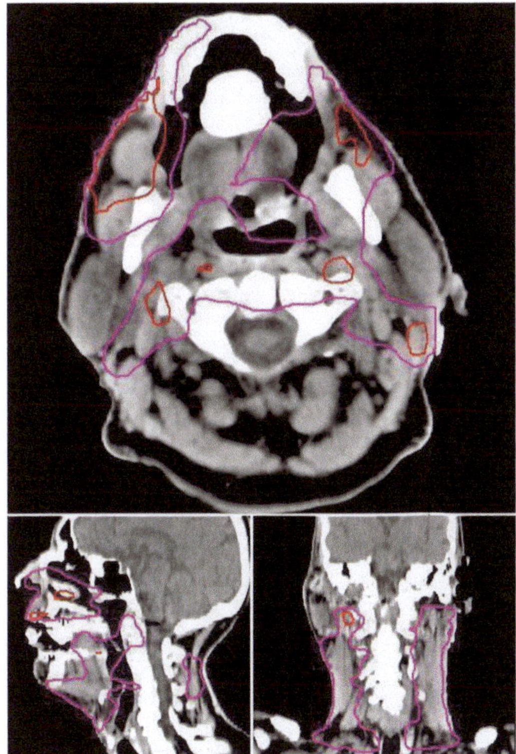

Fig. 9.5 Radiation therapy CT with dosimetry with isodose lines at 66 Gy (*red*) and 60 Gy (*pink*). *Top* (axial), *bottom left* (sagittal), and *bottom right* (coronal). The recurrent and progressing right-sided facial node was targeted for high doses of radiation therapy and showed a complete response by the end of treatment

The gross disease had resolved by the end of the radiation treatment and the patient remains in surveillance.

Example: Lower Extremity MCC

A 70-year-old man with a history of multiple, serious medical comorbidities noticed two nodules on the skin of his left lower leg, above the ankle. A biopsy revealed MCC. Dual-modality PET/CT showed a hypermetabolic focus in the medial left lower leg and a 1.2 cm left inguinal lymph node with FDG avidity. Fine-needle aspiration of the left inguinal lymph node was consistent with MCC. Ultrasound of the popliteal fossa did not reveal any suspicious nodal disease.

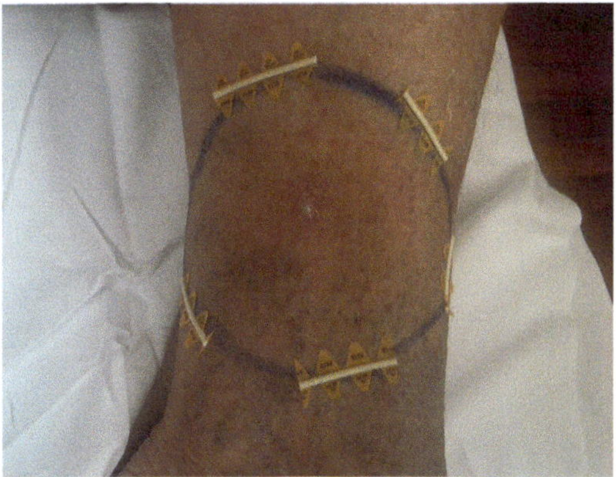

Fig. 9.6 Clinical setup for lower extremity MCC

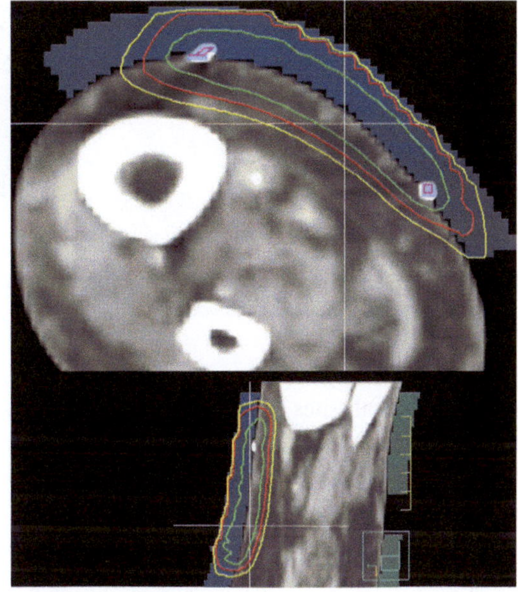

Fig. 9.7 Radiation therapy dosimetry with isodose lines delivered to the primary left lower extremity lesion. *Top*: axial slice. *Bottom*: sagittal

The patient was considered a poor candidate for surgery and after counseling, he opted for definitive RT. Treatment was carried out using electron therapy directed at a generous field surrounding the tumor on the left inner lower leg, shown in Figs. 9.6 and 9.7. Tissue equivalent bolus was placed on the skin to raise the dose to the surface of the tumor. The inguinal region was separately treated with a conformal photon plan

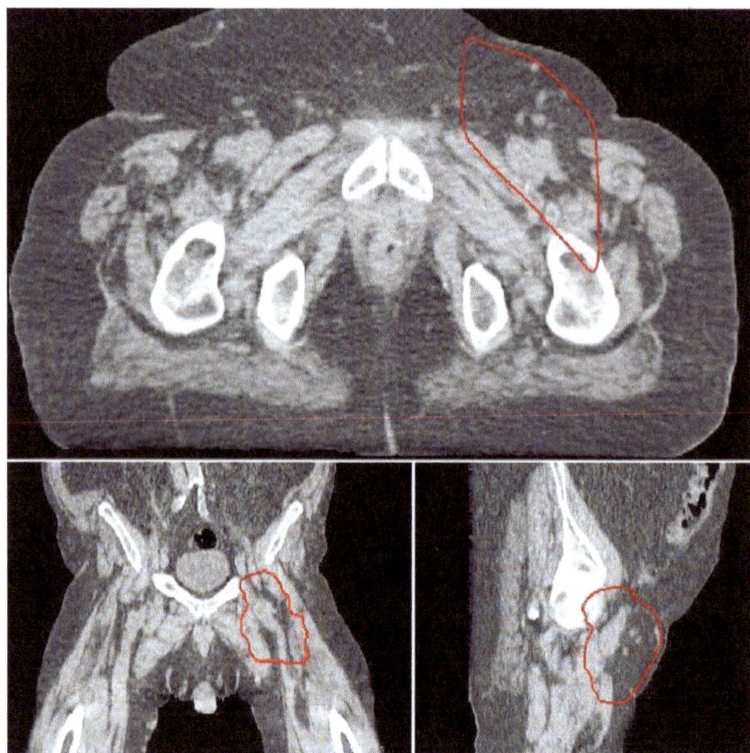

Fig. 9.8 Radiation therapy dosimetry with 100 % isodose line (*red*) delivered to the left inguinal lymph nodes. *Top* (axial), *bottom left* (sagittal), and *bottom right* (coronal)

(Fig. 9.8). Both sites received a dose of 56 Gy. The patient tolerated therapy well with moistness but not frank desquamation in the deep skin crease at the groin.

Treatment of Recurrent Carcinoma

When MCC is recurrent, a thorough restaging evaluation should be performed, as it is relatively uncommon for patients to experience an isolated local or regional recurrence. The vast majority of local or regional recurrences occur in concert with the development of distant metastasis. If the recurrence is confined to the local-regional area, the treatment of recurrent MCC is similar to that of primary MCC. Surgery is typically employed upfront, in a manner similar to the de novo setting. If further radiation is planned, a composite plan showing the previous and planned radiation dose distributions is used to evaluate the total dose distribution. Normal anatomic structures have cumulative lifetime radiation dose tolerances and these will limit the ability of the radiation oncologist to re-treat sensitive areas.

Treatment Techniques Under Development

Novel approaches are emerging to enhance the efficacy of RT for MCC. Here we describe a few novel methods such as brachytherapy, immunotherapy, hyperthermia, and lymphoscintigraphy that are under investigation.

Lesions of the lower extremities can be quite complicated to treat using conventional 3D or IMRT techniques. Cotter et al. [10] used surface mold computer-optimized high-dose rate brachytherapy for the treatment of multiple recurrent cutaneous nodules in the setting of a non-healing ulceration and a previously treated area in a 70-year-old man. Dose was easily delivered to the complex shape of the limb, limiting radiation delivery to unwanted areas.

It has been hypothesized that MCC is immunologically mediated. For example, in a case report describing a patient from the aforementioned brachytherapy series [6], an abscopal effect was observed in two untreated cutaneous nodules [11]. The abscopal effect refers to the resolution of distant, untreated lesions and is seen quite rarely in the medical literature. MCC has demonstrated the ability to regress spontaneously at both primary sites [12] and metastases [13]. Recently, the discovery of a polyomavirus associated with MCC has lent more credence to the role of the immune system in the development of the disease [14]. These observations have led to speculation about the possibility of immunotherapy combined with radiation. For example, a French report described the use of concurrent imiquimod [15] with RT for an unresectable patient who could not undergo chemotherapy due to comorbidities. The treatment was tolerated reasonably well and the patient had a complete response at 7 months after RT.

Hyperthermia is a technique that elevates the temperature of the tissues to be radiated, thereby increasing radiosensitivity. The technique has been used in conjunction with radiation for a variety of cancers. There have been a few cases of primary and recurrent MCC treated with radiation and hyperthermia with impressive response and outcomes [16, 17].

Finally, advances in imaging the regional lymphatics may assist in better defining the radiotherapy target volume. Lymphoscintigraphy, a technique used to map sentinel lymph nodes, has been used to help delineate RT planning for MCC [18]. In this technique, a radiolabeled substance is injected into or near the primary tumor. Draining lymphatics guide the radioactive material to the sentinel lymph node, which is then imaged at a later time. The rate of nonlocalization of the sentinel lymph node using preoperative lymphoscintigraphy was found to be 6.8 % in a series of head and neck melanoma and MCC patients [19]. Lymphoscintigraphy may enable more specific targeting of radiotherapy, thus offering the potential to reduce the morbidity of standard wide-field radiation treatment.

Evidence Basis for Therapy

Adjuvant radiation therapy delivered to the postoperative bed and residual gross disease has been proven to increase local control after surgical resection of the primary MCC. In addition, RT to the draining lymphatics has resulted in clear improvements in locoregional control. In situations when surgery is not possible, definitive radiation to the primary and regional lymphatics is a viable option for obtaining local and regional control. In this section, we discuss the evidence basis for adjuvant and definitive RT for MCC.

Adjuvant Radiation Therapy

Multimodal therapy, involving surgical resection of the primary tumor followed by adjuvant RT, is the standard of care for MCC. MCC can recur locally from unresected or residual microscopic disease and metastasizes via regional lymphatics. Unacceptably high local and regional recurrence rates after surgery combined with a relatively high radiosensitivity have led to the routine use of postoperative RT delivered to primary tumor bed and the regional lymphatics. Most retrospective studies over the past two decades have demonstrated the advantage of adjuvant RT for MCC, with excellent results for local and regional control as shown in the selected studies summarized in Table 9.1. Benefits to overall survival (OS) have been proposed, but may be less impressive due to the reliance on retrospective analyses and the rarity of the disease. Selected studies reporting survival metrics are shown in Table 9.2.

At a time when the primary method of treatment for MCC was wide local excision (WLE), Pacella et al. [20] reported excellent local control using RT, with a 100 % response rate in 19 patients with measurable disease. In sites that were prophylactically radiated, there were no failures. This strongly suggested that RT should play a role in the initial treatment of MCC. While

Table 9.1 Adjuvant radiation therapy: improved local and regional control

References	Year	Patients	Age (years)	Follow-up (years)	Treatment	Dose	Local and regional control	*p*
Ghadja et al. [35]	2011	180, 81 % L	73	5	S ± adjuvant RT	50 Gy	LRFS 93 % vs. 64 %	<0.001
							RRFS 76 % vs. 27 %	<0.001
Jouary et al. [36]	2011	83, 100 % L	79.9 (mean)	4.8	S + prophylactic RT to LN vs. S alone	50 Gy	Regional recurrence: 0 % vs. 16.7 %	0.007
Mendenhall et al. [34]	2011	40, 60 % L	69	3	S + adjuvant RT	60 Gy	5-year LC: 92 %, 5-year RC: 78 %	N/A
							5-year LR control: 79 %	
Hui et al. [7]	2011	176, 65 % L	79	2.2	S + adjuvant RT	50 Gy	LR recurrence rate 19 %	N/A
							5-year actuarial LRC 76 %	
							Dose ≥45 Gy predicts LR control	
Fang et al. [39]	2010	50, 100 % LR	N/A	1.5	Definitive RT vs. LN dissection ± adjuvant RT	N/A	Pathologic LN+: 100 % RC	0.8
							Clinical LN+: 2-year RRFS: 78 % for RT, 73 % for CLND ± RT	
Foote et al. [6]	2010	112, 56 % L, 11 % LR, 33 % DM	74	3.7	S + adjuvant RT	N/A	2-year LRC rate 75 %	N/A
							In-field local relapse rate: 3 %	
							In-field regional relapse rate: 11 %	
Lawenda et al. [43]	2008	36, 72 % L, LR, 28 % DM	71.6 (mean)	3.4	S ± adjuvant RT	54.5 Gy	19 % local recurrence overall	
							2-year LC: 95 % vs. 69 %	0.020
							2-year RC: 82 % vs. 60 %	0.225
Clark et al. [44]	2007	110, head and neck	68.6	1.8	S ± adjuvant RT	50 Gy	Improved LC & RC	0.009
								0.006
Lewis et al. [30]	2006	669, 85 % L	68 (mean)	2.4 (mean)	S ± adjuvant RT	N/A	LC: 23 % vs. 38 %, HR = 0.27	<0.001
							RC: 15 % vs. 44 %, HR = 0.34	<0.001
Jabbour et al. [28]	2006	82, 61 % L, 35 % LR	72	1.9	S (100 %) & adjuvant RT to primary (44 %) & LN (38 %)	50 Gy	Median time to first recurrence	
							Primary site: 24.2 vs. 11.8 months, HR = 0.62	0.18
							Regional LN: 46.2 vs. 11.3 months, HR = 0.42	0.01
							Any RT: increased time to recurrence	0.01
Allen et al. [27]	2005	251, 44 % L, 50 % LR	69	3.3	S ± adjuvant RT	N/A	Local recurrence 8 % w/ negative margin	0.76
							Primary site: LC 10 % vs. 8 %	0.13
							Regional recurrence: 13 % vs. 26 %	

Veness et al. [29]	2005	86, 55 % L, 22 % LR, 19 % R	75	2.6	S & adjuvant RT	50 Gy	Local relapse: 12 % vs. 14 % Regional relapse: 18 % vs. 37 %	NS
Boyer et al. [26]	2002	25, 100 % L	74	2.3	Mohs ± adjuvant RT	45–60 Gy	Local recurrence rates: 0 % vs. 16 %	0.12
Gillenwater et al. [25]	2001	66, 77 % L, 18 % LR	68.4 (mean)	>6 months	S ± adjuvant RT	N/A	Local recurrence: 12 % vs. 44 % Regional recurrence: 27 % vs. 85 %	<0.01 <0.01
Medina-Franco et al. [45]	2001	1,024, 73.4 % L	69	N/A	S ± adjuvant RT	46–50 Gy	Local recurrence 10.5 % vs. 52.6 %	0.00001
Meeuwissen et al. [23]	1995	80, 68 % L	74	1.7	S ± adjuvant RT	50 Gy	3-year RFS: 68 % vs. 0 % (mostly nodal) Time to recur (med): 16.5 vs. 5.5 months Local recurrence: 0 % vs. 16 %, Regional recurrence: 18 % vs. 71 %	RFS < 0.01
Boyle et al. [46]	1995	34, 58 % L	68	3	S ± adjuvant RT	>45 Gy	Response rate: 70 % (37 % CR, 33 % PR) Prophylactic nodal RT: 1/11 in-field fail	N/A
Yiengpruksawan et al. [22]	1991	70, 69 % L	66	2.3	S ± adjuvant RT	55 Gy	Local recurrence: 20 % vs. 16 % Regional recurrence: 9 % vs. 0 %	0.32 0.23
Shaw and Rumball [24]	1991	234, 91 % L	69	2.3	S ± adjuvant RT	N/A	Local recurrence: 26 % vs. 39 % Regional recurrence: 22 % vs. 46 %	N/A
Morrison et al. [21]	1990	54, 66 % L	70	3–8	S ± adjuvant RT, RT alone, various chemo	50–60 Gy	5-year FFR 56 % vs. 11 % Regional recurrence: 1 % vs. 46 % 1/31 in-field, 3/31 marginal recurrences	FFR 0.002
Pacella et al. [20]	1988	20, 10 % L	65	1.25	S & adjuvant RT	36–60 Gy	22/23 CR, 1/23 PR: 100 % response 0/13 failures with prophylactic RT	N/A

Note: Patients described as having local disease (L), regional disease (R), locoregional disease (LR), distant metastases (DM). Age and follow-up is given in median years unless specified. Treatment includes surgery (S) and radiation therapy (RT). Local control: local recurrence-free survival (LRFS), regional recurrence-free survival (RRFS), local control (LC), regional control (RC), locoregional control (LRC), completion lymph node dissection (CLND), recurrence-free survival (RFS), freedom from regression (FFR), complete response (CR), and partial response (PR). For comparisons in the local and regional control column: S + adjuvant RT vs. S alone

Table 9.2 Adjuvant radiation therapy: impact on survival

References	Year	Patients	Treatment	Survival	*p*
Hui et al. [7]	2011	176	S + adjuvant RT	5-year actuarial OS: 45 %	N/A
Mendenhall et al. [34]	2011	40	S + adjuvant RT	5-year OS: 36 % L vs. LR 5-year OS: 48 % vs. 18 %	0.0037
Ghadjar et al. [35]	2011	180	S ± adjuvant RT	5-year OS: 56 % vs. 46 % With negative margins, 5-year OS 66 % vs. 40 %	0.2 0.03
Reichgelt and Visser [33]	2011	808	S ± adjuvant RT	HR = 0.82	0.09
Mojica et al. [31]	2007	1,665	S ± adjuvant RT	MS: 63 vs. 45 months	0.002
Jabbour et al. [28]	2007	48	S ± adjuvant RT	MS: 53.9 vs. 25.2 months	0.033
Lewis et al. [30]	2006	669	S ± adjuvant RT	5-year OS 57 % vs. 50 %, HR = 0.78	0.16
Veness et al. [29]	2005	86	S ± adjuvant RT	5-year OS 47 % DFS (med): 10.5 vs. 4 months	<0.01
McAfee et al. [47]	2005	34	S + adjuvant RT	5-year OS for N0: 44 % 5-year OS for N+: 23 %	0.07
Poulsen et al. [48]	2003	53	S + chemoradiation	3-year OS: 76 %	N/A
Gillenwater et al. [25]	2001	66	S ± adjuvant RT	No differences in OS	>0.3
Morrison et al. [21]	1990	56	S ± adjuvant RT	5-year OS: 55 % vs. 28 %	N/A
Pacella et al. [20]	1988	20	S ± adjuvant RT	2-year actuarial OS: 63 %	N/A

Note: Surgery (S), radiation therapy (RT), overall survival (OS), median survival (MS), disease-free survival (DFS), local (L), locoregional (LR), node-negative (N0), node-positive (N+). For comparisons in the survival column: S + adjuvant RT vs. S alone

a variety of doses had been used prior to this study [1, 2], these authors were the first to provide evidence to support a working dose of 50 Gy divided into 25 fractions. A larger series from M.D. Anderson highlighted the unsatisfactory local and regional relapse rates with surgery alone [21] and showed a significant decrease in relapse rates with the use of adjuvant RT. In this series, a small number of marginal failures prompted the authors to suggest radiation fields to cover the primary tumor, tumor bed, and regional lymphatics with large margins using doses of up to 60 Gy for gross residual disease.

After surgical excision of a primary MCC, local failures and regional failures will occur in approximately 30 % and 50 % of patients, respectively. Adjuvant RT significantly reduces local and regional recurrence in MCC as can be seen in Table 9.1. While some earlier studies did fail to demonstrate significance [22], even in these series, response rates are notable and the rate of in-field failures is low.

Survival is still largely determined by the emergence of systemic disease, which is why some studies have shown a benefit in local and regional control without improvement in overall survival. For example, Boyle et al. treated a group of patients with surgery and adjuvant RT with successful local and regional control (no local failures and just one nodal recurrence). However, 63 % died of distant disease. These observations underscore the need for prompt use of definitive local therapies and the improvement of systemic therapy. Meeuwissen et al. [23] raised the question of whether obtaining local control earlier could alter the rate of disease dissemination, proposing a linkage between local-regional and distant outcomes. The presence of locoregional failure has been shown to be a negative prognostic factor for survival in the study by Shaw and Rumball [24].

An important retrospective study of 66 patients with MCC at M.D. Anderson demonstrated improvement in local and regional recurrence rates with adjuvant RT [25]. One group included 34 patients (82 % node-negative) treated with surgery alone and another group included 26 patients (90 % node-negative) treated with adjuvant RT and a final group of six patients treated with definitive RT. With adjuvant RT, local recurrence significantly decreased from 44 to 12 % and regional recurrence went from 85 to 27 %. Despite this encouraging improvement, overall survival and the development of distant metastases unfortunately remained unchanged, with half of all patients dying from disease within 3 years.

Margin status in the setting of adjuvant RT has also been investigated. Interestingly, the study by Gillenwater et al. [25], did not show a significant dependence of locoregional control or survival on the degree of surgical margins. The authors propose that this was likely due to the small number of patients.

Logically, the extent of resection should affect local and regional control. In order to help determine the utility of adjuvant RT in the setting of negative surgical margins by Mohs excision, Boyer et al. [26], compared Mohs with and without adjuvant RT for node-negative patients. They concluded that if complete excision were achieved, adjuvant radiation to the tumor bed was unnecessary. However, a close look at this data does not reveal a local recurrence rate of zero, even with negative margins in the best case scenario as determined by Mohs. Allen et al. [27] also suggested that adjuvant RT should not be routinely used in node-negative patients with negative surgical margins at the primary site, but that RT may be considered when negative margins cannot be obtained. However, this approach assumes a high level of confidence in the extent of excision, favorable surgical candidacy and anatomy, and low stage disease (i.e., early detection). Unfortunately, a significant percentage of patients do present with regional disease.

In contrast to the aforementioned studies, an Australian report of patients who were treated with adjuvant RT had twice the median time to recurrence compared to those treated with surgery alone (24.2 vs. 11.8 months, $p=0.18$) in patients who were primarily node-negative [28]. The authors also found a significant improvement in regional control and disease-free survival (DFS) in those who received any RT. They argued that the role for adjuvant RT is warranted regardless of stage and margin status.

Though adjuvant RT is clearly helpful in local and regional control, the benefits to overall survival have been less evident. Only a handful of studies have demonstrated improvements in survival metrics. Improved DFS was shown in a retrospective study by Veness et al. [29]. This retrospective study revealed that adjuvant RT more than doubled DFS from 4 to 10.5 months. Overall survival (OS) and local relapse rates were not improved, but regional relapse was significantly lower. In addition to improved local and regional control, Jabbour et al. [28] report a statistically significant benefit in MS from 53.9 vs. 25.2 months.

A impressively large meta-analysis, which included 333 reports with 1,254 patients, also showed an improvement in local and regional control with adjuvant RT for MCC, yet no difference was seen in overall or cause-specific survival [30]. Hazard ratios were reduced by RT: 0.27 for local recurrence and 0.34 for regional recurrence ($p<0.001$). The rate of disease progression from stage I to stage II was also significantly lower with postoperative radiation. A subgroup analysis including only comparative studies without case reports did show a significant improvement in cause-specific survival, HR=0.62, $p=0.04$ and overall survival, HR=0.63, $p=0.02$. The authors calculated that the study was underpowered to show survival benefit without these constraints. This study, despite its retrospective limitations, is the largest body of evidence supporting RT in the adjuvant setting.

The Surveillance, Epidemiology and End Results (SEER) registry was queried to review 1,665 patients treated for MCC [31]. Despite limitations on details of surgical treatment and RT, an improvement in overall survival was revealed. Surgery was performed in 89 % of the cases, with 40 % of the surgical cases receiving some type of RT. Overall, median survival was 49 months for all patients with a median follow-up of 40 months. However, median survival was 45 months for surgery alone and 63 months for surgery with RT ($p=0.0002$). The benefit of radiation was apparent for all size lesions, but even more so for those tumors greater than 2 cm with median overall survival improving from 21 to 50 months. The patients who received radiation were younger (median of 72 vs. 76 years), but they also presented with more advanced disease. Housman et al. [32] argue that the OS benefit no longer is statistically significant when accounting for the selection bias that keeps sicker patients from receiving RT and the inherent limitations of the SEER database. In another study from the Netherlands with a large number of patients (808), survival after surgery and adjuvant radiation therapy was "borderline" significantly better than surgery as monotherapy (HR = 0.82, $p = 0.09$) [33].

While the SEER study lacked details regarding radiation treatment, a recent study by Mendenhall et al. [34], gives a clear picture of what to expect in terms of local control, regional control, and survival for different stage MCC treated with multimodal therapy. In this study, the overall rates of 5-year local control, regional control, and locoregional control were 92 %, 78 %, and 79 %, respectively. Distant metastasis-free survival was 79 %. Cause-specific survival and overall survival were 45 % and 36 %, respectively. Comparing those patients with local and locoregional disease, locoregional control was comparable at 87 % and 67 %, respectively ($p = 0.16$). The problem of distant metastases with locoregional disease is made clear by the 5-year distant metastasis-free survival of 71 % vs. 37 % ($p = 0.0073$) for local vs. locoregional disease, respectively. Given the fact that most patients die of distant disease and that locoregional disease is fairly controlled in both local and locoregional patients with MCC, it becomes clear that the losing battle is a systemic one. Five-year overall survival is between local and regional was 48 % vs. 18 % ($p = 0.037$). Another recent retrospective study showed significant improvements in local and regional recurrence-free survival (LRFS and RRFS), but failed to reach significance with 5-year OS: 56 % vs. 46 % ($p = 0.2$) [35]. A subgroup of patients with negative margins had 5-year OS 66 % vs. 40 % ($p = 0.03$).

A prospective randomized study of prophylactic nodal RT to node-negative patients attempted to answer many questions, but was stopped early due the use of sentinel node dissection [36]. Patients were treated with a WLE followed by adjuvant RT to the tumor bed with and without prophylactic RT to the regional lymph nodes. No difference was noted in OS or progression-free survival (PFS). As has been shown before, regional recurrence rates were lower in the irradiated arm (0 %) compared to the observational arm (16.7 %) with $p = 0.007$.

Definitive Radiation Therapy

As discussed, there is considerable evidence that wide excision followed by local and regional RT is the treatment of choice. However, for some patients the tumor location makes surgery technically impossible, particularly those with tumors in the head and neck. Elderly patients are often medically unfit for surgery due to multiple comorbidities or they may simply deny surgery altogether. The benefits of radiation alone include improved aesthetics and the elimination of surgical risk. Disadvantages include potential undertreatment of significant bulk disease and a theoretical decrease in local control given the strong evidence supporting the efficacy of postoperative RT. However, offering the opportunity for cure with radiation monotherapy is not unreasonable. Radiation can certainly offer control of undesirable mass effect, pain control and high overall quality of life.

Several small retrospective series support the use of radiation monotherapy with impressive results (see Table 9.1). Mortier et al. compared 9 stage I patients treated with radiation alone and 17 patients treated with surgery followed by RT, with a median follow-up of 3.0 and 4.6 years, respectively [37]. This work found no difference in overall survival or disease-free survival. The median dose was 60 Gy to the primary site (range 50–78 Gy), with the majority of patients treated to the regional lymphatics. None of the patients treated with radiation alone progressed, while one patient in the postoperative group relapsed and another progressed and died.

In a small Australian retrospective series, RT alone for inoperable patients with node-positive MCC had an in-field control rate of 88 % [8]. An

Table 9.3 Definitive radiation therapy for inoperable MCC

References	Year	Patients	Age (years)	Follow-up (years)	Dose	Local and regional control
Pape et al. [40]	2011	25	80	2.8	55 Gy	92 %
Fang et al. [39]	2010	50	N/A	1.5	N/A	100 % RC for pathologic+LN Clinical+LN: 2-year RRFS: 78 % for RT, 73 % for CLND±RT
Veness et al. [38]	2010	43	79	3.25	51 Gy	75 %
Koh and Veness [8]	2009	8	82.5	1	50 Gy	88 % (single in-field failures)
Mortier et al. [37]	2003	9	81	3	60 Gy	100 %

Note: Age, follow-up and does are median values. Regional control (RC), regional recurrence-free survival (RRFS), completion lymphadenectomy (CLND)

impressive complete response in a large tumor was noted in one patient. Another Australian study reviewed 43 patients with MCC with a median follow-up of 3.25 years, 33 of whom had nodal involvement [38]. Overall survival at 2 and 5 years was 58 % and 37 %, respectively. Fang et al. [39], found that definitive irradiation provided excellent regional control for microscopic disease and compared well to completion lymphadenectomy with or without adjuvant radiation. Equivalent results between treatments were also found for those patients with clinically positive disease. A French retrospective study compared 25 inoperable patients treated with radiation alone to 25 patients treated with surgery and postoperative radiation with similar results [40] (Table 9.3).

Treatment of Recurrent Disease

Often, systemic therapy is part of the treatment for recurrent and metastatic disease. Radiation therapy is an option for most previously untreated areas. Eng et al. [41] reported on 46 patients with recurrent disease and found patients with distant disease had a median survival of just 12 months. However, the mean survival for those treated with combination therapy, including surgery and RT, was just over 3 years compared to 17.5 months for those treated with monotherapy. The authors recommend that when possible, soft tissue and nodal recurrences should be excised followed by adjuvant RT. Re-irradiation should be done when possible, respecting normal tissue tolerance. In another series, 12 of 68 patients with recurrence had a complete response to salvage therapy [42]. Unlike those with local or regional recurrence, most of the patients with distant metastases did not fare well.

Conclusions

- MCC is an aggressive, yet very radiosensitive cancer and is best treated with multimodal therapy including surgery and radiation therapy.
- Radiation therapy plays a critical role in the local, regional, and distant control of MCC.
- Adjuvant radiation therapy significantly increases local and regional control.
- Adjuvant radiation therapy has been shown to increase overall survival in some studies, though the benefit is less certain.
- Definitive radiation therapy can be employed as effective monotherapy for inoperable MCC.
- Radiation therapy also plays a role in the treatment of recurrent MCC.
- Delay in the start of radiation has been associated with disease progression.
- Acute toxicity from radiation therapy is expected and acceptable given the clear benefit of improved local and regional control.
- Palliative radiation therapy can help with mass effects and pain control as well as other oncologic emergencies including spinal cord compression.

References

1. Cotlar AM, Gates JO, Gibbs Jr FA. Merkel cell carcinoma: combined surgery and radiation therapy. Am Surg. 1986;52(3):159–64.
2. Raaf JH et al. Trabecular (Merkel cell) carcinoma of the skin. Treatment of primary, recurrent, and metastatic disease. Cancer. 1986;57(1):178–82.
3. Ashby MA et al. Primary cutaneous neuroendocrine (Merkel cell or trabecular carcinoma) tumour of the skin: a radioresponsive tumour. Clin Radiol. 1989; 40(1):85–7.
4. Leonard JH et al. Radiation sensitivity of Merkel cell carcinoma cell lines. Int J Radiat Oncol Biol Phys. 1995;32(5):1401–7.
5. Hansen EK, Roach M. Handbook of evidence-based radiation oncology. 2nd ed. New York: Springer; 2010. p. xviii, 786.
6. Foote M et al. Effect of radiotherapy dose and volume on relapse in Merkel cell cancer of the skin. Int J Radiat Oncol Biol Phys. 2010;77(3):677–84.
7. Hui AC et al. Merkel cell carcinoma: 27-year experience at the Peter MacCallum Cancer Centre. Int J Radiat Oncol Biol Phys. 2011;80(5):1430–5.
8. Koh CS, Veness MJ. Role of definitive radiotherapy in treating patients with inoperable Merkel cell carcinoma: the Westmead Hospital experience and a review of the literature. Australas J Dermatol. 2009;50(4): 249–56.
9. Tsang G et al. All delays before radiotherapy risk progression of Merkel cell carcinoma. Australas Radiol. 2004;48(3):371–5.
10. Cotter SE et al. Treatment of cutaneous metastases of Merkel cell carcinoma with surface-mold computer-optimized high-dose-rate brachytherapy. J Clin Oncol. 2010;28(27):e464–6.
11. Cotter SE et al. Abscopal effect in a patient with metastatic Merkel cell carcinoma following radiation therapy: potential role of induced antitumor immunity. Arch Dermatol. 2011;147(7):870–2.
12. Kayashima K et al. Spontaneous regression in Merkel cell (neuroendocrine) carcinoma of the skin. Arch Dermatol. 1991;127(4):550–3.
13. O'Rourke MG; Bell JR. Merkel cell tumor with spontaneous regression. J Dermatol Surg Oncol. 1986; 12(9):994–6, 1000.
14. Wong HH, Wang J. Merkel cell carcinoma. Arch Pathol Lab Med. 2010;134(11):1711–6.
15. Balducci M et al. Treatment of Merkel cell carcinoma with radiotherapy and imiquimod (Aldara): a case report. Tumori. 2010;96(3):508–11.
16. Muggianu M et al. Radiotherapy and hyperthermia in the treatment of primary Merkel cell carcinoma of the skin: a case report. Bull Cancer Radiother. 1994;81(3): 237–40.
17. Knox SJ, Kapp DS. Hyperthermia and radiation therapy in the treatment of recurrent Merkel cell tumors. Cancer. 1988;62(8):1479–86.
18. Hebbard PC et al. Lymphoscintigraphy as a means for planning radiation therapy in a case of Merkel cell carcinoma of the buttock. J Surg Oncol. 2006;94(2): 167–9.
19. Stadelmann WK, Cobbins L, Lentsch EJ. Incidence of nonlocalization of sentinel lymph nodes using preoperative lymphoscintigraphy in 74 consecutive head and neck melanoma and Merkel cell carcinoma patients. Ann Plast Surg. 2004;52(6):546–9; discussion 550.
20. Pacella J et al. The role of radiotherapy in the management of primary cutaneous neuroendocrine tumors (Merkel cell or trabecular carcinoma): experience at the Peter MacCallum Cancer Institute (Melbourne, Australia). Int J Radiat Oncol Biol Phys. 1988; 14(6):1077–84.
21. Morrison WH et al. The essential role of radiation therapy in securing locoregional control of Merkel cell carcinoma. Int J Radiat Oncol Biol Phys. 1990; 19(3):583–91.
22. Yiengpruksawan A et al. Merkel cell carcinoma. Prognosis and management. Arch Surg. 1991;126(12): 1514–9.
23. Meeuwissen JA, Bourne RG, Kearsley JH. The importance of postoperative radiation therapy in the treatment of Merkel cell carcinoma. Int J Radiat Oncol Biol Phys. 1995;31(2):325–31.
24. Shaw JH, Rumball E. Merkel cell tumour: clinical behaviour and treatment. Br J Surg. 1991;78(2): 138–42.
25. Gillenwater AM et al. Merkel cell carcinoma of the head and neck: effect of surgical excision and radiation on recurrence and survival. Arch Otolaryngol Head Neck Surg. 2001;127(2):149–54.
26. Boyer JD et al. Local control of primary Merkel cell carcinoma: review of 45 cases treated with Mohs micrographic surgery with and without adjuvant radiation. J Am Acad Dermatol. 2002;47(6):885–92.
27. Allen PJ et al. Merkel cell carcinoma: prognosis and treatment of patients from a single institution. J Clin Oncol. 2005;23(10):2300–9.
28. Jabbour J et al. Merkel cell carcinoma: assessing the effect of wide local excision, lymph node dissection, and radiotherapy on recurrence and survival in early-stage disease—results from a review of 82 consecutive cases diagnosed between, 1992 and 2004. Ann Surg Oncol. 2007;14(6):1943–52.
29. Veness MJ et al. Merkel cell carcinoma: improved outcome with adjuvant radiotherapy. ANZ J Surg. 2005;75(5):275–81.
30. Lewis KG et al. Adjuvant local irradiation for Merkel cell carcinoma. Arch Dermatol. 2006;142(6): 693–700.
31. Mojica P, Smith D, Ellenhorn JD. Adjuvant radiation therapy is associated with improved survival in Merkel cell carcinoma of the skin. J Clin Oncol. 2007;25(9):1043–7.
32. Housman DM, Decker RH, Wilson LD. Regarding adjuvant radiation therapy in Merkel cell carcinoma: selection bias and its affect on overall survival. J Clin Oncol. 2007;25(28):4503–4; author reply 4504–5.
33. Reichgelt BA, Visser O. Epidemiology and survival of Merkel cell carcinoma in the Netherlands.

A population-based study of 808 cases in 1993–2007. Eur J Cancer. 2011;47(4):579–85.
34. Mendenhall WM et al. Cutaneous Merkel cell carcinoma. Am J Otolaryngol. 2012;33(1):88–92.
35. Ghadjar P et al. The essential role of radiotherapy in the treatment of Merkel cell carcinoma: a study from the Rare Cancer Network. Int J Radiat Oncol Biol Phys. 2011;81:e583–91.
36. Jouary T et al. Adjuvant prophylactic regional radiotherapy versus observation in stage I Merkel cell carcinoma: a multicentric prospective randomized study. Ann Oncol. 2012;23(4):1074–80.
37. Mortier L et al. Radiotherapy alone for primary Merkel cell carcinoma. Arch Dermatol. 2003;139(12):1587–90.
38. Veness M et al. The role of radiotherapy alone in patients with Merkel cell carcinoma: reporting the Australian experience of 43 patients. Int J Radiat Oncol Biol Phys. 2010;78(3):703–9.
39. Fang LC et al. Radiation monotherapy as regional treatment for lymph node-positive Merkel cell carcinoma. Cancer. 2010;116(7):1783–90.
40. Pape E et al. Radiotherapy alone for Merkel cell carcinoma: a comparative and retrospective study of 25 patients. J Am Acad Dermatol. 2011;65(5):983–90.
41. Eng TY et al. Treatment of recurrent Merkel cell carcinoma: an analysis of 46 cases. Am J Clin Oncol. 2004;27(6):576–83.
42. Tai P et al. Multimodality management for 145 cases of Merkel cell carcinoma. Med Oncol. 2010;27(4):1260–6.
43. Lawenda BD et al. Analysis of radiation therapy for the control of Merkel cell carcinoma of the head and neck based on 36 cases and a literature review. Ear Nose Throat J. 2008;87(11):634–43.
44. Clark JR et al. Merkel cell carcinoma of the head and neck: is adjuvant radiotherapy necessary? Head Neck. 2007;29(3):249–57.
45. Medina-Franco H et al. Multimodality treatment of Merkel cell carcinoma: case series and literature review of 1024 cases. Ann Surg Oncol. 2001;8(3):204–8.
46. Boyle F, Pendlebury S, Bell D. Further insights into the natural history and management of primary cutaneous neuroendocrine (Merkel cell) carcinoma. Int J Radiat Oncol Biol Phys. 1995;31(2):315–23.
47. McAfee WJ et al. Merkel cell carcinoma: treatment and outcomes. Cancer. 2005;104(8):1761–4.
48. Poulsen M et al. High-risk Merkel cell carcinoma of the skin treated with synchronous carboplatin/etoposide and radiation: a Trans-Tasman Radiation Oncology Group Study—TROG 96:07. J Clin Oncol. 2003;21(23):4371–6.

Chemotherapy (Primary and Recurrent Disease)

10

Rupali Roy and Timothy M. Kuzel

The role of systemic chemotherapy for Merkel cell carcinoma (MCC) has been poorly defined as few prospective, and no randomized clinical trials have been conducted due to the relative rarity of this disorder. However, the literature regarding chemotherapy in MCC does provide evidence that this entity is chemosensitive. Thus, most of the data regarding chemotherapeutics comes from retrospective analyses at single institutions. Though most institutions consider chemotherapy and/or surgery and/or radiation therapy for stage IV disease as reasonable, the role in this setting and the use of chemotherapy in the neoadjuvant or adjuvant setting for early stage or node positive disease remains controversial.

Chemotherapy for Metastatic Disease

A number of single agent and combination chemotherapy regimens have been shown to be active in MCC. Two of the most commonly used regimens are cisplatin or carboplatin with or without etoposide and cyclophosphamide with doxorubicin (or epirubicin) and vincristine. Other agents that have been used alone or in combination successfully include ifosfamide [1], 5-fluorouracil [2], methotrexate [2], topotecan [3], dacarbazine [4], and liposomal doxorubicin [5]. Responses, however, are relatively short-lived, and toxicity is not negligible in a patient population where the median age at diagnosis is 69.

Voog et al. reviewed the literature and reported the outcomes of 107 patients with either locally advanced or metastatic MCC treated with chemotherapy [6]. Cyclophosphamide or ifosfamide-containing regimens were given to 56 % of patients, anthracycline-containing regimens to 49 %, platinum-containing regimens to 25 %, 5FU-containing regimens to 13 %, and other regimens to 12 %. The overall response rate (ORR) for first-line chemotherapy was 61 %. There was no significant difference in ORR between locally advanced and metastatic tumors, which was 69 % and 57 %, respectively. Though the response rates observed with the different types of chemotherapy regimens ranged from 43 % to 100 %, none was associated with significantly superior survival. The median duration of response was 8 months, and the median overall survival (OS) from the date of initiation of chemotherapy was 24 months for patients with locally advanced disease and 9 months for patients with metastatic disease. Overall survival was significantly better in patients who had locally advanced disease and in those patients who achieved a CR after first-line chemotherapy.

R. Roy
Division of Hematology/Oncology, Department of Internal Medicine, University of Michigan Hospital, C367 Med Inn Building, 1500 East Medical Center Drive, SPC 5848, Ann Arbor, MI 48109-5848, USA
e-mail: royrupali@gmail.com; rupalir@med.umich.edu

T.M. Kuzel (✉)
Division of Hematology/Oncology, Department of Medicine, Feinberg School of Medicine of Northwestern University, 676 N Saint Clair St Suite 850, Chicago, IL 60611, USA
e-mail: t-kuzel@northwestern.edu

M. Alam et al. (eds.), *Merkel Cell Carcinoma*, DOI 10.1007/978-1-4614-6608-6_10,

Among the 33 patients who received second-line chemotherapy, 45 % responded, while only 20 % of the 10 patients who received third-line chemotherapy responded. Seven patients did achieve a prolonged survival of over 24 months after beginning chemotherapy. Three of these patients had locally advanced disease, and four patients had metastatic disease but did not have visceral metastases. Nine treatment-related deaths (8.4 % of the patient population) were reported, five of which were due to septic shock with febrile neutropenia. The majority of patients who died of toxicity were older than 65.

Similar results have been observed in other retrospective reviews. Tai et al. reported on 204 patients with MCC who received chemotherapy either in the adjuvant setting or at the time of nodal or distant recurrence [7]. They observed that the two most commonly used regimens in their series were cyclophosphamide, doxorubicin (or epirubicin), and vincristine with or without prednisone (CAV or CEV ± prednisone) and carboplatin or cisplatin with etoposide. There was no significant difference in the response rates between the two regimens, which were 75.7 % and 60 %, respectively. Six definite toxic deaths (3 % of all patients) were reported in this series of patients who had a median age of 73. In another retrospective review of 27 patients who received a variety of chemotherapy regimens for locoregional disease, metastatic disease, or in the second- or third-line setting at the time of recurrence, the ORR was 69 % with a median duration of response of 6 months (range 1–71 months) [8]. Once again, decreasing response rates were observed with second- and third-line chemotherapies, and visceral metastases were much less responsive to treatment.

Chemotherapy in the Adjuvant Setting

From the data reported in the metastatic setting, it is acknowledged by most oncologists that MCC is responsive to chemotherapy. However, to date, there is no data to show that chemotherapy significantly improves disease-free or overall survival if applied earlier in the disease course.

In one review of 85 patients with local, locally advanced, or metastatic disease, all of whom were initially treated with surgical intervention, the addition of adjuvant therapy with radiation and/or chemotherapy in 51 % of the patients decreased recurrence rates but did not have an effect on survival [9]. The recurrence rate in patients treated with surgery alone was 52.7 % vs. 32.5 % in patients treated with surgery and/or radiation and/or chemotherapy ($p < 0.05$). The recurrence rates in patients treated with surgery and radiation vs. surgery and chemotherapy were comparable at 40.7 % and 40 %, respectively. The number of patients who actually received chemotherapy in this study was admittedly very small.

In another small retrospective study, the addition of adjuvant chemotherapy did not seem to benefit a group of 34 newly diagnosed MCC patients with stage I to III disease who were treated with curative intent [10]. After initial surgical management in 32 patients, all patients received radiation therapy, and 9 went on to receive adjuvant chemotherapy. At a median follow-up of 3 years, 56 % of those patients who had received adjuvant chemotherapy had developed distant metastases while only 32 % of those who had not received chemotherapy had metastasized.

Allen et al. assessed 251 patients with MCC treated at a single large comprehensive cancer center, 28 of whom were given adjuvant chemotherapy for local or regional disease [11]. Carboplatin and etoposide was the most commonly used adjuvant regimen and did not positively affect the development of distant recurrence in that 19 % of the patients who did not receive adjuvant chemotherapy developed distant recurrence while 32 % of the patients who did receive adjuvant chemotherapy developed distant recurrence ($p = 0.11$). When factors associated with survival were analyzed by COX regression, the only independent predictors of survival were pathologic nodal status and disease stage.

A larger retrospective study of 364 patients with stage I to III MCC treated at the same center was published in 2011 [12]. The majority of patients underwent margin-negative excision of the primary tumor, and approximately a quarter went on to receive adjuvant radiation therapy.

Chemotherapy was received by 53 patients (15 % of all patients) most of whom had stage III disease. An additional 27 received it concurrently with radiation therapy. At a median follow-up of 3.6 years, 30 % of patients had developed a recurrence. The majority of these recurrences (80 %) developed in patients who had clinically involved lymph nodes or in patients who did not undergo pathologic lymph node evaluation, and the incidence of distant recurrence was highest in patients with stage IIIB disease (32 %). In multivariate analysis, factors associated with recurrence included a synchronous or previous diagnosis of leukemia or lymphoma and increasing pathologic stage, but not adjuvant chemotherapy or even adjuvant radiotherapy. Patients who were selected to receive chemotherapy in this study were in fact more likely to develop distant recurrence at 2 years compared to those who were not selected (30.5 % vs. 15.4 %, $p=0.02$). However, these retrospective studies suffer from obvious potential biases as patients with adverse clinical features are often the patients selected to receive the additional chemotherapy.

Thus, retrospective data available to date does not provide evidence that chemotherapy improves clinical outcomes in MCC. Neither does the little prospective data that exists. The Trans-Tasman Radiation Oncology Group (TROG) study 96:07 is one of the few prospective phase II studies that have been conducted in patients with MCC [13]. In this study, 53 patients who had disease localized to the primary site and regional nodes and who had at least one high-risk feature were enrolled. Patients were considered high risk if they had one or more of the following: recurrence after initial therapy, involved nodes, primary tumor size greater than 1 cm, gross residual disease after surgery, or occult primary with nodes. Surgery was performed prior to referral and entry into the study. Radiation was delivered to the primary site and nodes to a dose of 50 Gy in 25 fractions over 5 weeks and synchronous carboplatin (AUC 4.5) and intravenous etoposide 80 mg/m^2 days 1–3 were given on weeks 1, 4, 7, and 10. The median age at the time of enrollment was 67 (range 43–86). Forty-one patients had never been treated before. Three-year OS, locoregional control, and distant control were 76 %, 75 %, and 76 %, respectively. No treatment-related deaths were reported, but 64 % had grade 3 or 4 skin toxicity, 57 % experienced grade 3 or 4 neutropenia, and 35 % febrile neutropenia. It was previously reported that quality-of-life scores fell rapidly after week 3 of treatment and had not returned to pretreatment baseline by week 13 [14]. Multivariate analysis indicated that the major factor influencing survival was the presence of nodes, not chemotherapy.

Poulsen et al. later compared 40 of the patients treated on the TROG 96:07 trial to 62 patients from their database who had been treated with surgery and radiation alone [15]. The inclusion and exclusion criteria for the 62 patients chosen from the database were identical to that for the TROG 96:07 study. Multivariate analysis revealed that adjuvant chemotherapy had no significant impact on any of the end points of interest including overall survival, disease-specific survival, local-regional control, and distant metastatic-free survival. The authors argued that given the wide confidence intervals, a favorable chemotherapeutic effect could not be definitely excluded and that the study size was not powered to detect small improvements in survival.

The same group later conducted another prospective phase II trial of 18 patients who again had high-risk stage I or II disease as in the TROG 96:07 trial [16]. The chemo-radiation regimen in this trial was altered with the goal of decreasing the toxicity observed in the original TROG trial. These patients received radiation to the primary site and nodes with weekly carboplatin AUC 2 followed by 3 cycles of carboplatin AUC 4.5 and etoposide 80 mg/m^2 days 1–3 every 3 weeks. In comparison to the 53 patients in the TROG 96:07 study, the rates of both febrile neutropenia and grade 3 skin toxicity were significantly decreased ($p=0.003$ and $p=0.006$, respectively). Of the 18 patients, 7 patients died. None were treatment-related. One patient had in-transit recurrence, four developed nodal metastases, and three developed distant metastases. Because of the small number of patients, direct comparison of efficacy of this regimen in comparison to the original TROG 96:07 chemo-radiation regimen could not be made.

Thus, like the retrospective data, the small amount of prospective data on chemotherapy in MCC available to date does not show a significant benefit in clinical outcome.

Chemotherapy in the Neoadjuvant Setting

Data regarding the use of neoadjuvant chemotherapy in MCC is scarce. Jouary et al. published a case report of two patients in 2009 who were treated with neoadjuvant etoposide, cisplatin, and cyclophosphamide (EPC) [17]. The first patient had newly diagnosed stage II MCC of the left cheek that was too large to operate on initially. Thus, this 72-year-old patient received 1 cycle of EPC, which resulted in a partial response (PR). He went on to have a wide local excision and regional neck node dissection followed by an additional cycle of EPC followed by radiotherapy, which resulted in a complete remission (CR) for 32 months. The second patient was treated with 2 cycles of EPC for recurrent node positive MCC after which he achieved a CR. This was followed by a groin lymph node dissection, radiotherapy, and one additional cycle of EPC. He maintained a CR for 2 months and then developed a cutaneous recurrence for which he was treated with 2 cycles of EPC followed by wide local excision. This 61-year-old patient subsequently maintained a CR for 5+ years.

Investigational Approaches

Alternate strategies have been employed in an effort to improve upon the above outcomes in MCC. Autologous stem cell transplantation after high-dose chemotherapy has yielded similar results to chemotherapy alone with a short duration of response of 6 months [18]. There have been reports of intra-tumor injection of human tumor necrosis factor yielding complete responses in two Japanese patients [19]. There has been a case of the immune-modulating dinitrochlorbenzol having been applied topically to an extensive inoperable MCC of the scalp with local and regional metastases resulting in a complete remission that lasted 1 year [20]. Isolated limb perfusion or infusion with chemotherapy (melphalan alone, melphalan with actinomycin D and/or nitrogen mustard and/or tumor necrosis factor-a) for in-transit MCC has allowed some patients to avoid amputation and has yielded responses with a mean duration of 21.8 months without serious complication [21].

The somatostatin analogs, octreotide and lanreotide, have both been utilized in the treatment of MCC. In one elderly patient not fit for either chemotherapy or radiotherapy, a complete response was achieved after 10 months of treatment with octreotide [22]. In another patient with metastatic MCC, lanreotide was well-tolerated and resulted in a partial response for 7 months [23]. There is one case report of a 177-lutetium-labeled somatostatin analog given in conjunction with the radiosensitizing liposomal doxorubicin that resulted in a mixed response [24].

Studies have revealed that MCC can express VEGF, VEGFR, PDGF, PDGFR, and c-kit, thus suggesting a possible role for multi-targeted receptor tyrosine kinase inhibitors in management. Results to date utilizing this approach have unfortunately been disappointing. The SWOG S0331 study was a phase II trial of imatinib in patients with metastatic or unresectable MCC, all of whose tumors expressed c-kit [25]. Imatinib was given at a dose of 400 mg orally daily in a heavily pretreated group of 23 patients with a median age of 77.1. Only one of the 23 patients responded with a PR that lasted only 1 month. In retrospect, despite the expression of CD117 or c-kit in the tumors of both patients, it was found that neither had activating mutations of c-kit, which is likely why imatinib had limited activity. In another trial, pazopanib was used to treat a patient with recurrent metastatic MCC [26]. This patient was c-kit negative but was VEGF positive and had a 1432T>C mutation in PDGFR-a. Pazopanib was given at 800 mg orally daily, and after 2 months, the patient achieved a PR that lasted 6 months.

In summary, chemotherapy has shown activity in MCC in the neoadjuvant, adjuvant, and metastatic/recurrent setting, but responses are not durable and toxicity is not insignificant, especially in a patient population where the median age at diagnosis is 69. The data available to date has not shown a benefit in disease-free or overall survival. However, there are several limitations when attempting to draw conclusions regarding the use of chemotherapy in MCC. First, the majority of data comes from retrospective analyses with limited numbers of patients per treatment center and significant bias with regard to patient inclusion. Randomized controlled studies would certainly be helpful, but this is difficult given the rarity of the disease. Second, there is heterogeneity within many of the individual studies in the stage of patients treated, how chemotherapy is administered (adjuvantly, concurrently with radiation, in a metastatic setting, or as second or third-line therapy), and in the chemotherapy regimens used.

For now, since the literature is not definitive, clinicians should decide on the use of chemotherapy in MCC on a patient by patient basis. Our personal preference is to reserve adjuvant therapy for those patients with lymph node involvement either at the time of initial surgery with sentinel node assessment or at the time of identification of clinical lymph node involvement. We have anecdotally seen improved outcomes with cisplatin as opposed to carboplatin containing regimens for patients appropriate to receive it. It seems reasonable to consider chemotherapy in patients with unresectable locally advanced or metastatic disease if they have an excellent performance status with either of the two most commonly used regimens, either cisplatin/carboplatin with etoposide or cyclophosphamide/doxorubicin/vincristine with palliative benefits in mind. Ideally clinical trials will be designed and patients preferentially enrolled to allow definitive conclusions to be made into the future.

References

1. Pectasides D et al. Cisplatin-based chemotherapy for Merkel cell carcinoma of the skin. Cancer Invest. 2006;24(8):780–5.
2. Fenig E. The use of cyclophosphamide, methotrexate, and 5-fluorouracil in the treatment of Merkel cell carcinoma. Am J Clin Oncol. 1993;16(1):54–7.
3. Tai P et al. Multimodality management for 145 cases of Merkel cell carcinoma. Med Oncol. 2010;27(4): 1260–6.
4. Bajetta E et al. 5-Fluorouracil, dacarbazine, and epirubicin in the treatment of patients with neuroendocrine tumors. Cancer. 1998;83(2):372–8.
5. Wobser M et al. Therapy of metastasized Merkel cell carcinoma with liposomal doxorubicin in combination with radiotherapy. J Dtsch Dermatol Ges. 2009; 7(6):521–5.
6. Voog E et al. Chemotherapy for patients with locally advanced or metastatic Merkel cell carcinoma. Cancer. 1999;85(12):2589–95.
7. Tai PT et al. Chemotherapy in neuroendocrine/Merkel cell carcinoma of the skin: case series and review of 204 cases. J Clin Oncol. 2000;18(12):2493–9.
8. Fenig E et al. The role of radiation therapy and chemotherapy in the treatment of Merkel cell carcinoma. Cancer. 1997;80(5):881–5.
9. Eng TY et al. Treatment of merkel cell carcinoma. Am J Clin Oncol. 2004;27(5):510–5.
10. McAfee WJ et al. Merkel cell carcinoma: treatment and outcomes. Cancer. 2005;104(8):1761–4.
11. Allen PJ et al. Merkel cell carcinoma: prognosis and treatment of patients from a single institution. J Clin Oncol. 2005;23(10):2300–9.
12. Fields RC et al. Recurrence after complete resection and selective use of adjuvant therapy for stage I through III Merkel cell carcinoma. Cancer. 2012;118(13):3311–20.
13. Poulsen M et al. High-risk Merkel cell carcinoma of the skin treated with synchronous carboplatin/etoposide and radiation: a Trans-Tasman Radiation Oncology Group Study—TROG 96:07. J Clin Oncol. 2003;21(23):4371–6.
14. Poulsen M et al. Analysis of toxicity of Merkel cell carcinoma of the skin treated with synchronous carboplatin/etoposide and radiation: a Trans-Tasman Radiation Oncology Group study. Int J Radiat Oncol Biol Phys. 2001;51(1):156–63.
15. Poulsen MG et al. Does chemotherapy improve survival in high-risk stage I and II Merkel cell carcinoma of the skin? Int J Radiat Oncol Biol Phys. 2006;64(1):114–9.
16. Poulsen M et al. Weekly carboplatin reduces toxicity during synchronous chemoradiotherapy for Merkel cell carcinoma of skin. Int J Radiat Oncol Biol Phys. 2008;72(4):1070–4.
17. Jouary T et al. Neoadjuvant polychemotherapy in locally advanced Merkel cell carcinoma. Nat Rev Clin Oncol. 2009;6(9):544–8.
18. Waldmann V et al. Transient complete remission of metastasized Merkel cell carcinoma by high-dose polychemotherapy and autologous peripheral blood stem cell transplantation. Br J Dermatol. 2000; 143(4):837–9.
19. Hata Y et al. Two cases of Merkel cell carcinoma cured by intratumor injection of natural human tumor necrosis factor. Plast Reconstr Surg. 1997;99(2): 547–53.
20. Hermann G et al. Complete remission of Merkel cell carcinoma of the scalp with local and regional metastases after topical treatment with dinitrochlorbenzol. J Am Acad Dermatol. 2004;50:965–9.

21. Zeitouni NC. In-transit Merkel cell carcinoma treated with isolated limb perfusion or isolated limb infusion: a case series of 12 patients. Dermatol Surg. 2011; 37(3):357–64.
22. Cirillo F et al. [Merkel cell tumor. Report of case and treatment with octreotide]. Minerva Chir. 1997; 52(11):1359–65.
23. Fakiha M et al. Remission of Merkel cell tumor after somatostatin analog treatment. J Cancer Res Ther. 2010;6(3):382–4.
24. Salavati A et al. Peptide receptor radionuclide therapy of Merkel cell carcinoma using (177)lutetium-labeled somatostatin analogs in combination with radiosensitizing chemotherapy: a potential novel treatment based on molecular pathology. Ann Nucl Med. 2012; 26(4):365–9.
25. Samlowski WE et al. A phase II trial of imatinib mesylate in Merkel cell carcinoma (neuroendocrine carcinoma of the skin): a Southwest Oncology Group study (S0331). Am J Clin Oncol. 2010;33(5):495–9.
26. Davids MS et al. Response to a novel multitargeted tyrosine kinase inhibitor pazopanib in metastatic Merkel cell carcinoma. J Clin Oncol. 2009;27(26): e97–100.

11 Treatment Algorithm

Douglas Winstanley and Seaver Soon

Summary

The approach to the treatment of Merkel cell carcinoma (MCC) presents a clinical conundrum. The lack of prospective evidence-based studies due to the rarity of the tumor results in a nebulous body of data that can be conflicting. More recently, mounting evidence has provided a framework in which the clinician can logically approach, and optimize, treatment for this very aggressive disease.

The treatment of local disease consists of surgical excision to obtain clear margins. In cases where tumor diameter ≤2 cm, surgical margins of 1 cm are reasonable. For tumors >2 cm, 2 cm margins are recommended. Due to the high rate of sentinel node positivity, sentinel lymph node biopsy (SLNB) should be performed in nearly every case of MCC, unless comorbidities or potential postoperative complications provide compelling reason not to do so. In cases where excision prior to identification of the sentinel lymph node (SLN) may compromise lymphatic channels and identification of the SLN, adjuvant radiation therapy (RT) to the primary site, nodal beds, and in-transit lymphatics should be considered. Patients with a positive SLN should undergo completion lymph node dissection (CLND) or radiation monotherapy to the regional basin. Regular surveillance should then be employed.

Multidisciplinary tumor boards are helpful in planning treatment for patients with regional or systemic disease. Treatment of regional disease consists of lymphadenectomy with or without adjuvant radiation, radiation monotherapy, or possibly adjuvant chemotherapy. Overall survival for metastatic MCC is low. Treatment of distant disease primarily consists of palliative chemotherapy, with the addition of radiation treatment and surgery where indicated.

Introduction

Developing an approach to the management of MCC is complicated by a paucity of rigorous, prospective trials, due largely to the rarity of this tumor. Evidence from institutional, retrospective studies, however, has recently provided a conceptual framework to inform treatment decisions related to local, regional, and distant disease. Treatment options for local disease include surgery—specifically, wide excision or Mohs micrographic surgery—or radiation, either as monotherapy or in the postoperative setting. Local disease management should almost always include assessment of the regional nodal basin by SLNB. Treatment of regional and distant disease should be considered within the context of a

D. Winstanley (✉) • S. Soon
Division of Dermatology and Dermatologic Surgery, Scripps Clinic, 10666 North Torrey Pines Road, MS112A, La Jolla, CA 92037, USA
e-mail: Winstanley.Douglas@scrippshealth.org; Soon.Seaver@scrippshealth.org

M. Alam et al. (eds.), *Merkel Cell Carcinoma*, DOI 10.1007/978-1-4614-6608-6_11,

multidisciplinary tumor board. Treatment options for regional disease include lymphadenectomy, with or without adjuvant radiotherapy, or radiation monotherapy. Options for distant disease include largely palliative chemotherapy, with or without surgery and radiotherapy. This chapter synthesizes the current body of literature relating to treatment approaches and outcomes to propose an algorithm that can be employed as a guideline in the clinical management of this aggressive tumor.

Patient Selection

Considerations in patient selection for management are disease stage, based on the American Joint Cancer Committee (AJCC) staging classification for MCC, and patient overall health status. As MCC presents primarily in an elderly population, comorbidities or poor functional status may exclude treatment options that might otherwise be considered. In addition, many patients present in a frankly or relatively immunosuppressed state, which may further complicate management. Consultation with a multidisciplinary tumor board is paramount in considering the many variables particular to a patient's presentation.

Treatment of Local Disease

Although many approaches exist for the management of local disease, the mainstay of treatment is wide excision, with or without adjuvant radiotherapy. In special circumstances, Mohs micrographic surgery or radiation monotherapy may be considered. In almost all cases, SLNB should be planned prior to treatment of the primary lesion to minimize disturbance to lymphatic drainage patterns.

Wide Excision

Current excision margin recommendations of the National Comprehensive Cancer Network (NCCN) are based on primary tumor size: tumors ≤2 cm require a 1 cm margin, whereas tumors >2 cm require a 2 cm margin. Excision should include tissue to the investing fascia of the muscle or pericranium with the intent of achieving clear histologic margins. The specimen should be submitted for permanent section evaluation of all peripheral and deep margins (comprehensive en face examination) to ensure complete extirpation of the tumor [1].

While no prospective controlled trials examine recurrence rates based on varying surgical margins, several retrospective studies have analyzed tumor margins [2]. Historically, recommended excision margins were 2–3 cm [3]. More recently, low local recurrence rates have been demonstrated with more conservative, histologically clear, margins. In a retrospective analysis of 251 patients at a single institution treated with an average excision margin of 1.1 cm, Allen et al. reported an 8 % recurrence rate with negative margins, compared to 18 % with positive margins ($P=0.31$) [4–6]. Surgical margins >1 cm were not associated with a significant decrease in recurrence rates. In 31 patients, Ott et al. reported no local recurrence in 7 patients treated with margins >2 cm, compared to 7 local recurrences in 24 patients with excision margins <2 cm. However, no statistical difference in survival was observed in this small cohort by excision margin [7]. Given that no recurrence or survival benefit is associated with wide (2–3 cm) excision margins, more conservative margins as recommended by NCCN provide acceptable local control rates while minimizing surgical morbidity.

Mohs Surgery

No data suggest Mohs surgery provides superior outcomes to standard wide excision for MCC; nonetheless, the margin control and tissue-sparing characteristics of Mohs surgery render it useful in the treatment of tumors near functionally sensitive areas, such as the nose, lip, or eyelid, where a 1–2 cm excision margin may be unacceptable. In a retrospective case series comparing Mohs surgery to standard excision, O'Connor reported local recurrence rates of 31.7 % in a group of 86 patients who underwent wide local excision (mean follow-up 60 months) compared to 8.3 % in 12 patients who underwent Mohs surgery (mean follow-up 36 months). Regional recurrence rates were 48.8 % for patients treated with WLE and 33.3 % for patients treated with Mohs surgery alone. No statistical analysis was provided however to demonstrate that this absolute difference may not be spurious [8]. Given these favorable outcomes, Mohs surgery may be employed on a case by case basis where primary tumor location on the face may require tissue-sparing technique while providing adequate margin control.

Adjuvant Radiation

Adjuvant radiation to the primary tumor bed following excision is associated with decreased local recurrence rate. This combination therapy should be considered particularly in tumors with high-risk features: (1) diameter >1.5–2 cm, (2) increasing tumor thickness, (3) perineural or vascular invasion, (4) positive margin excision, and (5) regional lymph node involvement [9]. In the setting of a negative SLNB, most schemes recommend treatment with a total of 45–60 Gy delivered in standard fractionations of 1.8–2.0 Gy to the primary tumor bed with a 4–5 cm margin. In the setting of a positive SLNB or of unknown nodal status, radiotherapy to the primary bed, in-transit lymphatics, and regional nodes should be considered. Tumors where adjuvant radiotherapy may be unnecessary include primary tumors <1–1.5 cm in diameter with clear surgical margin and no additional high-risk features [10, 11]. In a meta-analysis involving 1,254 patients, Lewis et al. reported a 3.7-fold increased local recurrence rate in patients treated with surgery alone vs. those treated with surgery and adjuvant radiation [12]. Further, a retrospective analysis of 1,665 patients treated for stage I–III in which 1,487 patients were treated surgically, with 40 % (477/1,487) of those patients having adjuvant radiation therapy. A median follow-up of 40 months was reported. Overall median survival for patients undergoing surgery and adjuvant radiation was 63 months, compared to 45 months in patients undergoing surgery alone [13]. These studies suggest that adjuvant radiation to the primary tumor bed following excision should be strongly considered in all but low-risk tumors.

Radiation Monotherapy

Definitive radiation therapy is generally reserved for poor surgical candidates or in cases where surgery would result in acceptable functional impairment or disfigurement. In a retrospective case series examining 25 patients treated with radiation monotherapy (65 Gy) compared to 25 patients treated with surgery and adjuvant radiation (55 Gy), Pape et al. reported two locoregional relapses in the radiation monotherapy group (median 3 years follow-up) and four in the combination therapy group (median 9 years follow-up). No statistical difference was observed in disease-free survival or overall survival [14]. In a retrospective analysis of 24 primary tumors undergoing definitive radiotherapy (median dose: 51 Gy; median follow-up: 39 months), Veness et al. reported in-field control rate of 75 %, with a 60 % relapse rate, predominantly outside of the treatment field. Overall survival at 2 and 5 years was 58 % and 37 %, respectively. These results suggest that radiation therapy can achieve good in-field control, but rates of relapse remain high [15]. Thus, while there is evidence that primary radiation can be used as a monotherapy, it should be reserved for nonsurgical candidates.

Sentinel Lymph Node Biopsy

Regardless of whether the primary tumor is treated by excision, Mohs surgery, or radiation therapy, management of local disease should, almost categorically, involve assessment of the regional nodal basin by SLNB, which informs not only prognosis but also therapeutic decisions [16–18]. A positive sentinel node is associated with increased recurrence and mortality risk. Gupta et al. published a meta-analysis of 122 patients, 30 of which were treated at the authors' institution and 92 of which were identified in the literature among 12 studies. At 3-year follow-up, the recurrence rate for patients with a positive sentinel node biopsy was 60 %, while it was 20 % for those with a negative SNLB. The 3-year relapse-free survival was reported as 40 % for patients with a positive SLNB vs. 80 % for those with negative SLNB ($P=0.03$) [19]. Hitchcock et al. showed that while only approximately 25 % of patients presented with clinically apparent nodal disease, 30–50 % of patients eventually developed nodal disease [20]. Indeed, reported rates of SLN positivity range from 15 % to 50 % [5, 17, 21, 22], exceeding that for intermediate thickness melanoma and suggesting that SLNB is necessary to detect a substantial proportion of patients with occult nodal disease [5]. In the largest review to date of the utility of nodal evaluation in the prognosis of MCC, Lemos et al. examined the overall survival difference in patients with clinical vs. pathologic node staging. In a review that included 4,427 patients with nonmetastatic disease, the overall survival of patients with clinically negative nodal disease was worse than patients with pathologic proven negative nodal disease, revealing 5-year relative survival rates of 59 % vs. 76 %, respectively (excess hazard ratio 1.80, 95 % CI 1.4–2.4, $P<0.0001$). For patients with clinical nodal disease, 5 year survival rates were worse than for those patients with pathologically proven nodal disease 26 % vs. 42 %, respectively (excess hazard ratio 1.48, 95 % CI 1.1–1.9, $P<0.004$) [18]. This suggests that a large number of patients who do not have pathologic staging of nodes are likely understaged due to unrecognized micrometastatic node involvement.

Further, recent data suggest that even small primary tumors carry significant risk for regional metastasis. In a retrospective study, tumors characterized by the following "small" or "low-risk" clinical features were nonetheless associated with a 23–36 % risk of SLN positivity: size <1 cm, horizontal dimension ≤3.75 mm, tumor thickness ≤2 mm, low mitotic rate <10 per mm^2, or circumscribed growth pattern. Lending more evidence is a study by Sarnaik et al., who reported positive SLNB in 5 of 12 sentinel nodes in tumors less than 1 cm with serial sectioning and immunohistochemistry [23].

Immunohistochemistry increases the sensitivity of detecting a positive SLN. Su et al. examined the use of immunohistochemical staining in 23 sentinel nodes removed from ten consecutive patients. While all nodes appeared histologically clear with standard hematoxylin and eosin staining, four of the ten patients demonstrated sentinel node positivity when examined with cytokeratin-20 and cytokeratin AE1/AE3 [24]. Immunostains facilitate the identification of micrometastases missed on routine staining. In this study, 95 patients who were clinically node-negative underwent SLNB of 97 tumors. SLNB was successful in 93 instances, and of these occurrences, 45.2 % (42 occurrences) were found to have at least one positive sentinel node identified through the use of CK-20, AE1, AE3, and CAM 5.2. While positivity rates were not beyond what has previously been reported in the literature, they were higher than other large case series reports, particularly Allen et al. (22 %) and Mehrany et al. (33 %) [4, 17]. The authors suggest that the use of immunostains facilitates the identification of micrometastases that may otherwise be missed on routine staining [25]. While the clinical relevance of single cell and micrometastases in the sentinel node is unclear, the high rates of regional and distant disease observed in MCC argue that patients with positive SLNB by immunohistochemistry should be treated similarly to those with micrometastases observed with traditional staining. In summary, SLNB with immunohistochemistry, including cytokeratin-20, -AE1/AE3, and CAM 5.2, is critical to the staging and management of MCC and should be considered in almost every patient who presents with a diagnosis of MCC [9–12]. Algorithms for assessment and treatment of patients with clinically negative nodal disease (Fig. 11.1) and clinically palpable nodal disease (Fig. 11.2) are presented below.

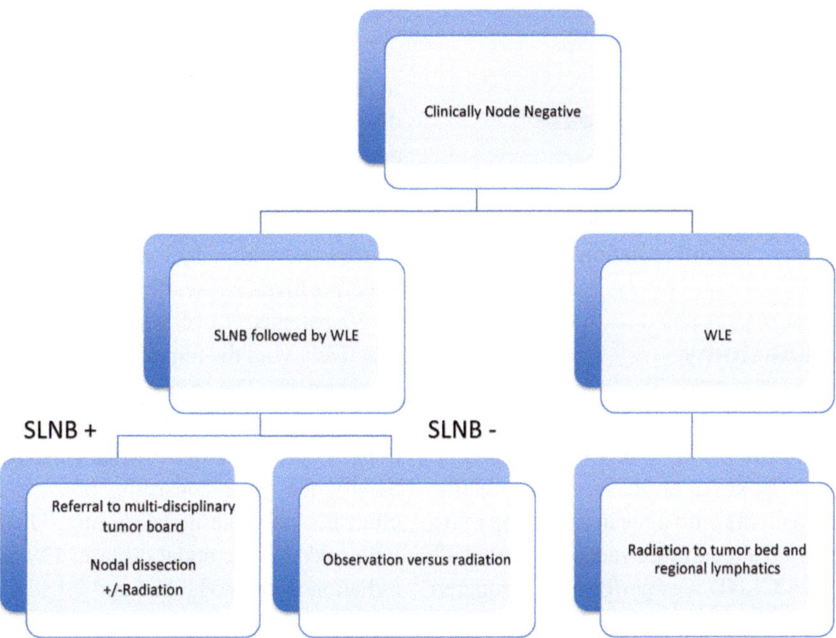

Fig. 11.1 Clinically node-negative Merkel cell carcinoma (MCC). Despite the higher rate of false-negative SNLB is head and neck MCC, the authors recommend sentinel lymph node biopsy (SLNB) in all cases of MCC. Cases which have been previously excised without SLNB should receive radiation therapy to the tumor bed and regional lymphatics. Frequency of clinical follow-up should be every 1–3 months for the first year and every 3 months for the second year after definitive management

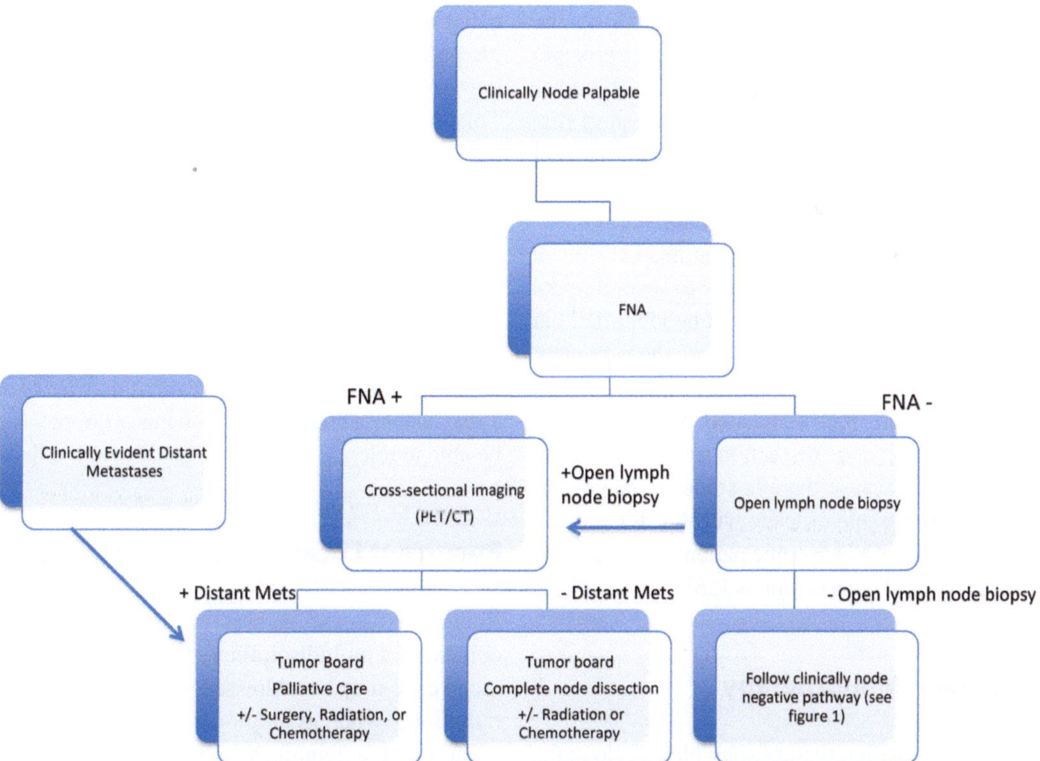

Fig. 11.2 Clinically palpable lymphadenopathy in MCC. A negative or indeterminate FNA should be followed by open lymph node biopsy. Frequency of clinical follow-up should be every 1–3 months for the first year and every 3 months for the second year after definitive management. Treatment of recurrence should be individualized to patient preference and the clinical scenario and should ideally take place within the context of a multidisciplinary tumor board

Treatment of Regional Disease

Treatment of regional disease consists of either lymph node dissection, with or without adjuvant radiation therapy, or with radiation monotherapy.

Lymphadenectomy

CLND effectively treats regional involvement, although associated with risk of postoperative complications. Kokoska et al., in a retrospective review of 35 patients with a mean follow-up of 31 months, reported a recurrence rate of 0 % (0 of 11 patients) when CLND was performed, compared to 91 % (20 of 22 patients) when CLND was not performed [26]. In the same study, a recurrence rate of 15 % (2/13) was reported for patients who had received regional XRT and 90 % (18/20) for those who did not. CLND may be a better option for patients with head and neck tumors when there is difficulty in localizing a sentinel node. The success rates of identifying a sentinel node in the head and neck are less than those of the trunk and extremities and are thought to be due to a number of possible factors: (1) the frequently short distance between the primary tumor and the draining nodal basin, (2) the rapid rate of dye migration in the head and neck, and (3) the relatively greater arborization of lymphatics in the head and neck that may lead to diffusion of dye to several nodal basins. If a sentinel node cannot be identified but a regional lymph node basin can, the option of elective lymph node dissection may be pursued [27]. However, the associated morbidities of regional lymph node dissection must be carefully considered. Because there is some evidence suggesting comparable efficacy with RT, RT may be favored over CLND in some patients to reduce the risk of surgical complications [28].

Radiation Monotherapy

Definitive radiation therapy may play a role in the treatment of nodal disease. To date, however, there is not a significant body of evidence to substantiate its efficacy as a primary therapy for regional disease. As previously discussed, most of the evidence for the use of radiation has examined its role as an adjuvant treatment for both local and regional disease. Fang et al. examined the largest group to date treated with radiation monotherapy for lymph node-positive disease. The study examined a total of 50 patients, 43 of whom were followed prospectively with the remainder being examined retrospectively. The group was divided into two cohorts, one group consisting of 26 patients with microscopic nodal disease that was established by SLNB, the other consisting of 24 patients with clinically palpable nodal disease. Of the patients with microscopic nodal disease, 19 had definitive radiation to the nodal bed and 7 had CLND (4 of whom also had adjuvant nodal radiation). At 2-year follow-up, there was no significant difference in the disease-specific survival between the two groups ($P=0.7$). For 24 patients with clinically apparent nodal disease, 9 underwent regional nodal radiation. Fifteen patients had CLND, 12 of whom had adjuvant radiation therapy. Of these patients, the disease-specific survival was 73 % for the group receiving definitive XRT and 59 % for the group undergoing CLND (± adjuvant XRT). This result also did not achieve statistical significance ($P=0.9$). The authors suggest, based on these results, that regional definitive XRT can achieve rates of locoregional control similar to those offered by surgery [29]. As there is a paucity of data regarding the efficacy of radiation monotherapy for regional disease, definitive recommendations regarding the benefits of radiation vs. surgery cannot be made. However, it may serve as a reasonable alternative for patients who may not be able to tolerate surgery.

Recurrent Local and Regional Disease

Recurrent disease is best managed within the context of a multidisciplinary tumor board. Local recurrence may be addressed with surgery and/or radiation, whereas regional disease may be treated with a combination of surgery and radiation or radiation alone. Enrollment in clinical trials should be encouraged.

Eng et al. examined the outcomes of recurrent disease in 46 patients in a retrospective case series. Twenty-one patients did not receive treatment because they succumbed to their disease at a median follow-up of 15 months. The remaining 25 patients underwent various treatments: excision; excision and radiotherapy; excision, radiotherapy, and chemotherapy; locoregional re-irradiation; surgery with adjuvant chemotherapy; radiotherapy and chemotherapy; and chemotherapy. At a median follow-up of 15 months, the overall survival of the 46 patients was 37 %. Specifically, 27 patients died of MCC, including 21 patients who did not receive any treatment for recurrent disease. Nine patients were alive with disease and eight had no evidence of disease after treatment for their recurrence. Two patients were lost to follow up [30].

Treatment of Distant Disease

Consultation with a multidisciplinary tumor board should be pursued to design management strategy in the setting of metastatic disease. Chemotherapy is the primary treatment for patients with metastatic or inoperable disease: the therapeutic goal is palliation or salvage of recurrent, locally advanced, and metastatic disease. Regardless of the modality employed, median overall survival for patients with metastatic disease is approximately 10 months [16].

Chemotherapy regimens for MCC have been based primarily on regimens for small cell lung carcinoma (SCLC) due to common histological features and their membership as part of the amine precursor uptake and decarboxylase (APUD) system [31]. The most common therapeutic regimen is cyclophosphamide/doxorubicin/vincristine with or without prednisone, with an overall response rate of 76 %. Etoposide with platinum-based agents was the next most common regimen, with response rates up to 70 % [32]. Second-line treatments consist of single-agent therapies, including topotecan, gemcitabine, irinotecan, or oral etoposide. Single-agent chemotherapies can be effective but are generally reserved patients with greater comorbidities and lower performance scores.

The greatest concern regarding chemotherapy is treatment-related toxicity. Neutropenic fever and sepsis are common. Voog et al. reported a toxic death rate of 7.7 % in a retrospective review of 101 patients with metastatic disease treated with various chemotherapy regimens. While the initial response rate was 61 %, the median survival for patients with distant disease was 9 months from the initiation of chemotherapy. For patients with locally advanced tumors, median survival was 24 months [33]. Because no data demonstrate that chemotherapy increases overall survival [5], alongside its known toxicity and potential mortality, chemotherapy should be used palliatively. The use of surgery and radiation in the setting of metastatic disease should similarly be palliative [34].

Follow-up

Close clinical follow-up comprising a complete cutaneous and lymph node examination should be performed every 3–6 months for the first 2 years, then every 6–12 months for life. The median time to recurrence is approximately 8 months. Laboratory and imaging evaluation should be performed based on clinical findings.

Evidence-Based Findings

The body of knowledge surrounding treatment for MCC is based on retrospective studies; thus, the level of evidence is considered to be II-3 as established by the US Preventive Services Task Force.

Conclusions

A summary algorithm for assessment and treatment is shown below (Fig. 11.3). The recommendations for the treatment of MCC are in evolution. The aggressive nature of this tumor mandates a systematic approach founded on best available evidence. The importance of SLNB with immunohistochemistry in the context of this disease has been established. Surgery, radiotherapy, and

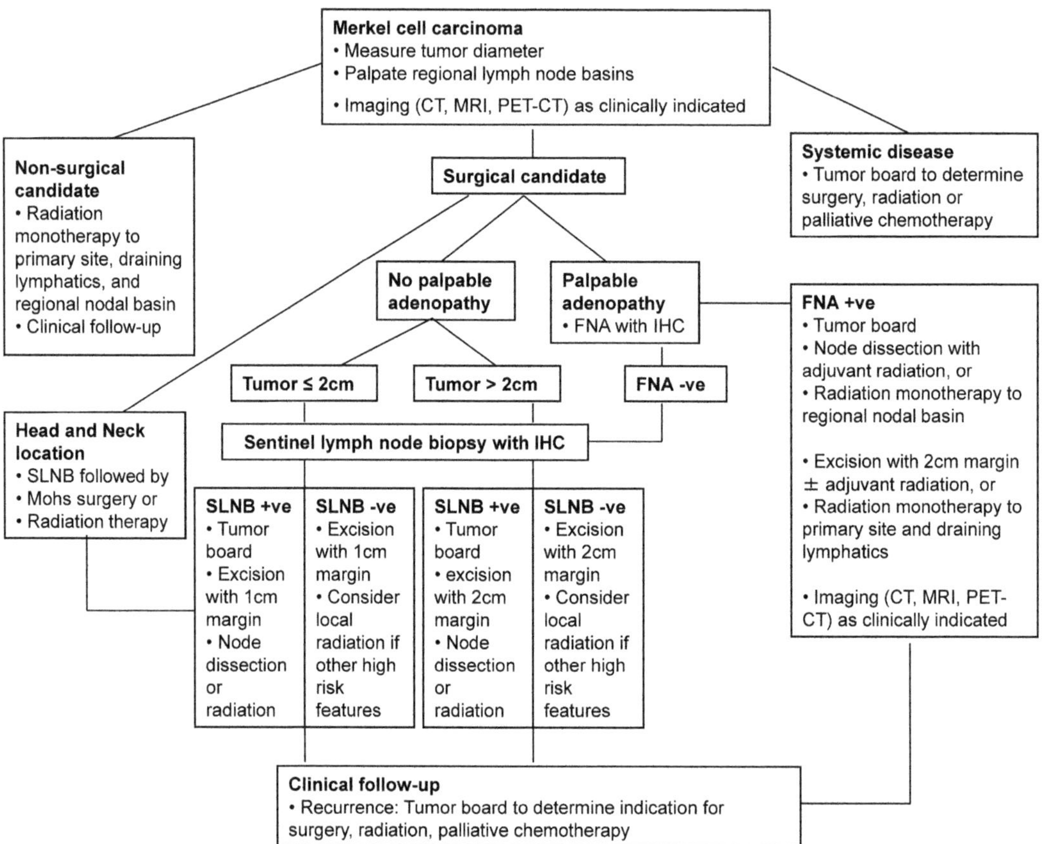

Fig. 11.3 Summary algorithm for assessment and treatment

palliative chemotherapy, alone or in conjunction will, for the near future, constitute the mainstays of treatment. Further understanding of the etiologic role of the Merkel cell polyomavirus, along with the identification of underlying genetic mutations, may open an avenue for targeted molecular therapy. Continuing efforts bring hope for effective treatments of this uncommon, devastating disease.

References

1. National Comprehensive Cancer Network (NCCN). NCCN clinical practice guidelines in oncology. Merkel cell carcinoma version 1.2011. 2011. http://www.nccn.org/professionals/physician_gls/pdf/mcc.pdf. Accessed 19 Oct 2012.
2. Gonzalez RJ, Padhya TA, Cherpelis BS, Prince MD, Aya-ay ML, Sondak VK, et al. The surgical management of primary and metastatic Merkel cell carcinoma. Curr Probl Cancer. 2011;34(1):77–96.
3. Shaw JH, Rumball E. Merkel cell tumour: clinical behaviour and treatment. Br J Surg. 1991;78(2):138–42.
4. Allen PJ, Busam K, Hill AD, Stojadinovic A, Coit DG. Immunohistochemical analysis of sentinel lymph nodes from patients with Merkel cell carcinoma. Cancer. 2001;92(6):1650–5.
5. Allen PJ, Bowne WB, Jaques DP, Brennan MF, Busam K, Coit DG. Merkel cell carcinoma: prognosis and treatment of patients from a single institution. J Clin Oncol. 2005;23(10):2300–9.
6. Medina-Franco H, Urist MM, Fiveash J, Heslin MJ, Bland KI, Beenken SW. Multimodality treatment of Merkel cell carcinoma: case series and literature review of 1024 cases. Ann Surg Oncol. 2001;8(3):204–8.
7. Ott MJ, Tanabe KK, Gadd MA, Stark P, Smith BL, Finkelstein DM, et al. Multimodality management of Merkel cell carcinoma. Arch Surg. 1999;134(4):388–92; discussion 392–3.
8. O'Connor WJ. Merkel cell carcinoma. Comparison of Mohs micrographic surgery and wide excision in eighty-six patients. Dermatol Surg. 1997;23:929–33.
9. Eng TY, Boersma MG, Fuller CD, Goytia V, Jones WE, Joyner M, et al. A comprehensive review of the treatment of Merkel cell carcinoma. Am J Clin Oncol. 2007;30(6):624–36.

10. Veness MJ. Merkel cell carcinoma (primary cutaneous neuroendocrine carcinoma): an overview on management. Australas J Dermatol. 2006;47(3):160–5.
11. Boyer J. Local control of primary Merkel cell carcinoma: review of 45 cases treated with Mohs micrographic surgery with and without adjuvant radiation. J Am Acad Dermatol. 2002;47(6):885–92.
12. Lewis KG, Weinstock MA, Weaver AL, Otley CC. Adjuvant local irradiation for Merkel cell carcinoma. Arch Dermatol. 2006;142(6):693–700.
13. Mojica P, Smith D, Ellenhorn JD. Adjuvant radiation therapy is associated with improved survival in Merkel cell carcinoma of the skin. J Clin Oncol. 2007;25(9): 1043–7.
14. Pape E, Rezvoy N, Penel N, Salleron J, Martinot V, Guerreschi P, et al. Radiotherapy alone for Merkel cell carcinoma: a comparative and retrospective study of 25 patients. J Am Acad Dermatol. 2011;65(5):983–90.
15. Veness M, Foote M, Gebski V, Poulsen M. The role of radiotherapy alone in patients with Merkel cell carcinoma: reporting the Australian experience of 43 patients. Int J Radiat Oncol Biol Phys. 2010;78(3): 703–9.
16. Bichakjian CK, Lowe L, Lao CD, Sandler HM, Bradford CR, Johnson TM, et al. Merkel cell carcinoma: critical review with guidelines for multidisciplinary management. Cancer. 2007;110(1):1–12.
17. Mehrany K, Otley C, Weenig R. A meta-analysis of the prognostic significance of sentinel lymph node status in Merkel cell carcinoma. Dermatol Surg. 2002;28(2):113–7.
18. Lemos BD, Storer BE, Iyer JG, Phillips JL, Bichakjian CK, Fang LC, et al. Pathologic nodal evaluation improves prognostic accuracy in Merkel cell carcinoma: analysis of 5823 cases as the basis of the first consensus staging system. J Am Acad Dermatol. 2010;63(5):751–61.
19. Gupta SG, Wang LC, Penas PF, Gellenthin M, Lee SJ, Nghiem P. Sentinel lymph node biopsy for evaluation and treatment of patients with Merkel cell carcinoma: the Dana-Farber experience and meta-analysis of the literature. Arch Dermatol. 2006;142(6):685.
20. Hitchcock CL, Bland KI, Laney RG, Franzini D, Harris B, Copeland EM. Neuroendocrine (Merkel cell) carcinoma of the skin. Its natural history, diagnosis, and treatment. Ann Surg. 1988;207(2):201–7.
21. Shnayder Y, Weed DT, Arnold DJ, Gomez-Fernandez C, Bared A, Goodwin WJ, et al. Management of the neck in Merkel cell carcinoma of the head and neck: University of Miami experience. Head Neck. 2008;30(12):1559–65.
22. Maza S, Trefzer U, Hofmann M, Schneider S, Voit C, Krössin T, et al. Impact of sentinel lymph node biopsy in patients with Merkel cell carcinoma: results of a prospective study and review of the literature. Eur J Nucl Med Mol Imaging. 2006;33(4):433–40.
23. Sarnaik AA, Zager JS, Cox LE, Ochoa TM, Messina JL, Sondak VK. Routine omission of sentinel lymph node biopsy for Merkel cell carcinoma. J Clin Oncol. 2010;28(1):e7.
24. Su LD, Lowe L, Bradford CR, Yahanda AI, Johnson TM, Sondak VK. Immunostaining for cytokeratin 20 improves detection of micrometastatic Merkel cell carcinoma in sentinel lymph nodes. J Am Acad Dermatol. 2002;46(5):661–6.
25. Schwartz JL, Griffith KA, Lowe L, Wong SL, McLean SA, Fullen DR, et al. Features predicting sentinel lymph node positivity in Merkel cell carcinoma. J Clin Oncol. 2011;29(8):1036–41.
26. Kokoska ER, Kokoska MS, Collins BT, Stapleton DR, Wade TP. Early aggressive treatment for Merkel cell carcinoma improves outcome. Am J Surg. 1997; 174(6):688–93.
27. Stadelmann WK, Cobbins L, Lentsch EJ. Incidence of nonlocalization of sentinel lymph nodes using preoperative lymphoscintigraphy in 74 consecutive head and neck melanoma and Merkel cell carcinoma patients. Ann Plast Surg. 2004;52(6):546–9; discussion 550.
28. Sian KU, Wagner JD, Sood R, Park HM, Havlik R, Coleman JJ. Lymphoscintigraphy with sentinel lymph node biopsy in cutaneous Merkel cell carcinoma. Ann Plast Surg. 1999;42(6):679–82.
29. Fang LC, Lemos B, Douglas J, Iyer J, Nghiem P. Radiation monotherapy as regional treatment for lymph node-positive Merkel cell carcinoma. Cancer. 2010;116(7):1783–90.
30. Eng TY, Naguib M, Fuller CD, Jones WE, Herman TS. Treatment of recurrent Merkel cell carcinoma: an analysis of 46 cases. Am J Clin Oncol. 2004;27(6): 576–83.
31. De Wolff-Peeters C, Marien K, Mebis J, Desmet V. A cutaneous APUDoma or Merkel cell tumor? A morphologically recognizable tumor with a biological and histological malignant aspect in contrast with its clinical behavior. Cancer. 1980;46(8):1810–6.
32. Tai PT, Yu E, Winquist E, Hammond A, Stitt L, Tonita J, et al. Chemotherapy in neuroendocrine/Merkel cell carcinoma of the skin: case series and review of 204 cases. J Clin Oncol. 2000;18(12):2493–9.
33. Voog E, Biron P, Martin JP, Blay JY. Chemotherapy for patients with locally advanced or metastatic Merkel cell carcinoma. Cancer. 1999;85(12): 2589–95.
34. Rockville Merkel Cell Carcinoma Group. Merkel cell carcinoma: recent progress and current priorities on etiology, pathogenesis, and clinical management. J Clin Oncol. 2009;27(24):4021–6.

Part IV

Expert Opinions and Future Directions

Case Study A: Multiply Recurrent Merkel Cell Carcinoma

12

Jerry D. Brewer

Description of Case

This patient is a 66-year-old gentleman that presented in March of 2000 after having noticed a superficial plaque on his left lower extremity a few months prior. The area was biopsied, and he was subsequently diagnosed with Merkel cell carcinoma May of 2000 (Fig. 12.1). The patient then underwent a wide excision with split-thickness skin graft and sentinel lymph node biopsy of his left inguinal base which was negative. He then received radiation therapy to the local area only. He developed a recurrence of Merkel cell carcinoma on his left lateral calf March of 2002 outside of the originally radiated area thought to be an in-transit metastasis. After a wide excision of the area, he developed another in-transit metastasis in October 2002, also located on the lateral calf area. A second wide excision of the left lateral calf area was performed with a split-thickness skin graft and a second round of radiation therapy was given between February and March of 2003. The patient was then scheduled to receive PET scans every 3 months to monitor for recurrence or systemic disease. On December 17, 2003, a new focus noted on a PET scan of the left upper medial calf overlying the gastrocnemius fascia was found and diagnosed as Merkel cell carcinoma, also thought to be an in-transit metastasis (Fig. 12.2). The patient then underwent wide local excision and postoperative radiation therapy for the third time, and was started on adjuvant Leukine (GM-CSF) therapy following the Spitler regimen of 250 μg delivered subcutaneously in 28 day cycles of 14 days receiving the injection, then 14 days of no injections. One year later, in December of 2004, a PET scan revealed a new nodule on the left lateral leg, which was diagnosed as Merkel cell carcinoma via biopsy. On December 13, 2004, this new focus of Merkel cell carcinoma as well as the previous two sites of recurrence was excised. In January of 2005 the patient underwent isolated limb infusion of chemotherapy at Sloan-Kettering in New York. A PET scan in April 2005 showed some new areas of nonspecific hypermetabolism above the left knee, but a follow-up MRI was normal. In August of 2006, however he developed another in-transit metastasis on the anterior tibia, followed by another in-transit metastasis of the posterior calf in October of 2006. At that point, he underwent circumferential radiation to the entire left lower leg below the knee December of 2006 and has been recurrence-free since then. The last PET scan was performed on June 15, 2011 and did not show any evidence of recurrence or metastatic disease.

J.D. Brewer (✉)
Department of Dermatology, Mayo Clinic,
200 1st street SW, E-5 Dermatology, Mayo Building,
Rochester, MN 55905, USA
e-mail: brewer.jerry@mayo.edu

M. Alam et al. (eds.), *Merkel Cell Carcinoma*, DOI 10.1007/978-1-4614-6608-6_12,

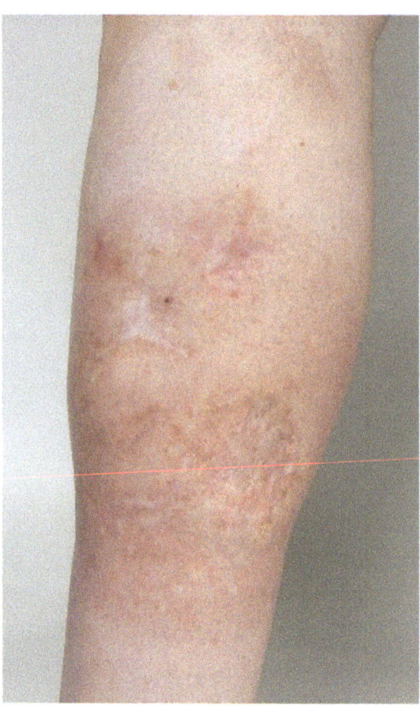

Fig. 12.1 Left lower leg status post-multiple in-transit metastases of MCC treated with surgery and localized radiation

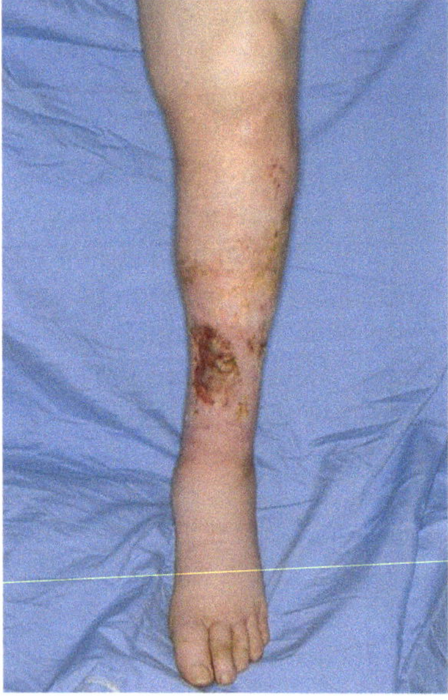

Fig. 12.2 Left lower leg after circumferential total let radiation below the knee

Commentary

This case highlights some interesting points regarding the treatment, follow-up, and adjuvant therapy in cases of MCC. This case also highlights the aggressive nature of MCC with a tendency for multiple recurrences in spite of aggressive combination surgery and radiation treatment measures. For diagnostic evaluation of MCC, CT scans, Octreotide scans, and PET scans are most often employed [1]. A recent report found that PET scans may be most beneficial in the evaluation of MCC, and specifically when evaluating the regional lymph node basin [2].

Due to the rare incidence of MCC, few if any prospective clinical studies have been performed to evaluate the effects of initial therapy or treatment approaches for multiple recurrences, however wide local excision with sentinel lymph node biopsy is generally accepted as the most appropriate initial treatment approach [3, 4]. Both radiation and chemotherapy (less studied) have been viewed as effective adjuvant or palliative therapies, and radiation therapy to the primary site and involved lymph nodes postsurgically has been shown to prevent local recurrence and may improve survival [3–7].

When multiple modalities are used to treat MCC (chemotherapy, radiation therapy, and surgery), it has also been shown that the overall survival rates are significantly higher compared to single modality therapy (average survival of 36.5 months compared to 17.5 months) [6]. Biologic agents, especially interferon and tumor necrosis factor have been used as therapeutic possibilities [1].

In this case, although multiple recurrences/in-transit metastases developed over a period of 6 years, the patient never progressed to stage III disease and none of the recurrences were above the knee. This patient ultimately underwent total (circumferential) leg irradiation to treat any occult disease that was being missed with focal surgery and spot radiation treatment sessions. Total leg irradiation has its risks which include compromised vasculature, non-healing chronic ulcerations, and a roughly 25 % chance of amputation. In spite of these risks, this patient has remained recurrence-free and did not need an amputation; however, he does have a non-healing ulcer in spite of multiple Apligraf applications.

References

1. Goessling W, McKee PH, Mayer RJ. Merkel cell carcinoma. J Clin Oncol. 2002;20:588–98.
2. Colgan MB, Tarantola TI, Weaver AL, et al. The predictive value of imaging studies in evaluating regional lymph node involvement in Merkel cell carcinoma. J Am Acad Dermatol. 2012;67(6):1250–6.
3. Eng TY, Boersma MG, Fuller CD, Cavanaugh SX, Valenzuela F, Herman TS. Treatment of Merkel cell carcinoma. Am J Clin Oncol. 2004;27:510–5.
4. Eng TY, Boersma MG, Fuller CD, et al. A comprehensive review of the treatment of Merkel cell carcinoma. Am J Clin Oncol. 2007;30:624–36.
5. Eich HT, Eich D, Staar S, et al. Role of postoperative radiotherapy in the management of Merkel cell carcinoma. Am J Clin Oncol. 2002;25:50–6.
6. Eng TY, Naguib M, Fuller CD, Jones III WE, Herman TS. Treatment of recurrent Merkel cell carcinoma: an analysis of 46 cases. Am J Clin Oncol. 2004;27: 576–83.
7. Medina-Franco H, Urist MM, Fiveash J, Heslin MJ, Bland KI, Beenken SW. Multimodality treatment of Merkel cell carcinoma: case series and literature review of 1024 cases. Ann Surg Oncol. 2001;8:204–8.

Case Study B: Radiation Monotherapy for Extensive Local and In-Transit Merkel Cell Carcinoma

13

Sherrif F. Ibrahim, Sue S. Yom, and Siegrid S. Yu

Presentation: A 93-year-old male presented to the dermatologist with multiple firm, deeply erythematous nodules covering the majority of the parietal scalp (Fig. 13.1). He stated that the nodules appeared rapidly, never bled, and were not painful. Punch biopsies were performed at two locations and both were shown to be consistent with Merkel cell carcinoma (MCC). His past medical history was notable for hypertension, hyperlipidemia, and coronary artery disease.

Initial workup included a full body PET/CT scan to determine the extent of local disease and the presence of regional lymph node involvement or distant metastases. The PET/CT revealed the known multiple scalp nodules, consistent with in-transit disease, and an incidental renal cell carcinoma; no evidence of lymph node involvement or metastatic spread was noted, categorizing him as having Stage IIIB disease. The patient's case was then presented at the multidisciplinary tumor board.

Representatives from dermatology, head and neck surgery, medical oncology, radiation oncology, and plastic surgery collectively felt that surgical management of the patient's disease was not in his best interest. His advanced age, medical comorbidities, and the degree of cutaneous involvement were factors raised to support this decision. Furthermore, it was felt that there would be a high risk of recurrence with surgery alone and an unacceptable delay of adjuvant therapy with such an extensive surgical procedure. Sentinel lymph node biopsy (SLNB) was likewise not recommended given the extent of disease at presentation, complicating the ability of the surgical team to correctly identify all associated draining lymph node basins. Given the known radiosensitivity of MCC to radiation therapy (RT), initial RT with the intent of local control was the favored treatment approach.

Once RT was decided upon, additional discussion was held to determine the extent of the primary treatment field and whether or not to incorporate elective treatment to the draining lymph node basins of the neck. The latter was declined by the patient and his family given the increased dose of radiation, entailing associated risks for greater acute xerostomia and mucositis. Furthermore, with the degree of cutaneous disease, radiation fields to comprehensively include the next echelon of draining nodes would be bilateral, further increasing morbidity of treatment

S.F. Ibrahim (✉)
Department of Dermatology, University of Rochester Medical Center, 400 Red Creek Drive, Suite 200, Rochester, NY 14623, USA
e-mail: Sherrif_Ibrahim@URMC.Rochester.edu

S.S. Yom
Department of Radiation Oncology, University of California, San Francisco, 1600 Divisadero Street, San Francisco, CA 94115, USA
e-mail: yoms@radonc.ucsf.edu

S.S. Yu
Department of Clinical Dermatology, UCSF Dermatologic Surgery & Laser Center, 1701 Divisadero Street, Third Floor, San Francisco, CA 94115-0316, USA
e-mail: YuS@derm.ucsf.edu

M. Alam et al. (eds.), *Merkel Cell Carcinoma*, DOI 10.1007/978-1-4614-6608-6_13,

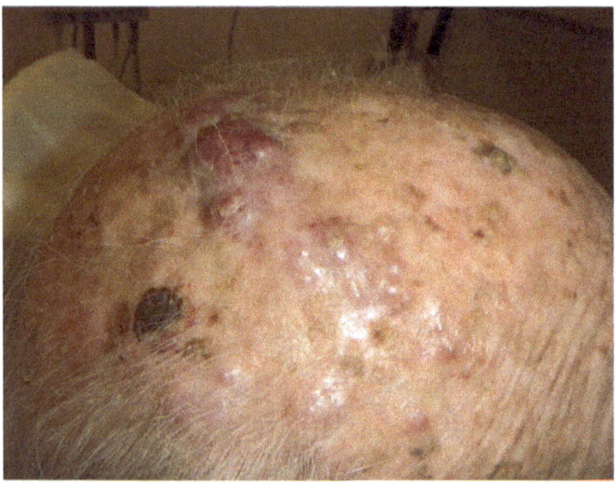

Fig. 13.1 Extensive multifocal Merkel cell carcinoma (MCC) seen at initial presentation

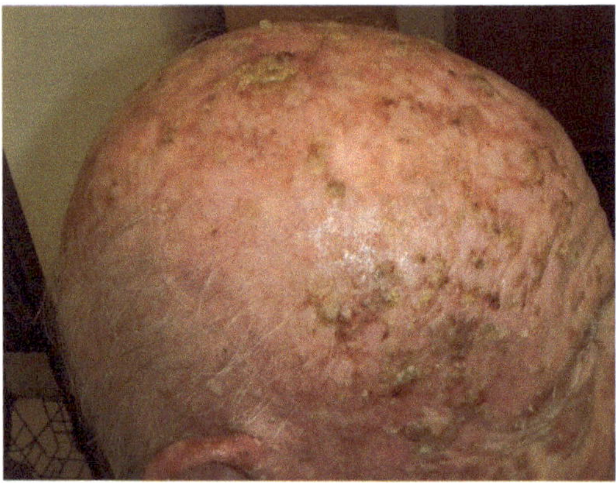

Fig. 13.2 Initial follow-up soon after completion of scalp radiation notable for desquamation and mild skin breakdown

and prolonging recovery time. Thus, the patient underwent scalp RT with wide margins to 6,400 cGy in 32 fractions over 53 days, delivered in conventional standard fractionation with intensity-modulated radiation therapy (IMRT) in order to fully cover the large surface area of the scalp while minimizing radiation dose to the brain. He did well with some areas of erythema, moderate crusting, and superficial ulceration of the vertex that resolved soon after treatment. Complete clinical regression was noted by 1.5 months (Fig. 13.2).

At 3 months post-RT, the patient underwent a follow-up full body PET/CT that demonstrated enhanced uptake within a right cervical lymph node but no evidence of distant disease.

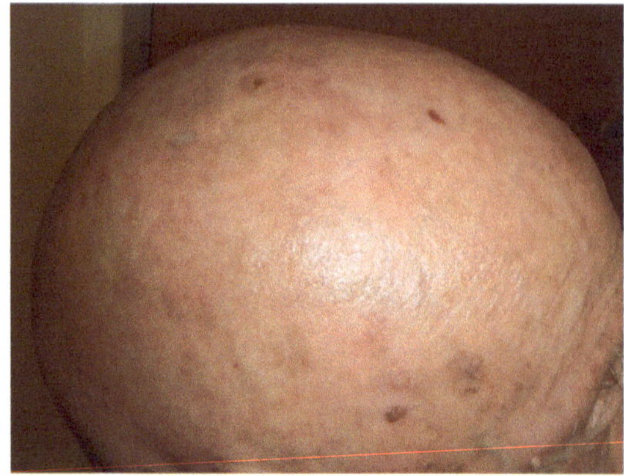

Fig. 13.3 Four-month follow-up post-radiation to the scalp with a remarkable and durable clinical response seen

Subsequent fine needle aspirate was consistent with MCC and the patient was again presented to the multidisciplinary tumor board. Surgical lymph node dissection was decided against given the inherent morbidity of the procedure, and it was felt that there was no supporting data indicating that lymph node dissection would impact survival. Chemotherapy was discussed, however, given his relatively poor performance status and the fact that he had small volume regional disease as opposed to widely metastatic involvement, directed therapy to the lymph node basin was still preferred. In light of his previous response to RT, the tumor board suggested additional radiation to the right neck and supraclavicular region. The right neck and right supraclavicular region received 5,000 cGy over 5 weeks, with the enlarged right neck lymph node boosted to 6,000 cGy. Resultant acute xerostomia improved within 2 months and he remained clinically disease-free (Fig. 13.3).

One month after the second course of XRT, a third PET/CT revealed a right axillary lymph node with an enhanced signal. Fine needle aspirate again demonstrated MCC and for reasons similar to those prior, it was recommended that he undergo RT to the right axilla. He was given 6,400 cGy in 32 fractions over 53 days to the right axilla with 3-dimensional conformal therapy delivered from mostly anteroposterior beam angles. Clinically, the patient remained disease-free; however, he was hospitalized numerous times with diagnoses such as aspiration pneumonia, urinary tract infection, and altered mental status. Although he was also noted to have progression of his renal cell carcinoma, now involving the perinephric fat, he remained clinically free of his MCC at 20 months since his initial presentation.

Eight months later, he was noted to have palpable right axillary lymphadenopathy and fine needle aspirate confirmed the presence of MCC. Restaging full body PET/CT was notable for extensive hypermetabolic multifocal soft tissue abnormalities of the neck, chest, abdomen, and brain. He succumbed to his disease 2 months later, 30 months from initial presentation.

Commentary

This case illustrates many of the challenges of managing.patients with MCC. Given this patient's age and extensive burden of disease at presentation, initial large-scale surgical approaches were deferred in favor of RT. With an initial tumor >5 cm but without evidence of deep tissue involvement and clinically negative lymph nodes, and given the presence of in-transit metastases, his cancer was classified as Stage IIIB by current staging criteria [1]. Patient's presenting with this stage of disease have a 1-year survival of 70 % and 3-year relative survival of 34 %, giving him a poor prognosis. His cutaneous lesions responded extremely well to radiation treatment and local control was durable, supporting the notion of MCC as a radiosensitive tumor. In fact, there are proponents of an RT-only approach for early stage MCC [2]. The decision to forego SLNB for this extensive scalp lesion was conditioned by the particular complexity of this anatomic location, when extensive disease limits the reliability of the technique, while PET/CT scan becomes a convenient and sensitive to survey the entire body both at initial presentation and at regular follow-up intervals [3]. In this case, PET/CT was able to detect nodal involvement on two occasions, supporting the utility of this imaging modality. As MCC is a metabolically active tumor, PET/CT allows for functional imaging of concerning foci with simultaneous anatomic localization. The renal cell carcinoma discovered on the initial PET/CT scan also demonstrates a scenario of incidental findings that may further confound management. The timing at which follow-up PET/CT should be conducted has not yet been established.

Once RT was decided upon as the primary treatment approach, the extent and dose of radiation was a complicated decision, ultimately rooted in the patient's wishes to minimize potential side effects and impact on quality of life. It is difficult to predict whether his outcome would have improved had RT been originally administered to the scalp as well as regional nodes, given that the neck was the first place for disease to recur. However, it is an extremely morbid endeavor to irradiate the bilateral neck and the patient's age might be considered a practical contraindication, with risk of mortality from such extensive treatment. At our institution, if patients are not deemed to be surgical candidates and RT is used as monotherapy, very strong consideration is given to elective treatment of the next echelon of nodes, as this is a common site for disease progression. For this patient, this dose and extent of RT would likely have resulted in side effects beyond what he was willing or able to endure.

This patient's schedule of radiation was an extended one, using standard conventional fractionation, which delivers between 1.8 and 2.0 Gy per weekday over several weeks. For situations in which rapid palliation is one of the primary goals, hypofractionated regimens may be used. These shorter schedules delivering higher amounts of radiation dose per day can be used very effectively for palliation in many other areas of the body. However, for extensive scalp lesions, because of the proximity of large amounts of brain tissue, hypofractionated schedules are usually avoided because of the potential for a higher risk of brain necrosis.

Another option for palliation is simply to reduce the total dose of radiation, with the intention to deliver just enough treatment to provide relief of major symptoms. For this patient, while there is no consensus on the optimal amount of radiotherapy dose required for control of advanced lesions, a fairly high dose of radiation was employed due to the bulk of disease, in an effort to achieve durable local control. Uncontrolled MCC on the scalp can become a hygienic issue and cause considerable pain and morbidity. In this case, the patient and his family opted for a relatively lengthy schedule with the hopes of obtaining some lasting relief of his symptoms. Arguably, a lower dose of radiation might have sufficed, but for large or thick lesions, many radiation oncologists would prescribe higher doses.

Unfortunately, this case demonstrates the aggressive nature of MCC and the propensity for the tumor to recur in draining lymphatic channels. It is important to note that recurrences tend to occur relatively soon after presentation, with head and neck primary tumors having the highest rates of recurrence [4]. Virtually all instances of recurrence occur within 24–36 months of initial presentation [5], as was the case with the current patient. This rapid nature of recurrence points to the need to follow MCC patients closely, both with routine full body skin and lymph node exams in addition to periodic imaging.

Lastly, this case is a prime example of the importance of multidisciplinary management of all MCC patients. Given the complexity of the patient's findings and clinical course, input from several medical specialties and discussion of these suggestions as a group was necessary for his management, and to respect his wishes to prioritize quality of life in the face of a very aggressive disease presentation.

References

1. Lemos BD et al. Pathologic nodal evaluation improves prognostic accuracy in Merkel cell carcinoma: analysis of 5823 cases as the basis of the first consensus staging system. J Am Acad Dermatol. 2010;63(5):751–61.
2. Pape E et al. Radiotherapy alone for Merkel cell carcinoma: a comparative and retrospective study of 25 patients. J Am Acad Dermatol. 2011;65(5):983–90.
3. Colgan MB et al. The predictive value of imaging studies in evaluating regional lymph node involvement in Merkel cell carcinoma. J Am Acad Dermatol. 2012; 67(6):1250–6.
4. Bichakjian CK et al. Merkel cell carcinoma: critical review with guidelines for multidisciplinary management. Cancer. 2007;110(1):1–12.
5. Allen PJ et al. Merkel cell carcinoma: prognosis and treatment of patients from a single institution. J Clin Oncol. 2005;23(10):2300–9.

Case Study C: Complete Spontaneous Regression of Merkel Cell Carcinoma Metastatic to the Liver

14

Natalie Vandeven and Paul Nghiem

Case History

A 58-year-old Caucasian man noted a small lesion on the right side of his neck in August of 2006. The papule, resembled an ingrown hair, was relatively uncomfortable and slowly increased in size. Three months later a reddish-purple nodule had grown to a diameter of 2 cm and was narrowly excised. Pathology revealed a nodular proliferation of atypical round cells with hyperchromatic nuclei displaying "salt and pepper" chromatin. Numerous mitotic figures were observed and there were both individual cell and en masse necrosis. Immunohistological staining indicated positivity for cytokeratin 7, cytokeratin 20 (in a perinuclear dot-like pattern), neuron-specific enolase, and focal positivity for chromogranin and synaptophysin. The tumor cells were negative for TTF1 and S-100. On the basis of these results, a diagnosis of an unusual (cytokeratin 7 positive) Merkel cell carcinoma (MCC) was made. Full body CT and Octreotide scans were performed 1 month later and showed no evidence of disease. The patient underwent a wide local re-excision and sentinel lymph node biopsy (SNLB) 1 month later. Two of three sentinel nodes were positive and the following month he underwent a lymphatic dissection of the neck. None of the 39 nodes removed were positive for MCC. Two months later, the patient began radiation treatment at the primary site and draining lymph node basin with a total of 5,000 rads in 25 fractions. A PET scan 2 months after the completion of radiation therapy showed no evidence of disease.

During regular follow-up 6 months after completion of therapy, a PET scan revealed a 1.2 cm lesion in the liver, which was confirmed by MRI. Fine-needle aspiration cytology of the lesion indicated histological features consistent with his primary MCC tumor. It was determined that surgery and radiation were not possible given the location of the tumor. Because of the relatively poor outcomes and significant side effects associated with chemotherapy treatment of MCC, the patient refused this standard approach.

The patient began exploring possible immune stimulating and alternative therapeutic options. These included seeing a medical intuitive at the Upledger Institute in Cumberland, Maine for "somato-emotional release" therapy. The patient began taking dietary supplements including vitamin C, a multivitamin, CoQ-10, turmeric, probiotics, and cod-liver oil. Twice daily he took 500 mg of a mushroom supplement (Stamets 7® mushroom formula produced by Fungi Perfecti). He also began using Flor Essence as a liver and

N. Vandeven
Department of Medicine, University of Washington, 1850 Republican Street, Brotman Room 242, Seattle, WA 98109, USA
e-mail: vandeven@uw.edu

P. Nghiem (✉)
Department of Dermatology Medicine, University of Washington School of Medicine & Fred Hutchinson Cancer Research Center, 815 Mercer Street, Box 358050, Seattle, WA 98109, USA
e-mail: pnghiem@uw.edu

M. Alam et al. (eds.), *Merkel Cell Carcinoma*, DOI 10.1007/978-1-4614-6608-6_14,

colon cleanser and markedly altered his diet by removing meat, eggs, and dairy and substituting organic brown rice, beans, and sautéed vegetables. The patient also drank freshly prepared juices of organic vegetables (carrots, spinach, beet greens, Swiss chard, kale, and a beet) twice daily.

In March of 2008, 5 weeks after beginning these alternative approaches, an MRI revealed complete remission of his liver metastasis. Since March 2008, he has remained asymptomatic (a total of 53 months) and his most recent scan in February of 2011 showed no evidence of disease. He has maintained this strict diet and use of all supplements in addition to regular consultations with the medical intuitive since his remission.

Comments

We report this case as an example of a rare, complete spontaneous remission of metastatic MCC and because of the patient's use of several alternative therapies. The patient was previously healthy, with no significant immune suppression or other medical problems. The Stamets 7® mushroom blend capsules taken by the patient is composed of seven mushroom species (Royal Sun Blazei, Cordyceps, Reishi, Maitake, Lion's Mane, Chaga, and Mesima) and was used to support general immunity. Mushroom extracts have previously been shown to elicit anticancer responses via an immune-mediated mechanism [1, 2]. Recently, a study in women with breast cancer showed that freeze dried mycelial powder from the *Trametes versicolor* mushroom enhanced natural killer (NK) cell activity [1]. In this study, *Trametes versicolor* mycelium capsules were taken at 6 and 9 g/day as an adjunct to chemotherapy and radiation. Patients who received these extracts had faster recovery of lymphocytes, enhanced NK cell activity, and increased numbers of CD8+ T cells and CD19+ B cells [1]. Polysaccharide-Krestin (PSK), an extract of *Trametes versicolor*, is believed to mediate many of these effects and has been shown to enhance NK cytolytic activity via a Toll-like receptor 2-mediated mechanism in both human peripheral blood mononuclear cells (PBMCs) and in an $HER2^{+}$ breast cancer mouse model [3]. Additionally, in a prostate cancer mouse model (TRAMP C2), in combination with the chemotherapeutic agent docetaxel, PSK resulted in a significant reduction in tumor burden as well as an increase in the number of tumor infiltration lymphocytes (TIL) [2].

In addition to the mushroom extract, fresh organic vegetable juice was a notable change to his diet. The World Health Organization indicates that diet is closely linked to cancer prevention and numerous epidemiological studies have suggested that dietary phytochemicals could provide an effective intervention in cancer development [2, 4]. Phytochemicals, such as resveratrol, (−)-epigallocatechin gallate (EGCG), [6]-gingerol, and myricetin, have been shown to directly alter molecular signaling pathways known to induce cancer cell death or to inhibit cancer cell proliferation, however, in most cases, the specific molecular and cellular targets have yet to be identified [5].

Although it is unclear which, if any, of these specific interventions may have promoted tumor regression, the patient has remained free of MCC for over 4 years. The present case represents one of 30 reported in the literature demonstrating a complete spontaneous regression of MCC and of those, it is one of only ten documenting complete spontaneous regression of a metastatic lesion [6–11].

References

1. Torkelson CJ, Sweet E, Martzen MR, Sasagawa M, Wenner CA, Gay J, et al. Phase 1 clinical trial of Trametes versicolor in women with breast cancer. ISRN Oncol. 2012;2012:251632.
2. Wenner CA, Martzen MR, Lu H, Verneris MR, Wang H, Slaton JW. Polysaccharide-K augments docetaxel-induced tumor suppression and antitumor immune response in an immunocompetent murine model of human prostate cancer. Int J Oncol. 2012;40: 905–13.
3. Lu H, Yang Y, Gad E, Inatsuka C, Wenner CA, Disis ML, et al. TLR2 agonist PSK activates human NK cells and enhances the antitumor effect of HER2-targeted monoclonal antibody therapy. Clin Cancer Res. 2011;17:6742–53.
4. Danaei G, Vander Hoorn S, Lopez AD, Murray CJ, Ezzati M. Causes of cancer in the world: comparative risk assessment of nine behavioural and environmental risk factors. Lancet. 2005;366:1784–93.

5. Lee KW, Bode AM, Dong Z. Molecular targets of phytochemicals for cancer prevention. Nat Rev Cancer. 2011;11:211–8.
6. Strub B, Moron M, Meuli-Simmen C, Grunert J. Merkel cell carcinoma of the right cheek and spontaneous regression – case report and literature review. Zentralbl Chir. 2012:22614233.
7. Val-Bernal JF, Garcia-Castano A, Garcia-Barredo R, Landeras R, De Juan A, Garijo MF. Spontaneous complete regression in Merkel cell carcinoma after biopsy. Adv Anat Pathol. 2011;18:174–7; author reply 177.
8. Ciudad C, Aviles JA, Alfageme F, Lecona M, Suarez R, Lazaro P. Spontaneous regression in Merkel cell carcinoma: report of two cases with a description of dermoscopic features and review of the literature. Dermatol Surg. 2010;36:687–93.
9. Wooff JC, Trites JR, Walsh NM, Bullock MJ. Complete spontaneous regression of metastatic Merkel cell carcinoma: a case report and review of the literature. Am J Dermatopathol. 2010;32:614–7.
10. Kubo H, Matsushita S, Fukushige T, Kanzaki T, Kanekura T. Spontaneous regression of recurrent and metastatic Merkel cell carcinoma. J Dermatol. 2007; 34:773–7.
11. Hassan SJ, Knox M, Griffin M, Kennedy MJ. Spontaneous regression of metastatic Merkel cell carcinoma. Ir Med J. 2010;103:21–2.

Case Study D: Evaluation of Multiple Merkel Cell Carcinomas in a Single Patient

15

Iris Ahronowitz and Siegrid S. Yu

A 69-year-old otherwise healthy Caucasian woman was evaluated for a small, asymptomatic, erythematous papule on her right infraorbital cheek. After 4 months, she developed a second red plaque on her left distal medial calf. Her past medical history included a left arm squamous cell carcinoma excised 5 years prior, hypertension, and dyslipidemia. She had no history of immunosuppression. Medications included lisinopril, hydrochlorothiazide, and lovastatin. She had a family history of a grandmother with melanoma and a grandfather with bladder carcinoma.

By the time of her initial presentation for care (9 months after she first noted the cheek lesion), the right infraorbital lesion had grown to a dome-shaped nodule approximately 3×3 cm in size. The patient had no lymphadenopathy on exam. The nodule was excised, and histopathology showed small malignant cells with hyperchromatic nuclei and scant cytoplasm (typical of neuroendocrine carcinoma) distributed diffusely in the dermis and in subjacent soft tissue and skeletal muscle. Immunohistochemical stains for neurofilament and CK20 antibody, chromogranin, and synaptophysin were positive, and MART-1, TTF-1 and S-100, CD20, CD45, MP63, and factor I were all negative, effectively eliminating the possibility of metastasis of a visceral neuroendocrine tumor or melanoma.

The patient presented for further evaluation 2 weeks after her initial excision. At this time, the left leg nodule was noted to have increased in size to 2.2 cm. The leg lesion was biopsied, with pathology demonstrating irregularly shaped masses of neoplastic cells in the dermis (including many mitotic figures and necrotic cells) with scant cytoplasm and large round nuclei with inconspicuous nucleoli. Perinuclear dot-like expression of Cam 5.2 and CK20, positivity for neuron-specific enolase, and negativity for S100 and TTF-1 were demonstrated by immunostaining, confirming again the diagnosis of MCC.

In light of the near-synchronous appearance of her right cheek and left leg nodules, our multidisciplinary tumor board felt that her presentation was suggestive of two distinct primary tumors. Therefore wide local excision and sentinel lymph node biopsy of both cheek and leg lesions was recommended. Preoperative full-body FDG-PET/CT demonstrated positive uptake at the site of the tumor of the left lower extremity, but no evidence of other metabolically active distant metastatic disease. The cheek lesion underwent wide local re-excision, which was found to be free of residual carcinoma. Right parotid sentinel lymph node biopsy showed a single negative node. The calf lesion also underwent wide local excision and

I. Ahronowitz
Department of Dermatology, University of California San Francisco, 1701 Divisadero Street, Third Floor, San Francisco, CA 94115, USA
e-mail: ahronowitzi@derm.ucsf.edu

S.S. Yu (✉)
Department of Clinical Dermatology, UCSF Dermatologic Surgery & Laser Center, 1701 Divisadero Street, Third Floor, San Francisco, CA 94115-0316, USA
e-mail: YuS@derm.ucsf.edu

M. Alam et al. (eds.), *Merkel Cell Carcinoma*, DOI 10.1007/978-1-4614-6608-6_15,

sentinel lymph node biopsy was negative in three femoral nodes.

Based on the available data the patient was staged at T2pN0M0, representing overall stage IIA disease [1]. Given the large size of her tumors, she underwent adjuvant radiation therapy with a total dose of 5,000 cGy administered to each of the two cutaneous sites (25 fractions of 200 cGy treated to the 90 % isodose line with 0.5 cm bolus every other day). The patient tolerated the surgeries and radiation treatment well. She developed post-radiation transient moderate to severe skin erythema without skin breakdown, and had no lymphedema, infections, paresthesias, or significant pain. Her postsurgical course was complicated only by a right lower eyelid ectropion that was surgically repaired.

In light of the patient's unusual presentation, array comparative genomic hybridization (aCGH) of each cutaneous lesion was performed, with results ultimately demonstrating that the two tumors were identical from a genetic standpoint. Both demonstrated identical distal amplification of chromosome 12p with loss of chromosomes 8p and 17p, essentially ruling out the possibility of two separate primary tumors. In other words, the data support the scenario that the patient had an initial primary (probably the infraorbital tumor) with a rapid, isolated cutaneous metastasis to the contralateral ankle via hematogenous spread. After consultation with medical oncology, the decision was made to clinically monitor the patient carefully, rather than initiate chemotherapy, given the absence of evidence for any other distant metastasis. Thirty-nine months after completion of adjuvant radiation therapy, and 46 months from the initial diagnosis of the cheek tumor, the patient has had no evidence of recurrence on physical exams or surveillance PET/CT imaging.

Commentary

In light of the near-synchronous appearance of the patient's two tumors, they were initially thought to be distinct primary cutaneous MCCs. Eight prior reports have been published in the English literature of multiple synchronous or near-synchronous cutaneous MCCs, some of which have been claimed as distinct primaries [2–9]. To our knowledge, only two have used genetic analysis to prove such a relationship [4, 7]. The first of these was highly unusual because the second tumor, in the palatine tonsil, appeared 7 years after an initial cutaneous tumor on the lip. Though by array CGH it showed a great deal of shared copy number variation with the initial tumor at over 40 sites, the second tumor showed significant differences in gene copy number at 31 distinct chromosomal locations. The similarity in areas of copy number variation between the two tumors strongly suggested a shared genetic lineage between the tumors; however, the many areas of difference also ruled out the possibility of the second tumor being a delayed metastasis of the first. The authors therefore arrived at the conclusion that the metachronous tonsillar tumor represented a "field primary," a special situation in which a new primary tumor arises within a genetically altered cell population surrounding the initial tumor, rather than a de novo unrelated distant primary. A more recent study used direct sequencing of Merkel cell polyomavirus DNA incorporated in tumor genomes to prove genetic distinctness between two tumors that appeared 6 years apart on the left upper arm, and then on the right forearm [7]. Of the other cases, none of which used genetic analysis to confirm tumor relationships, two cases had synchronous onset of in the same region of the body [2, 5], likely representing in-transit metastatic disease, while the others had contralateral appearance of a second tumor typically years later [3, 6, 8, 9], more consistent with the possibility of multiple primary tumors.

We have recently undertaken aCGH analysis of additional MCC patients at our institution with multiple tumors (unpublished data). In three patients with clinically apparent primary tumors and subsequent regional lymph node metastases, tumor specimens from the primary and metastatic sites were demonstrated to have identical genetic CGH profiles, consistent with the clinical presentation. Additionally, a patient who sequentially developed three subcutaneous nodular MCC tumors (of the left lower back, followed 9 months later by the left thigh, and then after a 15-month interval a third tumor of the right lower back) was seen at our clinic. Remarkably, CGH analysis of this patient's tumors revealed that the left lower back tumor demonstrated possible gain in chromosome 2q and clear loss in chromosomes 13 and 14q; the left thigh showed gain in 11 and 6q and loss in distal 3q; and the right lower back tumor showed gain in chromosome 5p and loss in chromosomes 3, 4, 5q, and 10q, proving three genetically distinct primary tumors, a phenomenon not previously reported in the MCC literature.

With respect to the initially described patient, as previously noted, her two MCC tumors were proven by aCGH to be genetically identical and therefore likely represent one primary (probably the infraorbital tumor) with a rapid, isolated cutaneous metastasis to the contralateral ankle via hematogenous spread, rather than two unique primary tumors. Although it is possible that these two cutaneous lesions could represent metastasis from an occult primary tumor, we find this scenario unlikely given the consistently negative comprehensive imaging studies on 46 months of follow-up from the time of diagnosis, as the great majority (91 % in a retrospective study of 102 patients) of nodal and distant metastases of MCC are known to appear within 2 years of diagnosis [10]. Our case demonstrates the concept of oligometastasis, in which cancer cells from a primary site travel to a single remote site [11], which has not been previously described in Merkel cell carcinoma. The most common sites of metastasis reported in Merkel cell carcinoma are skin—mostly "in transit" metastasis (28 %), lymph nodes (27 %), liver (13 %), lung (10 %), bone (10 %), and brain (6 %) [12].

The distinction between a multiple primary MCCs vs. an isolated, distant cutaneous metastasis is of great importance given its implications with regard to staging, treatment, and prognosis. In our patient, based on the larger of the two presumed primary tumors, her initial stage IIA disease (T2pN0M0) was later revised to stage IV (T2pN0M1a) cancer after the array CGH data became available. With regard to management, while a second primary would warrant local excision with sentinel lymph node biopsies at both sites, the demonstration of distant cutaneous metastasis necessitates a comprehensive search for other metastatic foci, possible tumor excision depending on extent of disease, and a possible role for palliative systemic chemotherapy. Our patient's initial workup and treatment were completed prior to the availability of the aCGH data. If cutaneous metastasis had been suspected at the outset, the patient would not have undergone sentinel lymph node biopsy at both sites, given that the leg lesion would not have been expected to show the same pattern of spread as a primary tumor. As for prognosis, our patient's case raises very important questions about atypical presentations of Stage IV Merkel cell carcinoma. Recent data shows a poor survival rate of 44 % at 1 year from diagnosis, rapidly dwindling down to 18 % at both 4 and 5 years [1]; however, these numbers are largely based on patients with a more classic lymphatic spread pattern and visceral organ involvement, who seem to be in a distinct category from patients like ours, in whom multiple genetically related tumors may not clinically behave like classic Stage IV disease. Regardless, staging remains the most important prognostic factor in Merkel cell carcinoma, and we feel that genetic analysis remains under-utilized in elucidating the relationship between multiple cutaneous tumors to accurately stage MCC and guide workup and management.

Acknowledgments This chapter describes patient cases from our institution, one of which was previously published as a full-length case report. [Text extract reprinted from Ahronowitz IZ, Daud AI, Leong SP, Shue EH, Bastian BC, McCalmont TH, Yu SS. An isolated Merkel cell carcinoma metastasis at a distant cutaneous site presenting as a second "primary" tumor. J Cutan Pathol 2011; 38: 801–807. With permission from John Wiley & Sons, Inc.]

References

1. Lemos BD, Storer BE, Iyer JG, Phillips JL, Bichakjian CK, Fang LC, et al. Pathologic nodal evaluation improves prognostic accuracy in Merkel cell carcinoma: analysis of 5823 cases as the basis of the first consensus staging system. J Am Acad Dermatol. 2010;63(5):751–61.
2. Taxy JB, Ettinger DS, Wharam MD. Primary small cell carcinoma of the skin. Cancer. 1980;46: 2308–11.

3. Rustin MH, Chambers TJ, Levison DA, Munro DD. Merkel cell tumour: report of a case. Br J Dermatol. 1983;108:711–5.
4. Nagy J, Fehér LZ, Sonkodi I, Lesznyák J, Iványi B, Puskás LG. A second field metachronous Merkel cell carcinoma of the lip and the palatine tonsil confirmed by microarray based comparative genomic hybridisation. Virchows Arch. 2005;446:278–86.
5. Satter EK, Derienzo DP. Synchronous onset of multiple cutaneous neuroendocrine (Merkel cell) carcinomas localized to the scalp. J Cutan Pathol. 2008;35:685–91.
6. Thakur S, Chalioulias K, Hayes M, While A. Bilateral primary Merkel cell carcinoma of the upper lid misdiagnosed as basal cell carcinoma. Orbit. 2008;27:139–41.
7. Schrama D, Thiemann A, Houben R, Kähler KC, Becker JC, Hauschild A. Distinction of 2 different primary Merkel cell carcinomas in 1 patient by Merkel cell polyomavirus genome analysis. Arch Dermatol. 2010;146:687–9.
8. Pollock J, Caranosos T, Polack EP. Metachronous Merkel cell carcinoma: a case report. Case Rep Dermatol. 2011;3(3):206–8.
9. Kamiyama T, Ohshima N, Satoh H, Fukumoto H, Katano H, Imakado S. Metachronous Merkel cell carcinoma on both cheeks. Acta Derm Venereol. 2012;92(1):54–6.
10. Allen PJ et al. Merkel cell carcinoma: prognosis and treatment of patients from a single institution. J Clin Oncol. 2005;23:2300–9.
11. Hellman S, Weichselbaum RR. Oligometastases. J Clin Oncol. 1995;13:8–10.
12. Voog E, Biron P, Martin JP, Blay JY. Chemotherapy for patients with locally advanced or metastatic Merkel cell carcinoma. Cancer. 1999;85(12):2589–95.

Case Study E: Multidisciplinary Management of Merkel Cell Carcinoma

16

Adam R. Schmitt and Jeremy S. Bordeaux

A 79-year-old white male with a history of multiple squamous cell and basal cell carcinomas presented to his dermatologist for routine follow-up. Upon examination, a 3×3 mm erythematous dome-shaped papule was noted on the left cheek, approximately 1.0 cm from the left lower eyelid. No palpable lymphadenopathy was found in the head and neck. Biopsy of the lesion revealed Merkel cell carcinoma that stained positive for AE1/AE3 and negative for CK20, TTF1, S100, HMB45, CD45RB, and melan-A. A chest radiograph showed no sign of lung malignancy. The patient was then referred to the author (JSB) for treatment and his case was presented at the University Hospitals Case Medical Center Multidisciplinary Cutaneous Oncology Tumor Board. Sentinel lymph node biopsy (SLNB) and Mohs micrographic surgery were recommended by the group. Mohs micrographic surgery was recommended due to the proximity of the tumor to the eyelid and the morbidity that would result from performing a 1–2 cm wide local excision around the tumor. Mohs micrographic surgery was performed in an outpatient setting under local anesthesia. One stage of Mohs surgery was required to obtain clear margins, resulting in an 8×10 mm surgical defect. The surgery did not interfere with the integrity of the eyelid. The resultant surgical defect was not repaired immediately and the patient subsequently underwent SLNB followed by linear repair of the surgical defect. The SLNB was performed successfully by otolaryngology and yielded one node negative for malignancy (the node stained negative for AE1/AE3). The patient was discussed once more at the University Hospitals Case Medical Center Multidisciplinary Cutaneous Oncology Tumor Board. The clinical size of the tumor was <2 cm (T1), the SLNB did not show any tumor (N0), and there was no sign of distant metastasis (M0). Based on AJCC staging criteria, the patient was staged as IA. The tumor board recommended that the patient see a radiation oncologist familiar with the treatment of Merkel cell carcinoma to discuss the advantages and side effects of adjuvant radiation therapy. After consultation the patient decided to undergo radiation therapy to the primary site. He received 50 Gy in 25 fractions of 2 Gy each to the left upper cheek and periorbital region. Though the patient developed erythema in the irradiated region through the entire treatment volume, he did not experience any erythema on the conjunctivae or eyelids, and the treatment was generally well-tolerated. The patient is now being seen every 3 months by his general dermatologist. He has been instructed to palpate the surgery site and

A.R. Schmitt
Case Western Reserve University School of Medicine, 10900 Euclid Avenue, Room T308, Cleveland, OH 44106-4920, USA
e-mail: adam.schmitt@case.edu

J.S. Bordeaux (✉)
Department of Dermatology, University Hospitals Case Medical Center, Case Western Reserve University, 11100 Euclid Avenue, Lakeside 3500, Cleveland, OH 44106-5000, USA
e-mail: Jeremy.Bordeaux@uhhospitals.org

M. Alam et al. (eds.), *Merkel Cell Carcinoma*, DOI 10.1007/978-1-4614-6608-6_16,

examine his head and neck for lymphadenopathy every month. Two years following diagnosis he is free of disease.

Commentary

- Our patient was an older Caucasian gentleman with a history of excess sun exposure and multiple non-melanoma skin cancers, all of which are risk factors for developing Merkel cell carcinoma [1, 2].
- Our patient's tumor was located on his face. The most common location for Merkel cell carcinoma is the head and neck [2–4].
- Our patient's tumor did not stain positive for CK20, but did stain positive for AE1/AE3. Although most Merkel cell carcinomas do stain positive for CK20, this is not universal [1, 3].
- Given the proximity of the tumor to the eyelid, Mohs micrographic surgery was performed. Our tumor board frequently recommends wide local excision with 1–2 cm margins unless this will result in significant morbidity to the patient. This allows the wide local excision to be performed at the same time as the SLNB (SLNB is recommended for all new cases of Merkel cell carcinoma that have not been previously treated). However, if significant morbidity will result from the wide local excision, the patient will have Mohs micrographic surgery and SLNB in separate surgical sessions.
- The sentinel lymph nodes should be examined with immunostains. Frequently they are stained for CK20; however, in our case the tumor was CK20 negative, so AE1/AE3 were used.
- The role of radiation therapy as an adjunctive therapy for small (<2 cm) tumors in the setting of a negative SLNB is controversial [1, 5, 6]. In this case the patient discussed the advantages and disadvantages of radiation therapy with a physician familiar with Merkel cell carcinoma. Our patient did decide to obtain therapy and tolerated it well.
- Our patient is under frequent surveillance (every 3 months) by his general dermatologist and also performs monthly self-skin exams and lymph node exams. He is currently free of disease.
- This case highlights the importance of multidisciplinary coordination of care. The expertise of the general dermatologist, dermatopathologist, Mohs micrographic surgeon, otolaryngologist, and radiation oncologist were put to use in order to maximize benefit to the patient and optimize his treatment.

References

1. Miller SJ, Alam M, Anderson J, et al. NCCN clinical practice guidelines in oncology (NCCN Guidelines™): Merkel cell carcinoma. http://www.merkelcell.org/usefulInfo/documents/NccnMcc2012.pdf. Accessed 30 Sept 2012.
2. Swann MH, Yoon J. Merkel cell carcinoma. Semin Oncol. 2007;34(1):51–6.
3. Heath M, Jaimes N, Lemos B, Mostaghimi A, Wang LC, Penas PF, et al. Clinical characteristics of Merkel cell carcinoma at diagnosis in 195 patients: the AEIOU features. J Am Acad Dermatol. 2008;58(3):375–81.
4. O'Connor WJ, Roenigk RK, Brodland DG. Merkel cell carcinoma. Comparison of Mohs micrographic surgery and wide excision in eighty-six patients. Dermatol Surg. 1997;23(10):929–33.
5. Jabbour J, Cumming R, Scolyer RA, Hruby G, Thompson JF, Lee S. Merkel cell carcinoma: assessing the effect of wide local excision, lymph node dissection, and radiotherapy on recurrence and survival in early-stage disease—results from a review of 82 consecutive cases diagnosed between 1992 and 2004. Ann Surg Oncol. 2007;14(6):1943–52.
6. Lewis KG, Weinstock MA, Weaver AL, Otley CC. Adjuvant local irradiation for Merkel cell carcinoma. Arch Dermatol. 2006;142(6):693–700.

17 Track and Attack: Emerging Prognostic and Therapeutic Approaches

Olga Afanasiev and Paul Nghiem

Introduction

Merkel cell carcinoma (MCC) is an aggressive skin cancer with increasing incidence, high mortality, and limited treatment options for progressive disease [1, 2]. The recent discovery of the Merkel cell polyomavirus (MCPyV) and its causal association with MCC [3, 4] has provided insight into MCC pathogenesis and underscored the importance of disease-specific immune responses. This chapter will explore emerging approaches to harness antitumor and antivirus immunity to track and treat MCC.

Association with Immune Suppression Leads to Merkel Cell Polyomavirus Discovery

Numerous lines of evidence suggest that the immune system is critical in preventing and controlling MCC. Epidemiologic data suggest that patients who are chronically immune suppressed by HIV infection, chronic lymphocytic leukemia, or medications after solid organ transplant have a 3–30-fold increased risk of MCC [5]. Although these cases represent fewer than 10 % of MCC patients, most patients have an apparently normal immune system. Instead, as discussed below, localized tumor-specific defects are likely at play. In addition, 29 cases of complete spontaneous regression of MCC have been reported [6] representing 1.4 % of all reported cases of MCC [7]. Many of these regressions followed improvement in immune function [8–10], thus suggesting a sudden recognition by the immune system leading to the clearance of MCC. This evidence raised the possibility of an infectious etiology for MCC. The discovery of Merkel cell polyomavirus in 2008 provided a missing link between MCC and immune suppression [3]. As detailed in Chap. 2, MCPyV is integrated into the host genome in approximately 80 % of MCC tumors, with a cumulative average among multiple studies from around the world recently summarized as 77 % (924 of 1,198 MCCs) [11].

Although infection with MCPyV is common (80 % seroprevalence [12], and the prevalence of MCPyV DNA isolated from cutaneous swabs is 40–100 % [12, 13]), the rarity of MCC can be explained by the requirement for several uncommon mutagenic events as well as escape from immune surveillance (Fig. 17.1). Ultraviolet (UV) radiation or other environmental mutagens may promote virus integration into the host genome and "oncogenic truncation" of the large

O. Afanasiev
Departments of Dermatology/Medicine and Pathology, University of Washington School of Medicine, 850 Mercer Street, Box 358050, Seattle, WA 98109, USA
e-mail: olga54@uw.edu

P. Nghiem (✉)
Departments of Dermatology/Medicine and Pathology, University of Washington School of Medicine & Fred Hutchinson Cancer Research Center, 850 Mercer Street, Box 358050, Seattle, WA 98109, USA
e-mail: pnghiem@uw.edu

M. Alam et al. (eds.), *Merkel Cell Carcinoma*, DOI 10.1007/978-1-4614-6608-6_17,

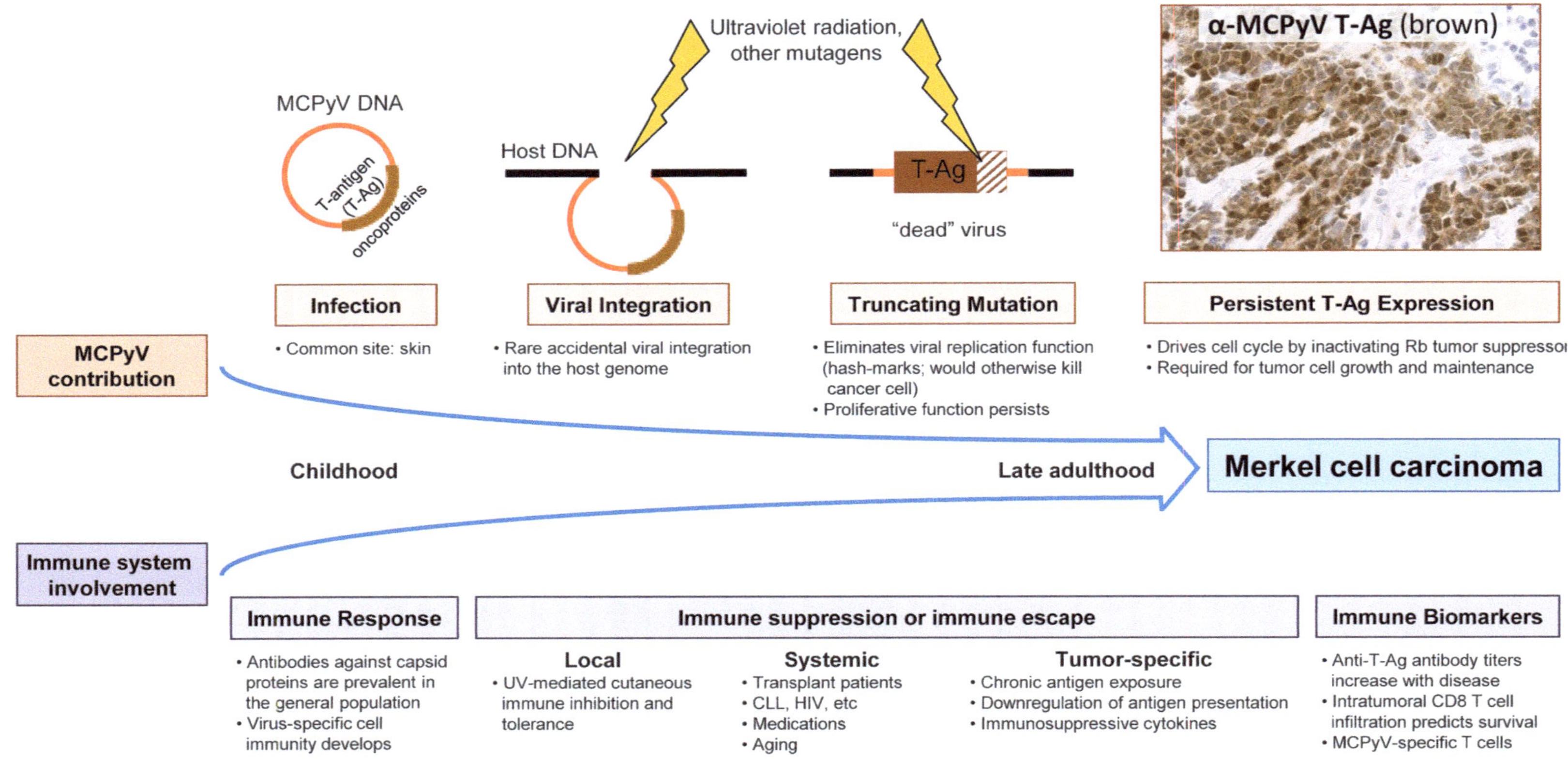

Fig. 17.1 If infection with Merkel cell polyomavirus (MCPyV) is so common, why is Merkel cell carcinoma very uncommon? Early childhood infection with MCPyV is extremely common, not known to be symptomatic, and induces antibody and cellular immune responses. Ultraviolet (UV) radiation and/or other mutagens likely contribute to virus integration into the host genome and large T (LT)-antigen truncation mutations. Persistent T-antigen expression (brown stain with IHC anti-LT antibody, CM2B4) plays a key role in Merkel cell carcinoma (MCC) pathogenesis. Furthermore, immune evasion at the local, systemic, or tumor-specific levels is also likely required for developing MCC. Immune biomarkers such as anti-T-antigen antibody levels and T cell infiltration into MCC tumors may aid in disease monitoring and prediction of outcome (adapted from Bhatia S. Immunobiology of Merkel Cell Carcinoma: Implications for Immunotherapy of a Polyomavirus-Associated Cancer. Current Oncology Reports 2011;13(6): 488–97. With permission from Springer Science + Business Media)

T-antigen. Such T-antigen truncation events are very common in MCC pathogenesis and important in that they preserve critical cell-cycle progression functions but eliminate cell-lethal viral DNA replication activities [14]. These rare genetic events result in persistent T-antigen expression that plays a key role in MCC pathogenesis [15]. Elimination of T-antigen from tumor cell lines results in inhibited growth or tumor cell apoptosis [4, 16]. Thus, the viral protein that drives MCC progression is an appealing target for disease tracking and therapeutic manipulation. As discussed below, disease progression can be effectively monitored via immune biomarkers such as anti-T-antigen antibody levels [17], and disease outcome can be predicted by the extent of tumor infiltration by CD8+ lymphocytes [18] that are presumably capable of eliminating MCC tumor cells.

Tumor Antigens: A Prerequisite for Immunologic Tracking and Treatment of MCC

All cells present "antigens" or molecules that can be surveyed by the immune system. The term was originally derived from the molecule's ability to be an "antibody generator" but now also refers to molecular fragments that can be recognized by T cells when presented by major histocompatibility complex (MHC, also known as human leukocyte antigen, HLA). The immune system is generally tolerant to "self" antigens but neutralizes "non-self" antigens (foreign and potentially harmful) via antibodies or kills infected cells via cytotoxic CD8 T cells. Tumor-associated antigens (TAAs), or molecules that can generate an antitumor immune response, were first described in mouse models in the 1950s [19] but have been intensively studied and therapeutically exploited in humans in the past two decades. A milestone in the history of human tumor immunology was the molecular characterization of the melanoma-associated antigen (MAGE) and its recognition by T cells [20]. The ever-increasing list of tumor antigens is unfortunately balanced by a lengthy list of reasons why their efficacy in eliciting an antitumor response leading to tumor shrinkage is still clinically unsatisfactory [23, 24]. However, unlike most cancers, MCC is causally associated with the expression of viral antigens that can serve as specific targets for the immune system.

MCPyV T-antigens are (1) foreign to the host, (2) permanently integrated into the cancer genome (3) persistently expressed, and (4) necessary for MCC tumor progression [21]. These concepts allow the immune system to battle MCC via its evolutionarily designated job of killing virus-infected cells. Importantly, MCC's "addiction" to viral oncoproteins makes it unlikely that immunologic pressure will cause the escape of virus-independent tumor cell variants. Indeed, unlike the oncoproteins, viral capsid proteins (VP1, VP2/3) offer no advantage for tumor progression and are typically lost in MCC tumors.

For the 20 % MCC tumors with no virus association, other nonviral proteins such as survivin [22], HIP1 oncoprotein that interacts with c-KIT [23] or CD56 might be considered as tumor-associated antigens. However, these TAAs would not be ideal targets for immunotherapy for several reasons. First, like most TAA, these are self-antigens that are not specific to the tumor tissue. For example, CD56 (also known as neural cell adhesion molecule) is expressed on many normal tissues including neurons, skeletal muscle, and natural killer immune cells. As such, during thymic education, T cells that are highly reactive to self-antigens are eliminated to prevent autoimmune disease development. Second, survivin, a protein that inhibits apoptosis and been found to be expressed in up to 100 % of MCCs [22], is also expressed on activated T cells, including those that themselves recognize survivin. Promoting a T cell response against survivin in fact leads to elimination of survivin specific T cells ("fratricide") [24]. In order to overcome these potential barriers, approaches are being developed to create drugs or even engineered T cells that are activated only by tumor microenvironment-specific cues such as tumor-induced hypoxia [25]. The discovery of MCC-specific antigens can lead to innovative advances in tracking MCC disease progression and creating novel rational therapies as discussed below.

T-Antigen-Specific Antibody Response Tracks with Disease Burden

The antibody response is critical in preventing many viral infections and is often an important component of infection resolution. When infected with MCPyV, antibodies are produced against both the outer viral capsid proteins (such as VP1, VP2/3) [12, 30, 31] and against the virus-encoded oncoproteins (such as the T-antigens) [17]. Interestingly, although the prevalence of antibodies to viral capsid proteins is high in the general population, the titer of antibodies to MCPyV capsid proteins is higher still in MCC patients (Fig. 17.2a) [12, 26, 31, 32]. Importantly, MCC patients and control subjects have no difference in antibody levels to capsid proteins derived from other polyomaviruses [26]. Increased MCPyV capsid antibody levels in MCC patients as compared to controls are not due to increased MCPyV viral capsid antigen production by tumor cells because MCC tumor cells typically do not express viral capsid proteins [14]. The higher capsid antibody titers may instead be due to

a

Capsid & T-Ag seropositivity

In MCC cases and controls

□ Control subjects ■ MCC cases

Percent seropositive

0
20
40
60
80
100

53%
88%
0.9%
40.5%

MCPyV VP1
MCPyV T-Ag

b

T-antigen titers:

Biomarker of MCC disease

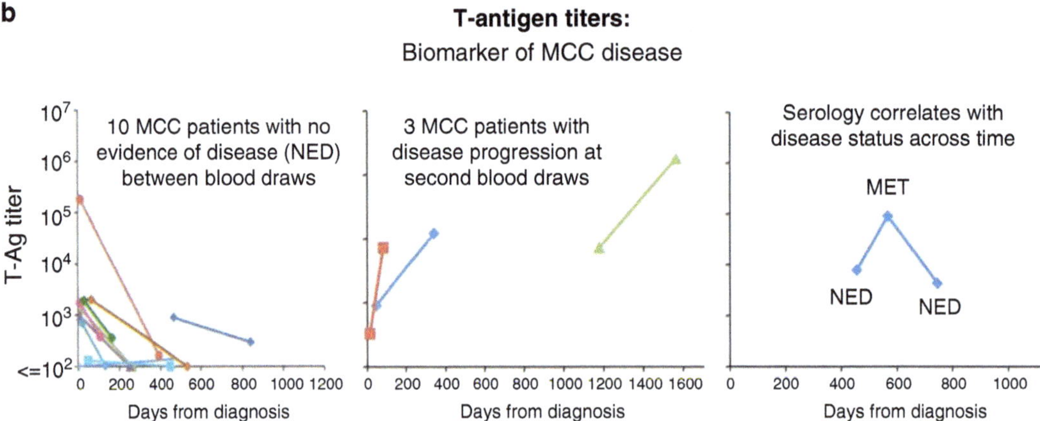

Fig. 17.2 Unlike capsid antibodies that are highly prevalent, antibodies against T-antigen oncoproteins are specific to MCC patients and are a useful biomarker of MCC disease burden. (**a**) Although antibodies against MCPyV capsid protein VP1 are higher in MCC patients compared to control subjects, these antibodies are prevalent in the general population. In contrast, seropositivity to T-antigen is highly specific to MCC patients. (**b**) T-antigen titers are dynamic and reflect the extent of disease burden. Each line represents a different MCC patient and each data point represents the T-antigen titer at the indicated time after diagnosis. *NED* no evidence of disease, *MET* metastasis/progression (adapted from [17, 26])

a higher burden of wild-type Merkel polyomavirus in MCC patients, which has been documented [13]. It remains to be determined if higher virus burden in patients was a predisposing factor for MCC development or, alternatively, if MCC results in MCPyV-specific immune tolerance leading to higher virus levels in MCC patients.

In contrast to antibodies to viral capsid proteins, antibodies to MCPyV T-antigen oncoproteins are rarely detected in the general population (<1 %) but appear to be present in a substantial proportion (~40 %) of patients with MCC (Fig. 17.2a) [17]. The apparent correlation between the humoral response to T-antigens and MCC disease burden is not surprising given the differences in T-antigen expression and biology between the normal MCPyV life cycle and its role in MCC tumors. In the normal virus life cycle, T-antigen oncoproteins are expressed in the infected cell nucleus only transiently, limiting exposure of this protein to the immune system. In contrast, T-antigen oncoproteins are persistently expressed in MCC tumor cells that rapidly proliferate and die, triggering antibody responses to the released intracellular proteins. Importantly, the antibody titers to T-antigen oncoproteins fluctuate dynamically in response to changing MCC disease burden (Fig. 17.2b). The antibody titer rapidly drops (~eightfold per year) after successful treatment of MCC tumors but rises with tumor progression (oftentimes prior to clinical detection or development of symptoms) [17]. Thus, antibody titers against T-antigen oncoproteins can serve as a biomarker of MCC disease burden and have indeed been used to detect occult MCC recurrences [18].

Cellular Immune Responses Against MCC Predict Survival and Can Be Used for Therapy

Cytotoxic T lymphocytes (also known as CD8 T cells) have the primary function of eliminating infected or damaged cells. The surprising high number of cases [29] of complete spontaneous regression of MCCs given its rarity [34, 35] supports the notion that MCC tumor cells may be susceptible to T-cell-mediated immunologic attack. Histologic analyses of MCC tumors revealed a variable presence of tumor-infiltrating lymphocytes (TILs) among MCC tumors [18]. Indeed, in a pattern similar to other cancers [27, 28], intratumoral (but not peritumoral) infiltration of CD8+ lymphocytes is an independent predictor of improved survival among MCC patients. Patients with robust CD8+ intratumoral infiltration ($n=26$) had 100 % MCC-specific survival as compared to 60 % survival among patients with sparse or no CD8+ intratumoral infiltration ($n=120$) (Fig. 17.3) [18]. These findings underscore the importance of the cellular immune response in the natural history of MCC and help explain the increased incidence of MCC in patients with cellular immune suppression.

Some of the key players mediating the antivirus and antitumor response likely include MCPyV-specific T cells. In fact, recent studies have identified virus-specific CD8 and CD4 lymphocytes present in the blood and tumors of MCC patients [29]. These viral epitopes could serve as tools to (1) isolate and track virus-specific T lymphocytes in MCC patients using an HLA/peptide tetramer (Fig. 17.4), (2) characterize immune evasion mechanisms and MCPyV-specific T cell functional status, and (3) develop tumor-specific therapies such as peptide vaccines or adoptive immunotherapy. Importantly, despite the association of infiltrating CD8 lymphocytes with improved survival and the presence of virus-specific T cells in blood and tumors of MCC patients, clinically apparent disease is likely the result of immune evasion by MCC tumors. Future research and clinical efforts will focus on immune system activation and reversal of tumor-mediated immune evasion.

Rational Treatment Strategies

Although surgery and/or radiation therapy (RT) may be curative for patients with locoregional MCC without clinically detectable distant metastases, relapses are common and often incurable [1]. The discovery of MCPyV and the importance of the immune system in cancer control support

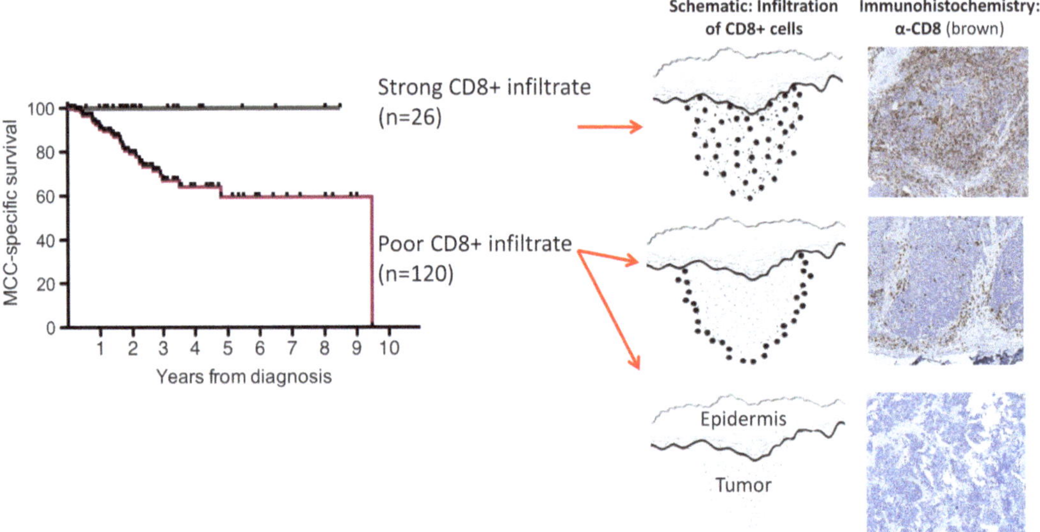

Fig. 17.3 Intratumoral CD8 lymphocytic infiltration is predictive of survival. Tumors with robust CD8+ infiltration are associated with excellent survival, as compared to those with cells that are stalled at the tumor-stroma border or those that lack CD8+ cells. CD8 lymphocytes are schematized as black dots or stained brown on IHC (adapted from Paulson KG, Iyer JG, Tegeder AR, et al. Transcriptome-Wide Studies of Merkel Cell Carcinoma and Validation of Intratumoral CD8+ Lymphocyte Invasion as an Independent Predictor of Survival. J Clin Oncol, 2011;20;29(12):1539–46. With permission from American Society of Clinical Oncology)

the pursuit of rational biology-driven therapies for MCC. The goals of the therapies discussed below are to stimulate the immune system and to establish a tumor microenvironment that favors immune system activation to mediate tumor regression.

Rethinking "Conventional" Therapies

Although radiotherapy and chemotherapy can effectively debulk tumors, they may, more importantly, mediate immunologic "side effects" that are critical in igniting the immune response to eliminate residual or therapy-resistant disease [30]. Even the mere removal of the tumor bulk can reverse cancer-induced immune tolerance to restore immune responses [31]. Radiation therapy can favor CD8-mediated cytotoxicity by upregulating HLA class I molecules and tumor antigens on the tumor cell surface [32], as well as by upregulating adhesion molecules (ICAM-I) and death receptors (Fas) [33]. Chemotherapy that leads to immune suppression associated with lymphopenia may mediate depletion of tumor-protective T regulatory cells and repletion of immune effectors that contribute to an anticancer response [30]. These anticancer therapies may also cause "immunogenic cell death" in which dying cells release antigens and produce immunostimulatory molecules [39, 42].

The dosing, fractionation, schedule, and selection of drugs may need to be optimized in order to best engage the immune system with conventional tools. For example, standard radiation therapy (RT) for MCC involves repeated administration of relatively low doses. Interestingly, studies in mice provide compelling evidence that single high-dose ("ablative") RT results in the rejection of local and distant tumors by engaging the immune system [34]. Specifically, these studies suggest that ablative RT activates myeloid dendritic cells in the primary tumor that ultimately result in vigorous priming and expansion of effector T cells in the draining lymph node. Importantly, these effects are abrogated by current fractionated radiotherapy perhaps because infiltrating T cells are eliminated by subsequent cytotoxic radiation doses. Notably, however, RT that involves high doses to multiple lymph node chains can lead to a decrease in nonspecific

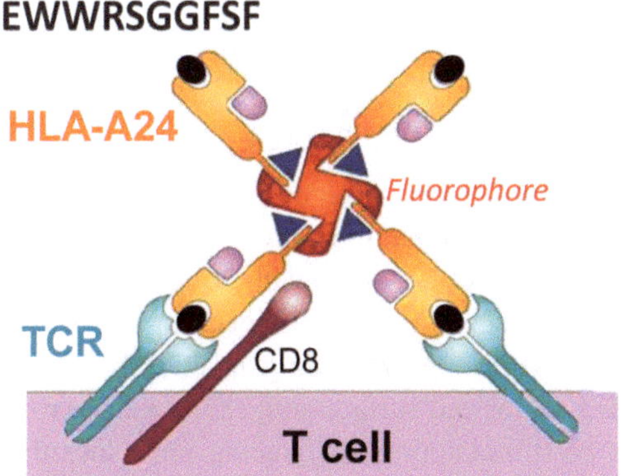

Fig. 17.4 A tool for tracking MCPyV-specific T cells. A synthetic human leukocyte antigen (HLA)/peptide molecule is called a tetramer or a multimer. Such tetramers can bind strongly to their corresponding MCPyV-specific T cells that have a T cell receptor (TCR) with a defined affinity for a particular viral peptide in context of its restricting HLA class I molecule. One such tool that can detect virus-specific CD8 T cells is shown above with an HLA-A24 (shown in *orange*)-restricted MCPyV peptide (shown in *black*) being recognized by a TCR (shown in *green*). These tetramers can be conjugated to a fluorophore that allows for detection by flow cytometry, for example (based on data from Iyer JG, Afanasiev OK, Mcclurkan C, et al. Merkel Cell Polyomavirus-Specific CD8+ and CD4+ T-cell Responses Identified in Merkel Cell Carcinomas and Blood. Clinical Cancer Research 2011;17: 6671–6680)

immune system responses that may remain suppressed several months following treatment [35]. Similarly, while sentinel lymph node biopsy is a sensitive test for detecting the spread of MCC [45], it could be important to preserve the sentinel lymph node, which constitutes the designated site of antigen priming.

Chemotherapeutics not only have variable clinical efficacy but also have broad effects on the immune system. Immunogenic cell death that favors immune activation can be induced by some chemotherapeutic agents (such as anthracyclines and oxaliplatin), while others (such as alkylating agents and cisplatin) fail to trigger such an immune reaction [36]. Furthermore, similar to radiotherapy administration, while a single cycle of chemotherapy-induced lymphodepletion may favor the repletion of T cells stimulated by tumor antigens, repeated cycles may deplete the expanding population of tumor-specific lymphocytes. These findings (rigorously studied in preclinical animal models) have important implications for the rational treatment of cancer in humans.

Overview of Immunotherapies

The immune system is extremely complex, multifactorial, and redundant; therefore, it is unlikely that a single silver bullet immunomodulatory therapy will cure the majority of MCC tumors. Nevertheless, we will introduce single modality therapies and then will discuss advantages of combination therapies that may offer durable cancer-specific effects.

Antigen-Targeted Immunotherapies

Adoptive T cell therapy uses a person's own T cells that have been selected, expanded, and sometimes even genetically manipulated to produce immune cells with augmented antitumor immune responses (Fig. 17.5). In contrast to tumor vaccination strategies, adoptive T cell therapy can offer far greater control over the magnitude and avidity of the targeted response by appropriate manipulation and selection in vitro of the T cells used for therapy [37]. In melanoma, adoptively transferred T cells persisted in vivo in response to low-dose IL-2, preferentially localized to tumor sites, and mediated an antigen-specific immune response characterized by minor, mixed, or stable responses in 8 of 10 patients for periods of 2–21 months [38]. T cell therapy may especially hold promise for MCC, a cancer that is highly dependent on immune control. As discussed above, 80 % of MCCs express a specific viral tumor antigen that can serve as a target for therapeutic T cells. Indeed, MCPyV-specific T cells, such as those that have been recently identified [29], can likely be used for T cell therapy in MCC patients. Virus-specific peptide-HLA tetramers can be used for isolation, enrichment, and monitoring of MCPyV-specific

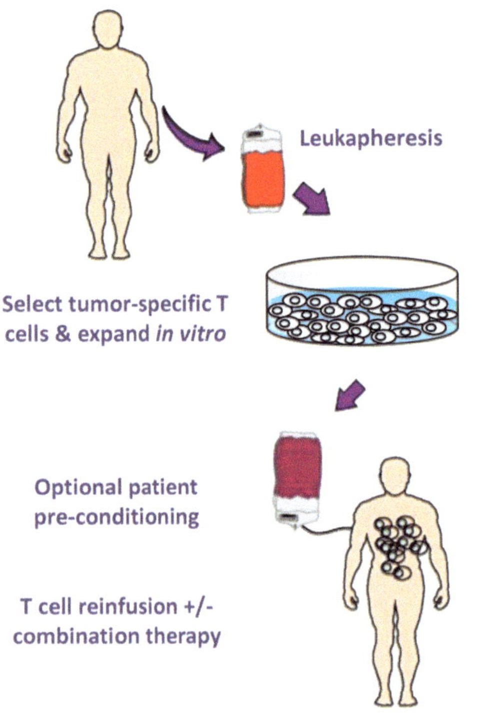

Fig. 17.5 Adoptive immunotherapy. In this approach, leukapheresis is commonly used to collect a patient's white blood cells. These white blood cells are then selected for antigen specificity (using a peptide-HLA tetramer for example) and expanded in tissue culture conditions that can skew or preserve a desired T cell phenotype. The patient can then undergo a preconditioning regimen prior to T cell infusion (such as chemotherapy to lymphodeplete and make "space" for infused T cells or radiotherapy to decrease tumor bulk and enhance tumor immunogenicity). After T cell infusion, additional treatments can be initiated

T cells among tumor-infiltrating lymphocytes and PMBC in MCC patients before, during, and after immunotherapy [29].

Importantly, MCC seems to be an immunogenic cancer regardless of whether or not it harbors viral T-antigen oncoproteins. Although intratumoral CD8+ lymphocyte infiltration is an independent prognostic factor in MCC, no relationship was observed between CD8 infiltration and virus status of the tumor [18]. In the 20 % of virus-negative MCCs with unknown tumor antigens, tumor-specific T cell therapy is still an option. Similar to promising reports in metastatic melanoma [39], tumor-infiltrating lymphocytes could be isolated directly from tumors, selected only for the CD8 marker (regardless of specificity), expanded to clinically useful numbers, and reinfused into the patient with appropriate pre-infusion conditioning (such as nonmyeloablative chemotherapy). In melanoma, this approach resulted in 19 of 33 patients (58 %) having an objective response by RECIST criteria, including three complete responders [39].

A recent immunotherapy breakthrough has been in the field of genetically modified T cells. One promising approach has been to engineer T cells to stably express binding moieties that recognize a tumor cell surface antigen, as well as various co-stimulatory and signaling molecules that enhance T cell activation, persistence, and antitumor responses. Using this chimeric antigen receptor (CAR) technology to target B cell surface protein CD19 that is expressed on malignant (and normal) B cells in chronic lymphocytic leukemia resulted in persistent expression of CAR T cells and complete remission of disease in two of three treated patients [40]. Healthy B cells were also targets of attack, resulting in hypogammaglobulinemia that could be mitigated with IVIG therapy. MCC also has potential targetable surface proteins (such as CD56), but activation of T cells targeting ubiquitously expressed self-proteins would need to be restricted to the tumor microenvironment.

Vaccines may help boost antigen-specific antitumor cellular immune responses by mediating T cell activation outside of the immunosuppressive tumor microenvironment. In HPV-associated vulvar intraepithelial neoplasia (VIN), synthetic long-peptide vaccination with incomplete Freund's adjuvant resulted in a 79 % (15 of 19) clinical response rate and a 47 % (9 of 19) complete response rate in women with HPV-16-positive high-grade VIN [41, 42]. This clinical response was attributed to efficient dendritic cell targeting to induce therapeutic CD8 and CD4 T cell responses.

Another approach increasingly used in a clinical setting involves preloading autologous dendritic cells (DC) ex vivo with appropriate tumor antigens. Such therapy (sipuleucel-T) has been approved by the FDA in 2010 to be used for the treatment of metastatic castration-resistant prostate cancer. Several phase III studies showed that treatment with sipuleucel-T resulted in a benefit in overall survival of about 4 months and improvement in the rate of 3-year survival (31.7 % for patients receiving sipuleucel-T, as compared with 23.0 % for those receiving placebo) [43, 44].

Taking Off the T Cell Brakes

The cellular CD8 lymphocyte response has evolved to fight virus-infected cells. As discussed above, in MCC, the presence of CD8 lymphocytes is associated with survival benefit [18]. Thus, MCC likely requires an immunosuppressive environment to progress. While clinically apparent immune dysfunction is present in 10 % of MCC patients, in the remaining 90 %, a wide spectrum of local immune evasion mechanisms may play a role. Some types of tumors effectively hide from the immune system by downregulating antigen presentation via MHC class I molecules, which is associated with worse prognosis [45]. Fortunately, this mechanism can potentially be therapeutically reversed using radiotherapy as discussed above [32] or cytokines (such as interferons and TNF-alpha) [46]. In contrast, chronic antigen stimulation can lead to T cell exhaustion characterized by progressive loss of T cell function [47]. In fact, the high antigenic burden of MCPyV proteins persistently expressed by MCC tumors strikingly resembles chronic infection of mice with lymphocytic choriomeningitis virus (LCMV). This mouse model was key in identifying the mechanisms (PD-1/PD-L1 pathway) by which antiviral T cell responses are circumvented in the context of chronic antigen exposure [48]. As mentioned above, it remains to be resolved if the high wild-type viral load in the skin of MCC patients contributes to T cell exhaustion predisposing to MCC pathogenesis or if it is the consequence of poor immunologic control by tumor-mediated T cell exhaustion.

There are several pathways that are important in immunoregulation of T cell responses (Fig. 17.6). Inhibitory pathways include programmed death (PD)-1 and its ligands PD-L1 and PD-L2, cytotoxic T-lymphocyte-associated protein 4 (CTLA-4), T cell immunoglobulin-, and mucin-domain-containing molecule-3 (Tim-3). Drugs inhibiting these pathways are already being investigated for their clinical utility in cancer. CTLA-4 receptor blocking agents such as ipilimumab are FDA approved for metastatic melanoma. These drugs, alone or in combination with other therapies, may be promising in enhancing T cell function in MCC patients.

Promoting T Cell Activation and Memory

An alternative or complementary approach to taking off the brakes to enhance T cell function is to provide pro-immunogenic T cell activation signals. Immunostimulatory cytokines such as interleukin (IL)-2, IL-12, IL15, and IL-21 or interferons could be delivered systemically or intratumorally to promote T cell activation or to counteract immune evasion strategies employed by MCC tumors. A phase II trial (NCT01440816) using intratumoral delivery of IL-12 plasmid DNA followed by in vivo electroporation of MCC tumors designed to lead to intratumoral persistent expression is underway. Other therapeutic agents that are appealing to investigate for MCC treatment include drugs targeting the co-stimulatory 4-1BB (CD137) pathway that can preferentially target CD8+ cells to enhance proliferation, survival, and cytokine production [49, 50].

"Treat Locally, Cure Systemically": Tumor-Targeted Drug Delivery

The immune system is under tight regulation. Disturbing the balance between immune cell activation and inhibition may result in intended anticancer effects in combination with undesirable off-target effects. Delivering therapy (chemotherapy, immunotherapy, etc.) directly to the tumor site offers an attractive alternative to systemic treatment that may allow for higher therapeutic doses to the tumor with fewer systemic side effects. Intratumoral and locoregional therapies have been used with many drugs (ranging

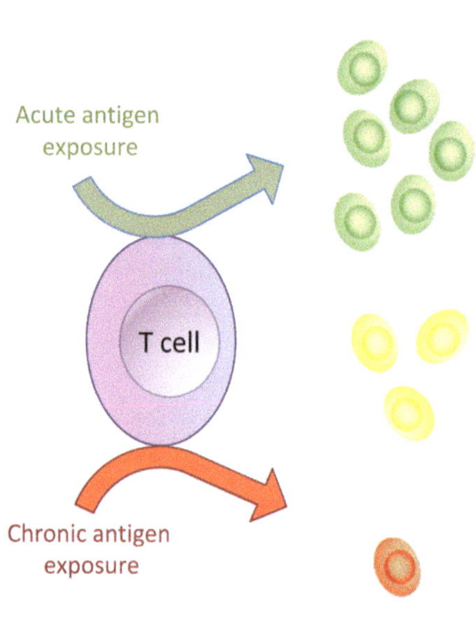

Activated cells, characterized by expression of:	
CD28	Co-stimulatory receptor (ligand: B7); required for T cell activation
CD69	Earliest inducible cell surface glycoprotein during T cell activation; plays a role in T cell proliferation
CD137 (4-1BB)	Member of TNF-receptor family; induced by T cell activation; important in T cell proliferation, cytokine secretion and cytotoxicity
CD38	Cyclic ADP ribose hydrolase; marker of T cell activation; functions in cell adhesion, signal transduction and calcium signaling
HLA-DR	MHC class-II surface receptor that is upregulated with T cell activation

Recently activated T cells, characterized by expression of:
Combination of activation and inhibition markers via appropriate immunoregulatory feedback mechanisms

Exhausted T cells, characterized by prolonged expression of:	
PD-1	Programmed death-1; inhibitory T cell receptor (ligands: PD-L1 (B7-H1), PD-L2 (B7-DC)); reduces T cell proliferation and effector functions
CTLA-4 (CD152)	Cytotoxic T-Lymphocyte Antigen 4; inhibitory receptor (ligand: B7); effectively competes for ligands with CD28 (which has lower avidity than CTLA-4), preventing T cell activation
Tim-3	T cell Immunoglobulin Mucin-3; inhibitory T cell receptor (ligand: galactin-9); leads to decrease in effector T cell function

Fig. 17.6 Antigen exposure can regulate T cell activation state. Acute antigen elicits appropriate immune response to provide a "go" signal to antigen-specific T cells (*greens cells*). Such activated T cells upregulate co-stimulatory or activation markers as indicated. In contrast, chronic antigen exposure results in a "stop" signaling cascade that can be identified by prolonged expression of multiple inhibitory receptors such as PD-1, CTLA-4, and Tim-3 (expressed on *red cells*). The presence of both activation markers and inhibitory receptors may indicate cells that were recently activated and are now entering a state of downregulation (*yellow cells*). Importantly, these states of activation and inhibition can be therapeutically manipulated using cytokines, receptor agonists, and receptor blockers

from chemotherapeutics to immunotherapeutics) in a wide number of tumors [51], including MCC. For example, intralesional bleomycin, a chemotherapeutic with pro-immunogenic properties, has been used in MCC in conjunction with conventional therapy with promising results [52]. Systemic treatment may be ineffective due to insufficient drug delivery to the tumor site or due to compensatory systemic immunoregulation. For instance, systemic interferon, often used as a broad-spectrum antiviral agent, has not been reported to be effective in inducing MCC regression [53]. However, two cases have been previously reported in which intralesional interferon-β injection has been successful as primary therapy for MCC [54, 55]. Similarly, cytokines have been delivered intratumorally in various cancers [51].

Many therapies are given systemically because metastatic tumors are often numerous, widely disseminated, and difficult to access. However, advanced techniques developed by interventional radiologists are limiting the inaccessibility of tumors. As discussed above, in mouse models, radiation treatment itself can provide an immunogenic stimulus to reduce or eradicate not only primary tumors but also distant metastases in a CD8+ T cell-dependent manner [34]. For tumors that are difficult to access, next-generation tumor-targeting molecules are being developed. For example, soluble T cell antigen receptor (STAR) reagents combine a T cell receptor with an exchangeable "warhead" to allow for tumor-specific immunohistochemistry (by coupling to biotin/peroxidase) or immunotherapy (by coupling drugs or cytokines) (Fig. 17.7) [56]. STAR molecules employ the TCR's ability to specifically recognize MHC-restricted, peptide-specific antigen targets on virus-infected or cancerous cells

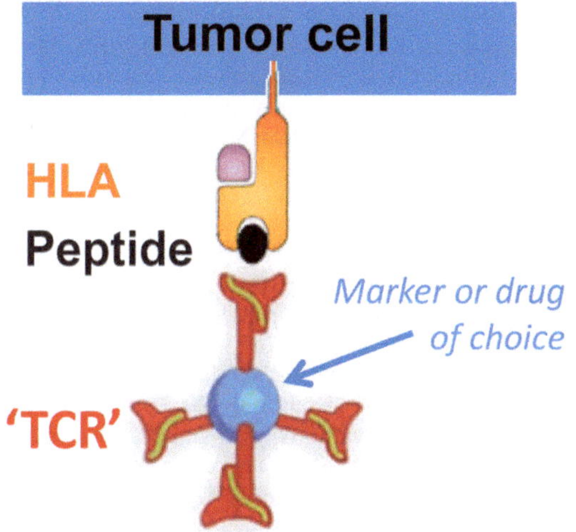

Fig. 17.7 Tumor targeting using soluble T cell antigen receptor (STAR) multimers. STAR multimers (*red*) are modified T cell receptor fusion proteins that can target a tumor cell expressing a specific HLA (*orange*) peptide (*black*) combination. The same multimer can be used for a variety of research/diagnostic (IHC staining) and therapeutic (drug delivery) applications by simply switching the attached "warhead" (schematized as a *blue circle*) (adapted from Wong, H. C. Company Profile: Altor BioScience Corporation. Biomarkers Med., 4: 499–504, 2010. With permission from Future Medicine, Ltd.)

[57]. With T cell clones recognizing specific MHC-peptide complexes already identified, this approach has the potential to offer "off-the-shelf" targeted drug delivery to MCC tumors. Local tumor targeting with treatments that can elicit an appropriate systemic antitumor immune response is promising in eliminating both metastatic and microscopic disease.

Customized "Immune Reconstitution Therapy"

Given the heterogeneity of MCC tumors and the variability of host immune responses, a combinatorial approach of immunotherapies along with conventional approaches will be necessary to improve MCC patient outcomes. While monotherapies may be appropriate early in the disease process, combinatorial approaches hold promise as a strategy for cancer therapeutics for more advanced disease. The possibilities, of course, are exponential, and the correct combination of therapies will need to be rigorously evaluated. Personalized combinations of treatments will likely be based on many parameters including, but not limited to disease status, tumor characteristics (including tumor-specific immune evasion strategies), and immune functional status.

The complexity of the immune system will require the use of multiple treatment modalities to trigger antitumor responses and reverse tumor-specific immune escape mechanisms. Importantly, conventional anticancer strategies can be combined with novel therapeutic advances for optimal treatment of patients. For example, while radiotherapy (RT) can be used to control local tumor growth, it is an ineffective tool to use for micrometastatic (undetectable) disease deposits. However, RT, even as monotherapy, is sometimes capable of mediating an "abscopal" effect (when local radiation has antitumor effects at a distant nonirradiated site) likely via activation of the immune system [58, 59]. RT in conjunction with immunotherapy may further synergize to exploit (1) radiation-induced tumor cell death as a source of antigens for immunotherapy and (2) postirradiation tumor cell modulation (i.e., increasing MHC-I, providing pro-immunogenic "danger" signals) that enhances immune cell access and T cell-mediated killing [33]. Similarly, chemotherapy has been combined with immunotherapies such as vaccines with promising results [60]. Future directions in clinical research and patient management will include the optimization of synergistic therapies with maximum efficacy, minimum toxicity, and integration with tumor-specific immune evasion strategies.

Conclusion

Merkel cell carcinoma (MCC) is an aggressive skin malignancy with an increasing incidence and high mortality rate. In the majority of MCC tumors, Merkel cell polyomavirus (MCPyV) oncoproteins appear to drive tumor progression and their ongoing expression is likely required. Thus, MCPyV is a promising tumor-associated target for disease tracking and immunotherapy. Indeed, virus-specific humoral and cellular immune responses are detectable in MCC patients, are linked to the natural history of the disease, and can be used for prognosis and early detection of disease recurrence. Learning how to therapeutically exploit the immune system to generate long-lasting and effective antitumor responses will be an ongoing challenge, but as our knowledge of the synergistic effects of therapies increases, the translational use of these strategies will be become more feasible for MCC patients.

References

1. Lemos BD, Storer BE, Iyer JG, Phillips JL, Bichakjian CK, Fang LC, et al. Pathologic nodal evaluation improves prognostic accuracy in Merkel cell carcinoma: analysis of 5823 cases as the basis of the first consensus staging system. J Am Acad Dermatol. 2010;63(5):751–61.
2. Albores-Saavedra J, Batich K, Chable-Montero F, Sagy N, Schwartz AM, Henson DE. Merkel cell carcinoma demographics, morphology, and survival based on 3870 cases: a population based study. J Cutan Pathol. 2010;37(1):20–7.
3. Feng H, Shuda M, Chang Y, Moore PS. Clonal integration of a polyomavirus in human Merkel cell carcinoma. Science. 2008;319:1096–100.
4. Houben R, Shuda M, Weinkam R, Schrama D, Feng H, Chang Y, et al. Merkel cell polyomavirus-infected Merkel cell carcinoma cells require expression of viral T antigens. J Virol. 2010;84:7064–72.
5. Heath M, Jaimes N, Lemos B, Mostaghimi A, Wang LC, Peñas PF, et al. Clinical characteristics of Merkel cell carcinoma at diagnosis in 195 patients: the AEIOU features. J Am Acad Dermatol. 2008;58:375–81.
6. Val-Bernal JF, García-Castaño A, García-Barredo R, Landeras R, De Juan A, Garijo, MF. Spontaneous complete regression in Merkel cell carcinoma after biopsy. Adv Anat Pathol. 2011;18:174–7; author reply 177.
7. Connelly T. Regarding complete spontaneous regression of Merkel cell carcinoma. Dermatol Surg. 2009;35:721.
8. Miller RW, Rabkin CS. Merkel cell carcinoma and melanoma: etiological similarities and differences. Cancer Epidemiol Biomarkers Prev. 1999;8:153–8.
9. Pan D, Narayan D, Ariyan S. Merkel cell carcinoma: five case reports using sentinel lymph node biopsy and a review of 110 new cases. Plast Reconstr Surg. 2002;110:1259–65.
10. Kubo H, Matsushita S, Fukushige T, Kanzaki T, Kanekura T. Spontaneous regression of recurrent and metastatic Merkel cell carcinoma. J Dermatol. 2007;34:773–7.
11. Van Ghelye M, Moens U. Merkel cell polyomavirus: A causal factor in Merkel cell carcinoma. Chapter 5 in Skin Cancers - Risk Factors, Prevention and Therapy. La Porta, C (ed). InTech (online publisher). p. 109–131. ISBN 978-953-307-722-2.
12. Schowalter RM, Pastrana DV, Pumphrey KA, Moyer AL, Buck CB. Merkel cell polyomavirus and two previously unknown polyomaviruses are chronically shed from human skin. Cell Host Microbe. 2011;7:509–15.
13. Foulongne V, Dereure O, Kluger N, Kluger N, Molès JP, Guillot B, et al. Merkel cell polyomavirus DNA detection in lesional and nonlesional skin from patients with Merkel cell carcinoma or other skin diseases. Br J Dermatol. 2010;162:59–63.
14. Shuda M, Feng H, Kwun HJ, Rosen ST, Gjoerup O, Moore PS, et al. T antigen mutations are a human tumor-specific signature for Merkel cell polyomavirus. Proc Natl Acad Sci U S A. 2008;105:16272–7.
15. Moore PS, Chang Y. Why do viruses cause cancer? Highlights of the first century of human tumour virology. Nat Rev Cancer. 2010;10:878–89.
16. Houben R, Adam C, Baeurle A, Hesbacher S, Grimm J, Angermeyer S, et al. An intact retinoblastoma protein binding site in Merkel cell polyomavirus large T antigen is required for promoting growth of Merkel cell carcinoma cells. Int J Cancer. 2012;130(4): 847–56.
17. Paulson KG, Carter JJ, Johnson LG, Cahill KW, Iyer JG, Schrama D, et al. Antibodies to Merkel cell polyomavirus T antigen oncoproteins reflect tumor burden in Merkel cell carcinoma patients. Cancer Res. 2010;70(21):8388–97.
18. Paulson KG, Iyer JG, Tegeder AR, Thibodeau R, Schelter J, Koba S, et al. Transcriptome-wide studies of Merkel cell carcinoma and validation of intratumoral CD8+ lymphocyte invasion as an independent predictor of survival. J Clin Oncol. 2011;29(12):1539–46.
19. Prehn RT, Main JM. Immunity to methylcholanthrene-induced sarcomas. J Natl Cancer Inst. 1957;18: 769–78.
20. Van Der Bruggen P, Traversari C, Chomez P, Lurquin C, De Plaen E, Van den Eynde B, et al. A gene encoding an antigen recognized by cytolytic T lymphocytes on a human melanoma. Science. 1991;254:1643–7.
21. Shuda M, Arora R, Kwun HJ, Feng H, Sarid R, Fernández-Figueras M-T, et al. Human Merkel cell polyomavirus infection I. MCV T antigen expression in Merkel cell carcinoma, lymphoid tissues and lymphoid tumors. Int J Cancer. 2009;125:1243–9.
22. Kim J, Mcniff JM. Nuclear expression of survivin portends a poor prognosis in Merkel cell carcinoma. Mod Pathol. 2008;21:764–9.
23. Ames HM, Bichakjian CK, Liu GY, Oravecz-Wilson KI, Fullen DR, Verhaegen ME, et al. Huntingtin-interacting protein 1: a Merkel cell carcinoma marker that interacts with c-Kit. J Invest Dermatol. 2011;131(10):2113–20.

24. Leisegang M, Wilde S, Spranger S, Milosevic S, Frankenberger B, Uckert W, et al. MHC-restricted fratricide of human lymphocytes expressing survivin-specific transgenic T cell receptors. J Clin Invest. 2010;120:3869–77.
25. Lalani AS, Alters SE, Wong A, Albertella MR, Cleland JL, Henner WD. Selective tumor targeting by the hypoxia-activated prodrug AQ4N blocks tumor growth and metastasis in preclinical models of pancreatic cancer. Clin Cancer Res. 2007;13:2216–25.
26. Carter JJ, Paulson KG, Wipf GC, Miranda D, Madeleine MM, Johnson LG, et al. Association of Merkel cell polyomavirus-specific antibodies with Merkel cell carcinoma. J Natl Cancer Inst. 2009;101: 1510–22.
27. Zhang L, Conejo-Garcia JR, Katsaros D, Gimotty PA, Massobrio M, Regnani G, et al. Intratumoral T cells, recurrence, and survival in epithelial ovarian cancer. N Engl J Med. 2003;348:203–13.
28. Pagès F, Berger A, Camus M, Sanchez-Cabo F, Costes A, Molidor R, et al. Effector memory T cells, early metastasis, and survival in colorectal cancer. N Engl J Med. 2005;353:2654–66.
29. Iyer JG, Afanasiev OK, Mcclurkan C, Paulson K, Nagase K, Jing L, et al. Merkel cell polyomavirus-specific CD8+ and CD4+ T-cell responses identified in Merkel cell carcinomas and blood. Clin Cancer Res. 2011;17:6671–80.
30. Zitvogel L, Apetoh L, Ghiringhelli F, André F, Tesniere A, Kroemer G. The anticancer immune response: indispensable for therapeutic success? J Clin Invest. 2008;118:1991–2001.
31. Danna EA, Sinha P, Gilbert M, Clements VK, Pulaski BA, Ostrand-Rosenberg S. Surgical removal of primary tumor reverses tumor-induced immunosuppression despite the presence of metastatic disease. Cancer Res. 2004;64:2205–11.
32. Reits EA. Radiation modulates the peptide repertoire, enhances MHC class I expression, and induces successful antitumor immunotherapy. J Exp Med. 2006;203:1259–71.
33. Hodge JW, Guha C, Neefjes J, Gulley JL. Synergizing radiation therapy and immunotherapy for curing incurable cancers. Opportunities and challenges. Oncology (Williston Park, NY). 2008;22:1064–70; discussion 1075, 1061–80, 1084.
34. Lee Y, Auh SL, Wang Y, Burnette B, Wang Y, Meng Y, et al. Therapeutic effects of ablative radiation on local tumor require CD8+ T cells: changing strategies for cancer treatment. Blood. 2009;114:589–95.
35. Belka C, Ottinger H, Kreuzfelder E, Weinmann M, Lindemann M, Lepple-Wienhues A, et al. Impact of localized radiotherapy on blood immune cells counts and function in humans. Radiother Oncol. 1999;50: 199–204.
36. Casares N. Caspase-dependent immunogenicity of doxorubicin-induced tumor cell death. J Exp Med. 2005;202:1691–701.
37. Yee C. Adoptive T cell therapy: addressing challenges in cancer immunotherapy. J Transl Med. 2005;3:17.
38. Yee C, Thompson JA, Byrd D, Riddell SR, Roche P, Celis E, et al. Adoptive T cell therapy using antigen-specific CD8+ T cell clones for the treatment of patients with metastatic melanoma: in vivo persistence, migration, and antitumor effect of transferred T cells. Proc Natl Acad Sci U S A. 2002;99:16168–73.
39. Dudley ME, Gross CA, Langhan MM, Garcia MR, Sherry RM, Yang JC, et al. CD8+ enriched "young" tumor infiltrating lymphocytes can mediate regression of metastatic melanoma. Clin Cancer Res. 2010;16: 6122–31.
40. Kalos M, Levine BL, Porter DL, Katz S, Grupp SA, Bagg A, et al. T cells with chimeric antigen receptors have potent antitumor effects and can establish memory in patients with advanced leukemia. Sci Transl Med. 2011;3:95ra73.
41. Kenter GG, Welters MJP, Valentijn ARPM, Lowik MJG, Berends-van der Meer DMA, Vloon APG, et al. Vaccination against HPV-16 oncoproteins for vulvar intraepithelial neoplasia. N Engl J Med. 2009;361: 1838–47.
42. Melief CJM, van der Burg SH. Immunotherapy of established (pre)malignant disease by synthetic long peptide vaccines. Nat Rev Cancer. 2008;8:351–60.
43. Higano CS, Schellhammer PF, Small EJ, Burch PA, Nemunaitis J, Yuh L, et al. Integrated data from 2 randomized, double-blind, placebo-controlled, phase 3 trials of active cellular immunotherapy with sipuleucel-T in advanced prostate cancer. Cancer. 2009;115: 3670–9.
44. Kantoff PW, Higano CS, Shore ND, Berger ER, Small EJ, Penson DF, et al. Sipuleucel-T immunotherapy for castration-resistant prostate cancer. N Engl J Med. 2010;363:411–22.
45. Bubeník J. Tumour MHC class I downregulation and immunotherapy (review). Oncol Rep. 2003;10:2005–8.
46. Bubeník J. MHC class I down-regulation: tumour escape from immune surveillance? (review). Int J Oncol. 2004;25:487–91.
47. Kim PS, Ahmed R. Features of responding T cells in cancer and chronic infection. Curr Opin Immunol. 2010;22:223–30.
48. Zajac AJ, Blattman JN, Murali-Krishna K, Sourdive DJ, Suresh M, Altman JD, et al. Viral immune evasion due to persistence of activated T cells without effector function. J Exp Med. 1998;188:2205–13.
49. Curran MA, Kim M, Montalvo W, Al-Shamkhani A, Allison JP. Combination CTLA-4 blockade and 4-1BB activation enhances tumor rejection by increasing T-cell infiltration, proliferation, and cytokine production. PLoS One. 2011;6:e19499.
50. Palazon A, Teijeira A, Martinez-Forero I, Hervas-Stubbs S, Roncal C, Penuelas I, et al. Agonist anti-CD137 mAb act on tumor endothelial cells to enhance recruitment of activated T lymphocytes. Cancer Res. 2011;71:801–11.
51. Goldberg EP, Hadba AR, Almond BA, Marotta JS. Intratumoral cancer chemotherapy and immunotherapy: opportunities for nonsystemic preoperative drug delivery. J Pharm Pharmacol. 2002;54:159–80.

52. Ely H, Pascucci A. Merkel cell carcinoma: treatment with bleomycin. Dermatol Online J. 2008;14:3.
53. Biver-Dalle C, Nguyen T, Touzé A, Saccomani C, Penz S, Cunat-Peultier S, et al. Use of interferon-alpha in two patients with Merkel cell carcinoma positive for Merkel cell polyomavirus. Acta Oncol. 2011;50:479–80.
54. Nakajima H, Takaishi M, Yamamoto M, Kamijima R, Kodama H, Tarutani M, et al. Screening of the specific polyoma virus as diagnostic and prognostic tools for Merkel cell carcinoma. J Dermatol Sci. 2009;56:211–3.
55. Matsushita E, Hayashi N, Fukushima A, Ueno H. [Evaluation of treatment and prognosis of Merkel cell carcinoma of the eyelid in Japan]. Nippon Ganka Gakkai Zasshi. 2007;111:459–62.
56. Wong HC. Altor BioScience Corporation. Biomark Med. 2010;4:499–504.
57. Card KF, Price-Schiavi SA, Liu B, Thomson E, Nieves E, Belmont H, et al. A soluble single-chain T-cell receptor IL-2 fusion protein retains MHC-restricted peptide specificity and IL-2 bioactivity. Cancer Immunol Immunother. 2004;53:345–57.
58. Demaria S, Ng B, Devitt ML, Babb JS, Kawashima N, Liebes L, et al. Ionizing radiation inhibition of distant untreated tumors (abscopal effect) is immune mediated. Int J Radiat Oncol Biol Phys. 2004;58: 862–70.
59. Hood L, Rowen L, Galas DJ, Aitchison JD. Systems biology at the Institute for Systems Biology. Brief Funct Genomic Proteomic. 2008;7:239–48.
60. Nisticò P, Capone I, Palermo B, Del Bello D, Ferraresi V, Moschella F, et al. Chemotherapy enhances vaccine-induced antitumor immunity in melanoma patients. Int J Cancer. 2009;124:130–9.

Index

M. Alam et al. (eds.), *Merkel Cell Carcinoma*, DOI 10.1007/978-1-4614-6608-6,

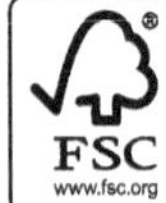

MIX
Papier aus verantwortungsvollen Quellen
Paper from responsible sources
FSC® C105338

If you have any concerns about our products,
you can contact us on
ProductSafety@springernature.com

In case Publisher is established outside the EU,
the EU authorized representative is:
Springer Nature Customer Service Center GmbH
Europaplatz 3, 69115 Heidelberg, Germany

Printed by Libri Plureos GmbH
in Hamburg, Germany